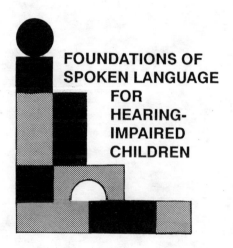

FOUNDATIONS OF SPOKEN LANGUAGE FOR HEARING-IMPAIRED CHILDREN

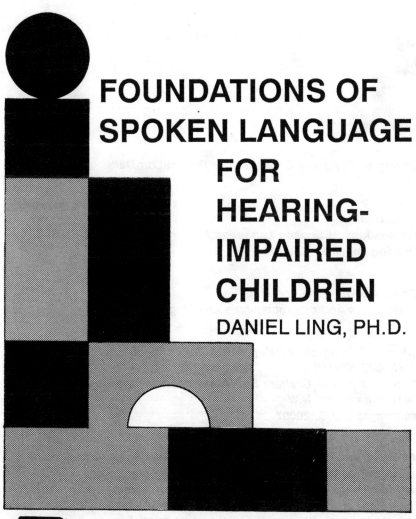

FOUNDATIONS OF SPOKEN LANGUAGE FOR HEARING-IMPAIRED CHILDREN

DANIEL LING, PH.D.

Alexander Graham Bell Association for the Deaf, Inc.
3417 Volta Place, N.W., Washington, D.C. 20007-2778

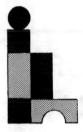

Library of Congress Cataloging in Publication Data

Ling, Daniel
Foundations of Spoken Language for
Hearing-impaired Children

Cover design: Jane Lee Ling
Illustrations and diagrams: Jane Lee Ling

Library of Congress catalog card number 89-060542
ISBN 0-88200-165-5
©1989 Alexander Graham Bell Association for the Deaf
3417 Volta Place, N.W.
Washington, D.C. 20007

Printed in the United States of America
10 9 8 7 6 5 4

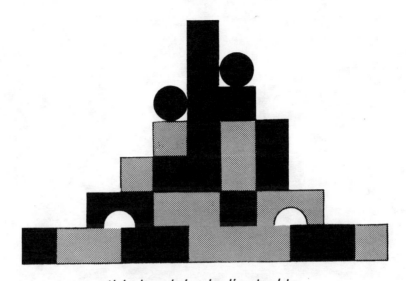

this book is dedicated to

Philip, Alister, Ken, And Brendan

and

to the many colleagues and children

who have contributed to my

learning and teaching

preface

In this text, I have attempted to present, in a step-by-step manner, the information necessary for helping hearing-impaired children to develop spoken language. My goal has been to present each topic in simple yet accurate terms, and to promote understanding of the essentials by avoiding unnecessary details and technicalities. At the same time, I have tried to write every chapter in such a way that it will provide insights into the processes involved in fostering the acquisition of spoken language by hearing-impaired children. To assist readers for whom this material is completely new, a glossary (Appendix D) defines all the special terms that are used. For those who find some parts too technical in spite of my efforts, I can only plead that the material is complex, and that to over-simplify would be to mislead. Most of those for whom this book is intended will, I am sure, find it reasonably easy to read. Those who want more detail than this text provides, may refer to the books and journals listed at the end of each chapter as suggested further reading. These, together with discussion and workshops on the various topics, are strongly recommended as sources for more advanced information.

This book has been written for the variety of people who are concerned with hearing-impaired children: students, educators, professionals engaged in providing support services, physicians, parents, and interested lay persons. The students I have in mind are those preparing to work as teachers of the hearing-impaired, audiologists, and speech-language pathologists. This text should be particularly helpful to teachers working in special and regular education who are likely to have hearing-impaired children integrated into their classes. The book should also be useful to practitioners who wish to focus more intensively on the development of spoken language. Several of the chapters inevitably contain material that will be more familiar to certain readers than to others. All the information presented is, however, essential for providing hearing-impaired children with the help they need in learning to communicate optimally through the spoken word.

Twelve years have passed since the publication of *Speech and the Hearing Impaired Child* (Ling, 1976). While that text will continue to be a useful reference, this one will be additionally helpful to those seeking to make the best use of recent advances in linguistic knowledge and relevant technology. Ten years ago, there were no wearable digital hearing aids, no children wearing cochlear implants or tactile devices, and few homes or classrooms with computers. Such technological tools now have widespread acceptance. They have led, and are continuing to lead, to new ways of harnessing a hearing-impaired child's sense modalities for the perception and production of spoken language. This book sets out to discuss such recent advances and suggest how they can be integrated with established practices of proven validity to promote truly effective perceptual-oral teaching. Strategies are outlined that can be used both to elicit new speech patterns and to take them beyond their phonetic level development into words and their everyday use in spoken language. In short, it deals with both principles and practices.

This text emphasizes the role of informal learning as well as the use of formal teaching. Systematic help of either sort can prevent common errors previously found in the speech of hearing-impaired children, improve incorrectly produced patterns, and enhance intelligibility.

Many reasons are provided for making an early start on building spoken language skills. One of the most obvious is that very young children really have nothing better to do in their first five years than to spend most of their waking time gaining an understanding of their physical and social world, and learning to communicate through speech. However, not all discussion is focused on how to create environments rich in experience and spoken language for very young hearing-impaired children. Certainly, such early childhood environments can increase the chances that a child will acquire a large proportion of his or her spoken language before formal schooling is begun. It is, however, stressed throughout the text that an abundance of opportunities for older children to learn spoken language and highly effective speech communication skills can also be provided.

As certain topics are considered, it will become apparent that more data are required if an adequate understanding of them is to be reached. The pursuit of further knowledge however, cannot be left entirely to those who specialize in university-based research. Much of the information necessary for future advances can only be generated by reflective practitioners - teachers, clinicians, parents, and other caregivers - who regard the effective application and refinement of emerging knowledge as an ongoing challenge. It is hoped that this text will be a stimulus to such individuals.

A small problem in writing about English speech is that several sounds represented by digraphs (two letters = one sound) in our everyday writing are represented by a single symbol in phonetic script. Because many readers of this text are likely to be unfamiliar with phonetic script, all sounds that have orthography and phonetic script in common will be presented between slash marks as, for example, with /b/, /d/, and /f/. Digraphs or other sounds that cannot be represented in this way will be underlined. These will, for example, include sounds such as j in the word *judge*, ch as in *cheese*, ah as in *father*, sh as in *sheep*, and ng as in *bang*. Italicized key words (as shown) also will be used to provide examples of how most people produce them. This arrangement, although novel, appears to be a simple and effective way to specify exactly what sounds are being talked about.

Caregivers of any sort (mothers, fathers, older peers, professionals), as well as the children themselves, as far as possible, are referred to throughout the text in the plural form in order to avoid the confusion of grammatical gender conventions with stereotypical sex roles. Where singular forms are more appropriate, the adults have been referred to as *she* in recognition of the high regard the writer has for the many mothers and female professionals with whom he has had the privilege of sharing his working life. The text recognizes that children come in both formats. They are often referred to in the plural as *they*, and sometimes symbolized in the singular as *he or she* and *him or her*, but just as often they are given names such as *Johnny* and *Joan* - all hypothetical children with wonderful personal attributes that hearing impairment could never tarnish.

Daniel Ling
Walkerville, Australia, March, 1988.
London, Ontario, Canada, October, 1988.

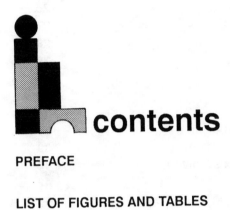

contents

figures and tables

Figure 1-1. A mother entertaining neighborhood children in her garden as a means of ensuring that her hearing-impaired child is happily and communicatively involved with hearing children of the same age. While the children are playing, she is noting their interests and language.**6**

Figure 1-2. A grandparent providing ongoing commentary as the hearing-impaired child is looking at some flowers. The proximity of the two ensures that the speech being addressed to the child has optimal clarity.**7**

Figure 1-3. A hearing-impaired child and his normally hearing brother being engaged in one of the many routine situations that abound in a home. In this case, the preparation of a meal provides the opportunity to relate spoken language to an ongoing activity. Note that only perceptual-oral commentary can be provided while a parent's hands are occupied.**10**

Figure 1-4. A profoundly hearing-impaired child being helped to produce a fricative through formal teaching. Touch is being used to convey the continuant property of the sh, a sound that could not be developed through the use of informal learning strategies.**18**

Figure 2-1. A diagram of the vocal tract showing the principal organs involved in speech.**29**

Figure 2-2. A narrow-band spectrogram showing the harmonics of voice. Time is represented on the horizontal axis, frequency on the vertical axis, and intensity by shading. The more intense the sounds, the darker the mark levels. On this spectrogram, the harmonics, multiples of the fundamental frequency, can be seen as a series of parallel horizontal bars. Vocal tract resonances make some harmonics stronger than others.**31**

Figure 2-3. A diagram depicting the approximate tongue configurations for production of the three vowels ah, oo, and ee, and (above) broad-band spectrograms showing the formants of these vowels as produced by the writer. Because broad-band spectrograms sample frequency bands that are twice as wide as those in narrow-band spectrograms (as in Figure 2-2), they highlight formants rather than harmonics.**34**

Figure 2-4. A chart showing the approximate center frequencies of the first and second formants of the three vowels oo, ah, and ee, as spoken by the writer. The points at which a vertical line drawn from any word would intersect the two lines in the diagram permit one to read off the approximate F_1 and F_2 center frequency values of the intermediate vowels.**35**

Figure 2-5. A broad-band spectrogram showing CV and VC transitions - the interaction of vowels and consonants. The transitions (rapid changes in formant frequency) shown are those created by saying the words *pier* and *tier*.**36**

Figure 2-6. The vocal tract in relation to place of consonant production. The shape of the lips and the tongue, as well as the point of contact or close approximation of the various organs (specified in each diagram), will vary considerably according to vowel context. The speech organs approximate and leave these positions dynamically as the various consonants release, interrupt and arrest the various vowels.**40**

Figure 3-1. A diagram showing the main components of the human auditory system.**49**

Figure 3-2. a. A diagram of the middle ear and cochlea. Part of the vestibule and part of the cochlea have been cut away, to show how the fluid contained in the cochlea moves as sound causes the stapes to vibrate. **b.** A diagram depicting the cochlea as if it has been unrolled, showing how frequency perception relates, in part, to distance from the stapes. The fluid movement, depicted by the arrows in both diagrams, results in maximal displacements of the structures in the inner ear at different points along the length of the cochlea, depending on the rate at which the stapes vibrates. Such displacement results in patterns of receptor cell stimulation that permit analysis of a sound's frequency.**50**

250 Hz plus or minus a half-octave are eliminated, differences in the remainder of the sounds are difficult to see. Similarly, if amplification in this frequency band is insufficient, differences in the remainder of the sounds could be difficult for severely and profoundly hearing-impaired children to discriminate. Because too little amplification would render the nasal murmur inaudible to them, they would probably be unable to distinguish between nasal and non-nasal sounds.**92**

Figure 4-3. a. Alan's aided (A−A) and unaided (O−O and X−X) thresholds in relation to the CLEAR zone (the approximate zone in which the conversational level elements of speech are present in the acoustic range normally created by a speaker at a distance of two yards). Only one response appears within this zone - the one at 1000 Hz. This permits Alan to hear only one of the elements of The Five-Sound Test, namely the vowel ah. **b.** The improvement in Alan's aided thresholds following adjustment of the hearing aid and the fitting of new earmolds. Only the /s/ and other sounds in the octave band centered on 4000 Hz cannot be amplified sufficiently, and remain inaudible to him.**100**

Figure 4-4. Audiograms showing Barbara's hearing levels and the effects of amplification on the intensity levels of speech she received:**a.** Barbara's thresholds in relation to how speech components in the CLEAR zone were amplified by her hearing aids. **b.** The satisfactory outcome of appropriate earmold selection: all significant components of speech including high-frequency cues, have been rendered detectable.**105**

Figure 4-5. Carleen's unaided (left ear) thresholds in relation to normal sound field thresholds (dB SPL re. 20 microPascals): **a.** with the CLEAR zone as amplified by her hearing aid. (Note inadequate amplification at 250 Hz.) **b.** The satisfactory outcome of hearing aid adjustments. (Note thresholds at all frequencies are in the CLEAR zone.)**106**

Figure 4-6. Dawn's unaided (left ear) thresholds in relation to normal sound field thresholds (SPL re. 20 microPascals): **a.** Dawn's responses together with the (unamplified) clear zone. Note that all her thresholds (X−X) lie above this zone and that she can, therefore, hear nothing of conversational level speech at a distance of two yards without her hearing aids. The response of the hearing aids selected for her (H−H) lies between her thresholds and her loudness discomfort level (LDL). **b.** The levels to which the CLEAR zone has been amplified by the hearing

Figure 8-1. The major stages of speech acquisition. The process of speech acquisition follows seven relatively distinct stages, each having both phonetic (motor speech) and phonologic (spoken language) components.**225**

Figure 9-1. An audiogram of a profoundly hearing-impaired boy named Sean. Note that his aided audiogram provides substantial amplification at 250 Hz. Because Sean has no hearing beyond 1000 Hz, there is no fear of upward spread of masking that could affect high-frequency acoustic cues. The increasing amount of shading in the CLEAR zone depicts the reduction of cues on voice and vocalization as frequency increases.**260**

Figure 10-1. The approximate frequency and intensity of F_1 and F_2 of the back and central vowels, and F_2 of the front vowels, depicted on an audiogram at the approximate hearing levels they would reach when produced at a conversational level by a talker speaking at a distance of about two yards.**290**

Figure 10-2. A spectrogram showing the similarity between the F_1 trajectories of the diphthongs in the words *eye* and *ow* - words that sound very different indeed to the normal listener. Cover the frequencies above 1000 Hz, and then study the patterns that remain. The lower portions of the spectrograms indicate how easily one of these sounds could be mistaken for the other by a listener with no hearing beyond that frequency.**309**

Figure 12-1. An audiogram showing the frequency band within the CLEAR zone in which the main cues on place of consonant production occur in conversational level speech from a distance of two yards, and the unaided and aided thresholds of Jim, a profoundly hearing-impaired child who through aided audition alone, could discriminate between some consonants differing only in place. Most severely hearing-impaired children (those with less restricted aided audition in the high-frequency range) can be expected to perceive most place distinctions through the use of hearing under good acoustic conditions.**341**

Figure 13-1. Spectrograms of the /w/ and j in the context of ah, indicating the similarity of the F_1 components of these semi-vowels. Children with no aided hearing beyond 1000 Hz may readily confuse them through audition alone. The temporal differences (j̱ as in ya being the longer) are not consistent in everyday speech.**365**

Figure 13-2. The position in which hands can be placed to provide an analogy for teaching the /k/ or /g/. The upper hand represents the palate, and the lower hand, the tongue.**369**

Table 5-1. The components of speech that can be detected wholly (Y), in part (Y_p), or not at all (N) through useful residual audition that extends up to, but not beyond 1000 Hz, normal vision, and the two together. Note that residual audition and vision together yield most of the available information on speech.**127**

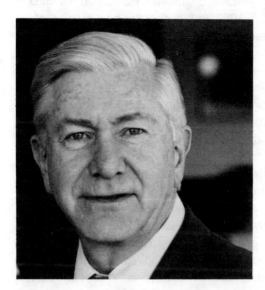

about the author

Daniel Ling was born in England. Following Royal Air Force service in radar and communications, he received his professional training as a teacher at St. John's College, York, and in Audiology and Education of the Deaf at Manchester University. He worked for four years as a class-room teacher of the deaf in Sheffield from 1951-55, and directed special educational services for hearing-impaired children in Reading, Berkshire, from 1955-63. While employed in Reading, he undertook research in various areas of speech, hearing, and educational audiology at Cambridge Institute of Education, and later in the Department of Psychology at Reading University. As a teacher in Reading, he established the first comprehensive services outside London for the mainstream education of hearing-impaired children, provision that included diagnostic and audiological services, a parent-infant program, special-class education within regular schools and itinerant supervision of fully integrated children. This provision served as a model for the establishment of similar work by many other Local Education Authorities throughout the British Isles.

Ling moved to Canada in 1963. He first served as Principal of the Montreal Oral School for the Deaf, and later directed the McGill University Research Project for Hearing-Impaired Children. He earned his Ph.D at McGill University, Montreal, in 1968 and, during the continuation of his work as Director of the Research Project, became a professor in the School of Human Communication Disorders. While at McGill University, Ling served for several years as Chairman of the Department and directed speech and audiology services in two Montreal hospitals. He accepted his present appointment as Dean of the Faculty of Applied Health Sciences at the University of Western Ontario, in 1984.

Ling has helped to establish education and habilitation for hearing-impaired children in many different countries. He has contributed over two hundred articles and six books to the literature related to hearing impairment in childhood. He is a Fellow of the American Speech-Language-Hearing Association, and has received several honors, including the Jonas Award of the New York League for the Hard of Hearing. He also received the Teacher of the Year Award from the International Organization of Educators for the Hearing Impaired (IOEHI), a section of the Alexander Graham Bell Association for the Deaf, in 1981 and served as President of that Association from 1984-86.

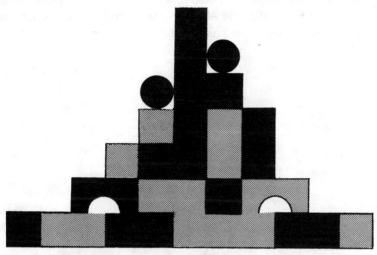

acknowledgements

The writer is grateful to Peter Blamey, Graeme Clark, Terry Nien-huys, and Field Rickards (University of Melbourne), who contributed ideas in the early stages of drafting this text. George Pittman (also from Australia) suggested several of the examples used in Chapter 7. Donald Doehring and Doris Leckie (McGill University) commented on early drafts of this book, which was begun in Australia during a study leave granted to me by the University of Western Ontario. Sos Brown floated some excellent ideas by me during the early stages of writing. Changes suggested by my son Philip, and my friends and colleagues Gillian Clezy, Robert Leckie and Bruce Casselman improved the clarity of the text. I am particulary indebted to my good friend and colleague Sandra North, whose reviews of repeated drafts made important contributions to every chapter. My thanks are also due to Marlene Pavey and Susan Schonfeld, both talented parents, for the helpful reviews and comments they provided. Timely, generous and thoughtful responses to my requests for technical criticisms were made by members of my Faculty at the University of Western Ontario - Jean-Paul Gagné, Shane Moodie, Kevin Munhall and Richard Seewald.

All illustrations and figures in the text were created with love and care by my wife, Jane, whose enthusiasm for helping and sharing was a constant encouragement and joy during the preparation of this text.

Lastly, this manuscript was edited in its entirety by Lucy Cuzon du Rest, Director of Publications at Alexander Graham Bell Association for the Deaf, with whom the writer enjoyed a close collaboration.

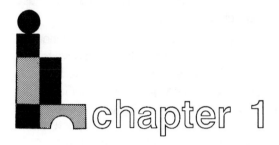

chapter 1

speech communication

People usually communicate through at least one spoken language. Each such language is a different code - a different way of using verbal patterns to convey meaning. The majority of people learn their mother tongue without conscious effort as young children and then, as adults, speak and understand it automatically. Most people are, therefore, unaware of the complexity inherent in talking and listening. But many children, particularly those who are profoundly hearing-impaired, need our help in learning to communicate through spoken language. In order to give that help, we must first become more fully aware of the tasks involved.

production and perception of speech

To produce spoken messages we, as talkers, have to go through a series of at least five distinct steps: we select words from a vocabulary stored in memory; arrange them in an order that will readily be understood by listeners who share our linguistic code and the implicit rules of grammar we and they have derived from experience; activate the

1

muscles that put the speech mechanism in motion; create the various speech sounds that make up our words and sentences; listen to ourselves as we talk to ensure that the message is produced as we intended; plan future sentences as we are speaking and, at the same time, assess the effect of what we are saying on the listener's behavior. Each activity, each aspect of the process, consists of many component skills. These will be discussed in subsequent chapters.

Speech perception is no less complex than speech production. To understand spoken messages in face-to-face situations, we have to sort out the words from background noise; separate and identify sounds and words in the stream of speech (for they are all joined together in natural utterances); note the talker's pronunciation and mood; recognize the form (grammar) of the sentences; attend to the talker's body posture and movements; deduce the person's reason for talking; search the words and sentences for their meaning; examine what has been or is being said and simultaneously predict what may be said next; and, if the message is being understood, signal the fact to the speaker. "Listeners," as they are described in this book, do more than use their ears. They search a message for meaning with all of their senses and certainly use their brains to interpret what is said. Given the complexity of the tasks in speech perception, it is amazing that most children can understand quite a lot of speech by (or soon after) their first birthday.

The characteristics of the human nervous system are such that speech production and speech perception, in spite of their complexity, come naturally to most of us and are mastered very readily by all but a few children at an early age. This fact is on our side in teaching hearing-impaired children to talk. Successful development of their spoken language can usually be promoted when we take the necessary steps to develop their perceptual-oral language skills - when we make it possible for them to become good listeners through aiding their residual hearing or providing other sensory aids, and when we provide them with sufficient experience of communication through spoken language.

speech and spoken language

The several features of a spoken message (the components of speech and the various aspects of language) are in fact inseparable.

However, to deal with them adequately, they often have be treated separately. One can talk about speech apart from language just as one can discuss the respiratory system, for example, as if it were a distinct part of one's anatomy. But, as everyone knows, if the lungs were truly taken out of the body, both the lungs and the body would quickly die. So it is with speech and the different aspects of spoken language. Speech can only be meaningful when it is used in communication. True, one can help a child to develop certain sounds outside the context of language (and most children, as infants, do develop their repertoire of speech sounds in this way) but spoken language will never develop from such activity alone. To elicit speech patterns in a non-linguistic context is often the most efficient strategy for developing a child's spoken language skills, but they would be lost in as brief a time span as it would take to elicit them unless they are quickly employed in purposeful communication.

Speech, then, is an intrinsic part of spoken language. While it carries meaning in interpersonal messages efficiently, it is not in itself meaningful. We become very aware of this when we listen to an unfamiliar foreign tongue, for the talker and listener must both know the underlying code - the language - if the meaning of a spoken message is to be communicated. But speech is more than merely a medium for conveying an encoded linguistic message. Speech helps to form the language that it carries (for example, many words are onomatopoeic; they contain sounds that reflect the noises they represent, like "bang," "bubble," and "hiss"). Even the typical length of clauses and sentences, as well as their intonation patterns, are, to a considerable extent, determined by breath supply. Speech also serves as an aid in the recall of spoken messages, for one frequently rehearses words such as names or shopping lists by "saying them to oneself" in order to remember them.

That speech and language are not one and the same is also demonstrated by the fact that a message in a given language can be conveyed through writing. The written form is, however, based on the spoken word in most languages. Thus a word like "dog" has both three sounds (phonemes) and three letters (graphemes). Although our spelling does not always correspond with the spoken pattern, it usually does so. This is a great help in learning to read, because new words can, for the most part, be "sounded out" from their written form and often thus recognized. This advantage is not shared by those who speak Chinese or communicate by sign, because the elements of these languages do not correspond closely to the written forms such individuals are expected to use.

Spoken language has been defined most simply as words and the way we use them. Such a definition implies that we must consider not just a vocabulary, but the rules by which words are constructed and are then put together to form sentences and the collections of sentences that are used in discourse. Of course, vocabulary is an important facet of language. We can no more communicate effectively without a vocabulary than we can build houses without construction materials. Nor can we communicate effectively without a thorough (though perhaps unconscious) knowledge of the basic rules of language.

learning communication skills in infancy

A great deal more is known about speech and language now than was known only a few years ago. Even so, adults are generally still not as good at language teaching as children are at language learning. Indeed, universally poor standards of spoken language communication would exist if children were not so good at acquiring it through adequate exposure to everyday discourse. Informal learning permits most children to speak fluently and to listen effectively by age four, and to achieve mastery over their basic speech and language skills by the time they are seven or eight years old. Children appear to be both biologically and socially programmed to learn most of their communication skills in their early years. During infancy, they give it a great deal of their time and attention, and these are essential ingredients for success. Such success can grace the lives of most hearing-impaired children, too, if they are helped to perceive - and are expected to produce - the spoken word from an early age.

Since the beginning of the twentieth century, numerous technological developments have increased the potential for hearing-impaired children to acquire spoken language from an early age. Today, as never before in our history, the use of technology provides rich opportunities for such children to become adept in all aspects of speech communication. To take advantage of such opportunities, professionals must consistently seek to incorporate modern technology into well established oral habilitation practices. With the insightful application of present day knowledge and the selection and use of appropriate electronic devices, most hearing-impaired children, regardless of the extent of their impairments, can be helped to acquire fluent perceptual-oral language skills that can enable them to communicate, compete, and conform with the majority of their hearing peers.

home conditions and verbal learning

Verbal learning - the acquisition of all aspects of language - will occur only if suitable conditions are present in a child's environment. The best conditions for verbal learning by young hearing-impaired children are usually those that are provided in the home. Hearing aids can now be fitted during the first few months of life (see Chapter 4), and parents can be helped by well-qualified professionals to ensure that their hearing-impaired babies receive at least as much exposure to spoken language as their normally hearing peers. The children who develop the best speech communication skills are usually those who have developed them under home conditions during their early years.

Knowledgeable parents or other caregivers are the best possible providers of spoken language for young children. Parents can also do much to stimulate the growth of speech communication skills by ensuring that their child has abundant social contact and interaction with hearing peers. To promote such contact, many parents put on simple parties, obtain indoor toys and outdoor equipment such as sand trays, swings, and slides (see Figure 1-1), and thus attract neighbors' children to their homes. They can also arrange outings involving other parents and their children. Watching what normally hearing children of the same age do, listening to what they say during play, and noting how other parents talk and sing to them, are productive ways for parents of hearing-impaired children to obtain excellent guidelines for activities and the use of language that will be at an appropriate interest level.

Progress in learning to talk often begins from the time hearing aids are used all day and every day. Because that time is so important, many professionals refer to the months or years that have elapsed from that time as a child's "hearing age." Children who can make good use of their residual hearing - including some profoundly hearing-impaired children - may be helped to communicate fluently and intelligibly through natural sounding speech. Even children with total or near total deafness can, with the help of other types of sensory aids, also benefit from the informal yet intensive speech communication experiences provided through family living (see Chapter 5).

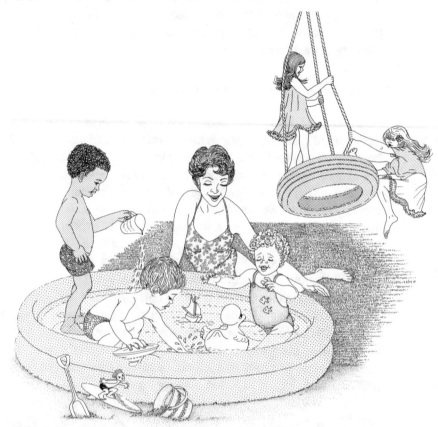

figure 1-1. A mother entertaining neighborhood children in her garden as a means of ensuring that her hearing-impaired child is happily and communicatively involved with hearing children of the same age. While the children are playing, she is noting their interests and language.

Communication by speech is normally rooted in the pre-verbal communication that occurs between children and their caregivers as they interact with each other long before the children's first words are uttered. Such pre-verbal communication is just as essential for children who are hearing impaired as for those who have normal hearing. Important components in pre-verbal communication are the adult's and child's shared attention to each other and to the same objects and events, and the adult's spoken commentary on them. Grandparents often make excellent caregivers and, as suggested by Figure 1-2, the time that a grandparent shares with a young child can be a joy and benefit to both.

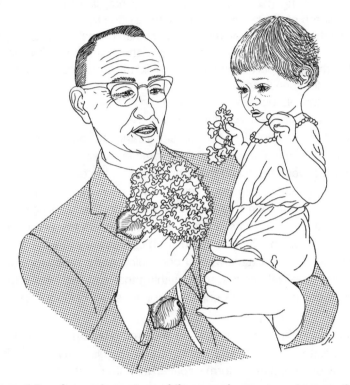

figure 1-2. **A grandparent providing ongoing commentary as the hearing-impaired child is looking at some flowers. The proximity of the two ensures that the speech being addressed to the child has optimal clarity.**

Parents, clinicians, and teachers are unlikely to succeed in establishing spoken language among hearing-impaired children if they have not already learned to interact with them through eye contact, touch, body posture, shared attention to external objects and events, and through the satisfaction of their needs as they are expressed other than in words.

Several different non-verbal behaviors may be developed to sophisticated levels by young hearing-impaired children who are over a year old and ready to learn how to communicate through speech. They include positive acts such as pointing, smiling, pulling, pushing, touching, hugging and kissing, and equally as many negative ones such as turning the head away, covering the eyes, throwing objects, kicking, and even biting. The important element in establishing communication from such behaviors is for the adult to recognize and acknowledge them in some way. Non-compliance is often intended as communicative behavior rather than as misbehavior. Young hearing-impaired children are, like many normally hearing children of the same age, much more often frustrated by adults' inability to interpret their pre-verbal behaviors than by their own inability to talk. Mothers who most successfully interpret their infant's primitive vocal and non-verbal attempts to communicate build the firmest foundations for that child's later speech communication. It is through parents' attempts to understand and encourage them during the first few years of life that hearing-impaired children also develop "oral intent" - the drive to talk.

Words are symbols that take on significance for normally hearing children over many months as they are uttered in the course of experiences shared between them and their caregivers. In the earliest stages of adult-child interaction, the adult talks about whatever is happening regardless of whether or not a baby can understand. Such talking makes babies aware of speech as an extension of the adult's presence - something that "keeps them in touch" with caregivers even when they are out of sight. This extensive and continuing early experience with normal adult vocalizations is also something that can, with the help of appropriate sensory aids, be enjoyed by almost all hearing-impaired children.

Knowledge that a child is hearing impaired often drives parents to seek immediate remedies; and teachers and clinicians try to provide them. The widespread use of formal speech teaching strategies with very young children who have not acquired any approximations to adult forms of language is an example. Speech skill acquisition in a special setting for hearing-impaired children should never be allowed to take precedence over language learning at home. Certainly a young child should be encouraged to vocalize and develop different sound patterns - but always in the course of what youngsters regard as play, and never without it being part of a fun activity. Few, if any, formal speech teaching strategies should be employed before children use speech patterns that approximate adult forms of utterance (see Chapter 7). One should not attempt to develop a specific speech or language pattern through formal teaching procedures until a child has failed, after having been given ample opportunity, to develop the looked-for pattern informally. Nothing can replace the opportunity to acquire a given language pattern spontaneously in home conditions and at an appropriate stage of acquisition.

So far as possible, it should be the children's search for meaning and clarity of expression, rather than procedures that adults impose, that guides the development of their communication skills.

Sadly, some parents stop talking to children when they are diagnosed as hearing impaired. Mistakenly, they reason "why talk if the child can't hear?" But most hearing-impaired children can learn to listen and function mainly through hearing if provided with appropriate hearing aids. Parents should, therefore, be encouraged to fit their children with hearing aids (and/or other sensory aids if more appropriate) and to continue talking to them, for at no time in a child's life are the physical and acoustic conditions as favorable for listening as in early infancy. The young child is frequently within touching distance, so that speech is heard well above most background noises. Home conditions also minimize the reflection and reverberation of sound. To talk to hearing-impaired children in the home, during early infancy, is to establish communication at a developmental stage when hearing speech and being in acoustic contact with adults have their most positive effects on later learning. It is during infancy that normally hearing children grasp the meaning of words that they hear clearly with very little repetition. The less clearly children hear what is said to them (and around them), the more experience of spoken language they must be given before they can comprehend and begin to use it.

activity-based learning

The routines in which babies first hear speech are highly repetitive as well as enjoyable for the baby. They are, of course, those connected with caregiving activities such as washing, dressing, feeding, and other forms of care, including play. Particularly as babies become aware of the variety of objects and events around them, caregivers generally start to use more slowly articulated utterances with exaggerated intonation patterns and sentences that fit more and more with what they think a child might understand. They share a baby's attention to objects and events more often than they expect a baby to look at or play with something that interests them as adults. The child tends to lead the adult in exploration of the world rather than the reverse. As they share attention with their baby, adults comment and explain the salient features of whatever the child is looking at. They do not normally pressure a child into responding by demanding imitations or insisting on answers to questions. Once speech communication is beginning to emerge, good parenting demands that, when questions are asked, the children are given adequate time to formulate a reply. Activities in and around the home that are accompanied by comments, explanations, descriptions, and other forms of verbal and non-verbal interaction with parents and siblings not only provide the foundations for language learning, but transmit the family's cultural values. The mother involving her hearing-impaired child and his normally hearing brother in the preparation of a meal (see Figure 1-3) provides a good example of a parent using a routine situation to provide ongoing commentaries on shared activities.

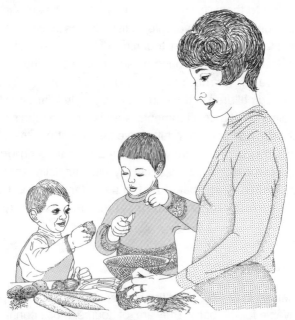

figure 1-3. **A hearing-impaired child and his normally hearing brother engaged in one of the many routine situations that abound in a home. In this case, the preparation of a meal provides the opportunity to relate spoken language to an ongoing activity. Note that only perceptual-oral commentary can be provided while a parent's hands are occupied.**

infancy: an optimal or a critical learning period?

The early years of a child's life can be an exceptionally fruitful period for spoken language development for several reasons. First, as mentioned above, young children have nothing better to do than discover as much as they can about their world and learn to communicate effectively through speech as they grow. Second, they can be the sole object of an adoring adult's attention for at least some, and often much of their time, and can be spoken to at close range. Third, the interaction between the caregiver and the child can focus, often exclusively, on meeting the child's unique needs and addressing the child's personal interests. Fourth, the acoustic environment, buffered against undue reflection and reverberation of sounds by carpets, drapes, and other soft furnishings, can approach the ideal. Of course, it is possible to turn homes into noisy, unsuitable places for hearing-impaired children to learn. The clatter of pots and pans, radios or television sets turned to high volume, and a few other children shouting as they bang toys against hard surfaces can make it impossible for anyone to hear speech and understand it. The best way for parents to determine what sound conditions are like for their child is for them to listen to their own and other's speech through their child's hearing aids. They should do this in different rooms in the house, and under both quiet and noisy conditions.

Parents should not despair of their child's chances to acquire speech communication skills if, for various reasons, they have missed opportunities to help them during the first few years. All is not lost if hearing-impaired children make a later-than-ideal start. Certainly, progress tends to be more rapid if attention is given to the development of speech communication in early infancy. However, the writer has successfully helped many profoundly hearing-impaired children to establish intelligible and natural sounding speech communication. Among them were those who did not begin their education (and hence did not begin to pronounce their first words) until they were between five and nine years old. Even work with young adults who wished to improve the quality of their unintelligible speech has been successful. Thus, the early years cannot be considered as a *crucial* or *critical* period for acquiring effective speech communication skills, but they are most certainly *optimal* for such learning.

alternative modes of communication

sign language

It is, of course, possible for hearing-impaired children to learn to communicate by sign rather than through spoken language. Sign language is usually recommended, by those who advocate its use, as the principal means of language development in total communication programs - those that use any or all possible means of communication. The essential difference between most oral programs and most total communication programs is that oral programs set out to teach spoken language *and to use it as the primary means of social and educational communication*, whereas total communication programs tend to rely principally on sign language for these purposes. This book is concerned with the essential bases of spoken language. Sign language and sign systems will not, therefore, be discussed except in relation to the right of parents to choose the communication system they prefer to use with their young children, and what modes of communication are open to older children in exercising their right to communicate as they wish with their peers. These issues will be briefly addressed in Appendix B.

Cued Speech

An alternative to sign language and auditory-oral programs is offered by Cued Speech, a system of hand cues designed to take some of the guesswork out of speech reception through speechreading. Some of the sounds of speech, such as /p/, /b/, and /m/ look alike on the lips. The hand configurations and hand positions used in Cued Speech can prevent confusion between such sounds and thus help those whose speechreading cannot be supplemented adequately by hearing aids, tactile devices or cochlear implants. Cued Speech has been successfully used to develop spoken language among children who are totally and near-totally deaf. Its possibilities and limitations are explored in considerable detail in Chapter 5.

choosing among modes of communication

The communication mode to be used by a child should be chosen by the parents once they have been informed of, and have observed, exemplary programs of all kinds. Parents should not be over-ready to accept the promises or advice given by advocates of any mode of communication, by the representatives of any educational system, or by the professionals in any program. Instead, they should insist on seeing and talking with children who are the representative products of intervention through the different modes of communication - children who have a similar background, and much the same type and degree of hearing impairment as that of their own child. In this way they can reliably determine what sort of preparation for life the various modes of communication would offer. They can then ask themselves whether they would be happy if their own child were to have similar communication skills and educational attainments some years down the road, whether a recommended program could meet their aspirations for their children, and whether they, themselves, could respond comfortably to the demands of the program. To make such judgements is a necessary, but difficult task for parents who are having to adjust to the fact that their child has impaired hearing. *It is important that the choice be theirs, however, for it is they and their child, and not the professionals or other advocates of a system, who will have to live with the results.*

It is often wise to avoid making the choice of communication mode immediately following diagnosis. Many parents give themselves time to consider the implications of choice by first enrolling their child in an early intervention program geared to spoken language development. They realize that decisions on the relative merits of the various modes can be rational only when they are related to the clearly defined needs and proven potential of individual hearing-impaired children. Valid diagnoses of a child's needs and potentials cannot be specified through clinical examinations; they can be adequately established only through ongoing evaluation in the course of treatment. Early (preferably parent-oriented) auditory-verbal programs can best assess a child's potential for acquiring speech communication skills because only such programs can offer the whole-hearted commitment that is optimal for developing them.

To begin an auditory-verbal approach with their child during infancy, parents should seek the guidance of, and work closely with, competent and experienced professionals. Close collaboration between caregivers and professionals can do more than help the majority of hearing-impaired children to establish excellent standards of spoken language and lay the foundations for academic success. Such collaboration can also help caregivers to learn and to share in diagnostic teaching activities. In this way, they can participate in the process of deciding whether or not there is a need to introduce supplementary or alternative forms of communication. This approach reduces parental anxieties and fears that they will make errors affecting the child's future. This is important, for supplementary and alternative types of information provided by Cued

Speech and sign language can end up retarding or supplanting rather than augmenting spoken language development if they are introduced when there is no need for them. Parents should be aware, however, that many school boards offer a limited range of options for hearing-impaired children, and though most are under an obligation to provide a free and appropriate education, many resist offering spoken language instruction (oral) programs. Advice on how to approach such problems with school boards can be obtained through contacting the Department of Professional Programs and Services at the Volta Bureau, the headquarters of the Alexander Graham Bell Association for the Deaf.

why spoken language?

Most professionals concerned with hearing impairment, even those who also use sign language, recognize that children who acquire spoken language have many advantages over those who do not. Because spoken language communication is the normal means of social interchange, the effective use and understanding of speech permits hearing-impaired individuals to interact easily with the majority of people in the community at large. As a result, ability to speak and understand speech affords hearing-impaired children optimal opportunity for independence and permits them a wide range of educational, social, and vocational choices. Learning to read is also enhanced by speech, because the correspondence between the spoken and the written form helps in the development of word attack skills. Speech also plays an important role in various memory processes, including the rehearsal and recall of verbal material. Note, for example, how many people say new words over to themselves in order to remember them. These reasons alone suggest that no hearing-impaired child who has the potential to learn to communicate through spoken language should be denied the opportunity to achieve it.

acquiring spoken language skills after infancy

The emphasis in this chapter so far, has been mainly on the enhancement of children's spontaneous learning through their immersion in home environments that emphasize speech communication from the outset. Given appropriate sensory devices such as hearing aids, tactile aids or cochlear implants, as well as caregivers who encourage learning through the dynamic and informed use of these devices in the context of everyday growth and living, most hearing-impaired children will spontaneously acquire a great deal of spoken language. Even such enlightened use of technology, however, will not be sufficient to lead all children to develop adequate speech communication skills through informal learning opportunities alone. While the main focus must always be on meaningful communication within language-rich living, some children will also need direct and formal teaching. For such teaching to be successful, it must never be regarded as a substitute for spontaneous spoken language development but rather as a supplement to it.

Older and later-starting children are often faced with situations that may not optimally enhance the acquisition of spoken language. Once past infancy, children are expected to learn other things, such as arithmetic, reading, writing, and other academic subjects that may be presented in such a way that they compete with, rather than promote speech communication. In school, teaching is usually geared to several children rather than to a single child. Learning to communicate as a member of a group requires a different and a vastly more difficult range of skills than learning to communicate as one of a dyad. The teacher or clinician, however caring, cannot achieve the quality of bond that is shared between parent and child. The acoustic conditions are far from ideal in most schools, where noise is less likely to be prevented by carpeting or absorbed by soft furnishings, and more likely to be created because there are more people to produce it.

The greatest disadvantage for later starters lies, not in the environmental features of school versus home, but in the fact that they have, over the years, acquired habits that hinder verbal learning - habits that must be overcome. Children who do not, during infancy, learn to communicate through spoken language as they acquire basic concepts of the world around them *do not just fail to learn spoken language; they learn to do without it.*

Older hearing-impaired children may have to receive remedial teaching in order to overcome certain deficiencies in spoken language that have occurred as a result of delay in their receiving assistance. Remedial teaching strategies are those that create and exploit age-appropriate situations that lead to mastery of specific skills that are normally acquired at an earlier age. Remedial work may demand the use of formal teaching rather than the informal enhancement of a child's opportunities for early, spontaneous learning (see Chapter 7). Inevitably, late starters must be helped to substitute new patterns of interaction for less desirable ones that may have become habitual. It is not surprising, then, that remedial strategies leading to meaningful use of spoken language in communication are more difficult and time consuming than those employed to develop it well from the beginning (see Chapter 9).

Speech communication must surround and involve hearing-impaired children who are in the process of learning spoken language. In order for them to learn to communicate through spoken language after infancy has passed, they must, either consciously or unconsciously, become aware of the advantages that accrue from effective speech communication, consistently experience success, and gain pleasure in the course of their verbal interactions with caregivers and peers. This being so, they require an environment where spoken language is an (if not the) accepted form of everyday communication among and between both adults and other children. Any formal procedures used to develop speech and language skills should be speedy, effective, and fun. Moreover, speech and language behaviors that are targeted for formal teaching procedures should, once elicited, be quickly targeted for use by the child in meaningful communication in school and at home.

Once children are in school, the most important variable in the development of their spoken language is the expectation that, with appropriate help from caregivers and professionals, they can achieve it. Unless effective speech communication is an expected outcome of an educational program, it will never occur. Not only must children enrolled in a given program become increasingly motivated to improve their speech communication skills through achieving satisfaction from the use of spoken language, their teachers must also be motivated by the children's successes to extend their knowledge of language acquisition processes and improve the techniques through which they promote them. Motivation is discussed more extensively in Chapter 9.

teaching speech communication skills

To fulfil its function in communication, a child's speech must be intelligible not only to family and teachers, but also to strangers. In order for such a standard of speech production to be achieved by severely and profoundly hearing-impaired children who have acquired little or no spoken language during infancy, a developmental model for speech acquisition, such as that described in Chapter 8, must be followed throughout the school years, so that gains are consistently realized and consolidated as the children move from class to class. Such a program can only be provided if each of the teachers in the school is completely familiar with the developmental model and can automatically select and employ whatever strategies are required to elicit and foster the communicative use of all speech patterns. Ideally, the children's caregivers should also be familiar with the speech development model and be able to support the school's initiatives in using it.

Children enrolled in schools that focus primarily on formal speech teaching must be provided from the outset with optimal opportunities to succeed. They must have hearing aids or other sensory aids that compensate as fully as possible for their hearing impairment, and a program designed to ensure that every activity undertaken with the child is one that provides optimal opportunity for them to understand speech and to learn to talk intelligibly. This means that any speech skills that are elicited through formal strategies should continue to be developed through the use of further informal learning stategies applied in the course of various ongoing school activities.

Direct, formal teaching of speech and spoken language usually involve situations in which a child is required to sit down and learn a particular pattern through conscious effort and through the use of visual and tactile strategies (see Chapter 7). Highly skilled teachers and clinicians favor working through natural, preferably auditory, strategies to the greatest extent possible, and they fall back on such formal teaching only when informal work alone does not yield the desired results. A teacher working with formal strategies in order to obtain a fricative from a profoundly hearing-impaired girl is depicted in Figure 1-4. Informal auditory strategies had led this child to acquire fluent spoken language that was marred by inadequate fricatives. This child had no hearing beyond 2000 Hz.

Unnecessary frustration is likely to be experienced by both adults and children when formal teaching of speech is introduced either at too early or too late a stage in a child's communicative development. Many normally hearing children cannot pronounce certain sounds by three years of age but will go on to master them without therapy. Hearing-impaired children can also fail to make certain sounds during their early years, not because they cannot hear them but because they are not developmentally ready to produce them. Children and their needs differ. It is, therefore, difficult to specify an appropriate age for beginning to focus on formal teaching strategies but, by and large, it is not to be recommended below age three. Nor, if formal strategies need to be adopted, should they be introduced too late, for both correct and incorrect patterns, when used frequently, tend to become habitual. Most children who need formal teaching should begin receiving it between three and eight years of age.

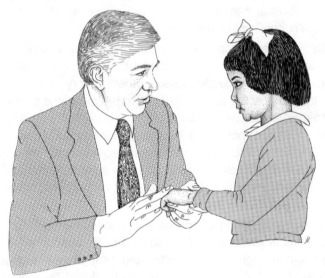

figure 1-4. **A profoundly hearing-impaired child being helped to produce a fricative through formal teaching. Touch is being used to convey the continuant property of the** sh, **a sound that could not be developed through the use of informal learning strategies.**

By age three, many hearing-impaired children who have been enrolled in appropriate early intervention programs are talking fluently, and would not, therefore, require formal teaching or special school education. Their needs are for support services within mainstream educational settings. Others, similarly treated, continue to benefit more from informal learning opportunities than from formal teaching beyond age three, and even beyond age five. There are two sorts of children in this age range who require formal spoken language teaching within a special school environment: those who have not benefitted sufficiently from auditory-verbal or other forms of early intervention, and those who are late starters. The upper limit of eight years for beginning formal spoken language training is suggested because, if children by this age have not already acquired a substantial amount of speech communication skill, they will either have learned to do without spoken language, have learned an alternative system of communication, or have handicaps in addition to hearing impairment that impede spoken language acquisition.

While it is possible *to improve* well-established speech skills after age eight, and indeed into adult life, it is extremely difficult for children to develop intelligible speech when they are expected *to begin* learning to talk so late. Progress in teaching severely or profoundly hearing-impaired children to talk when they have no functional speech communication skills by the middle of their elementary school years is extremely slow. It becomes almost impossible to attain reasonable levels of spoken language if one begins such work as late as age eleven. Decisions as to whether a child should have the opportunity to acquire fluency in spoken language skills (not just token sounds and words) should, therefore, be made early on, and preferably before formal schooling begins. *Nature does not leave open the option to learn effective speech communication until children are old enough to choose it for themselves.*

school-based speech communication specialists

Some schools that are strongly committed to the development of spoken language among their pupils employ speech communication specialists. These are usually speech/language pathologists who have had some special courses in, or experience relating to, speech development in hearing-impaired children, or teachers of the hearing-impaired who have a particular interest in developing spoken language communication. Such personnel can be a very great help in developing the speech communication skills and the spoken language of hearing impaired children within many school situations. Their work is often difficult to define and their schedules are by no means simple to organize. The following list of activities they commonly undertake makes this clear.

Speech specialists are usually expected to:

1. collaborate with the teacher(s) so that they keep themselves and the teacher(s) informed of the content of each other's work with all children;

2. work effectively with a sufficiently large number of children, in groups or individually, to make a difference to the standards within the school;

3. schedule their work so that the children are not taken from lessons that they should be sharing with others;

4. plan their work with each child so that each session contains not only speech, but meaningful spoken language targets, because speech targets are quickly achieved in the hands of an expert, boring to the children if continued for more than a minute or two, and of little relevance unless immediately placed in the context of meaningful language;

5. carry out appropriate evaluations with each of their children (see Chapter 8);

6. keep records of the speech and spoken language development of each of their children;

7. respond to the class teachers' requests for suggestions on strategies that may help them deal with unusual speech or communication problems;

8. provide ideas, as they are requested by the class teacher, on how best to integrate speech and spoken language development into each aspect of the school's academic program;

9. coordinate the speech programs of individual children as they move up through the school, from class to class, so that no ground is lost as a result of academic progression;

10. create effective liaisons with other support personnel and facilities that play an essential role in the children's lives (for example, audiologists, otolaryngologists, pediatricians, and leaders of clubs that the children may join).

Clearly, the role of speech communication specialists will vary from school to school. In most programs they serve as support personnel - specialists whose job it is to assist the teachers. In that role, they may or may not be involved with counselling parents or maintaining a liaison with teachers in regular schools where former pupils have been enrolled for part-time or full-time mainstream education. To be successful in such a support role, these specialists must not only be excellent practitioners;

they must also have a special blend of independence and interpersonal skills that will ensure smooth, high-quality collaboration with teaching staff whose personalities are likely to differ considerably. Additionally, speech specialists have to enjoy what they are doing, for this is the sort of work where achievement must often be rewarding in itself; speech specialists are not usually part of a system attended by promotion or other rewards.

teaching to ensure carry-over

The purpose of teaching speech communication to hearing-impaired children is to provide them with the necessary skills to engage in discourse through the use of spoken language. Many steps can be taken to ensure carry-over from a teaching situation to real-life communication. The most important of these is, without doubt, to ensure that teaching situations reflect, as closely as possible, the conditions that will prevail in real life. For example, if the procedures adopted for teaching sessions involve apparatus that is not met in real life communication, then little or no carry-over to interactive situations in real-life can be expected unless further procedures are introduced to bridge the gap between the two conditions. Such bridging can be achieved by eliciting the particular speech patterns again in the absence of apparatus, making sure that the child establishes feedback control over production either through the use of hearing aids or other sensory devices, as well as through articulatory sensation.

Spoken language patterns learned through everyday experience will automatically be practised, but those learned through direct teaching are likely to need scheduled attention, so that the elements taught are rehearsed in communicative situations until accuracy, speed, economy of effort, and flexibility of production and comprehension are achieved. Planning is required to extend the context of production of speech communication patterns into familiar, conversational language that can be used to describe, explain, tell, or question something that is truly of interest to the child. In short, the more unlike real-life communication the teaching is, the more carry-over may need to be programmed Phonologic level evaluation (determining how well speech patterns are used in meaningful speech) that is based on the sampling of the several aspects of conversation is of particular importance in discovering whether carry-over from teaching to everyday, real-life conditions is being achieved (see Chapter 7).

One of the most important real-life areas in which children can apply the speech communication skills they have learned in school is in the school itself. Each lesson, each subject, and each teacher, can offer a multitude of important opportunities for spoken language development. Specific speech lessons are not always required to develop awareness and provide practice in the use of specific speech patterns. Teachers of subjects can, in fact, have the most pervasive influence in speech communication development of anyone in the schoolchild's environment. With very little extra thought and effort, children's teachers can make speech and its intelligibility assume a reality for them that it will otherwise lack. They can, in fact, make the difference between whether children perceive speech as a subject that is taught or as a communication skill they would like to use. Speech communication specialists should do their utmost to bring this realization to any classroom-based colleagues so that they provide their children with abundant activity-based opportunities for spoken language exchange.

Carry-over, to reiterate a basic point, is very much more likely to occur spontaneously if optimal use is made of whatever residual hearing children possess, not just in specific lessons, but at all times. If children have too little residual hearing to benefit from hearing aids, then alternative devices that optimize speech detection should be used to keep the children aware of the speech around them (see Chapter 5). The incentive to communicate by speech is greatly enhanced when children can be helped not only to perceive spoken language that is addressed directly to them, but to be aware of speech communication around them.

Just as it is possible to identify procedures and situations that will enhance carry-over, so is it possible to identify obstacles in children's environments that inhibit it. Obstacles that commonly impede the carry-over of speech to everyday discourse include:

- undue emphasis on another language or another mode of communication;
- failure to use spoken language as a major, if not the most frequent vehicle of instruction;
- failure to encourage speech communication in everyday life;
- speech training that does not relate to everyday communication;

- professionals who have insufficient confidence or competence to develop spoken language skills;
- parents who have not been helped to learn how to cope with the language-learning problems of their children;
- professionals and parents who have not required children to accept increasing responsibility for making themselves understood.

The list could go on. The professionals responsible for a child's development of speech must find ways of overcoming obstacles, and accept the responsibility of seeing that the child is given every opportunity to achieve carry-over. If they do not, then they may justifiably be viewed as promoting their children's failure.

Carry-over can be promoted through ensuring that information commonly required of children is rehearsed until it can be produced intelligibly. Such information (that can also serve their security) includes names, addresses, parents' occupations, telephone numbers, age, birthday dates, favorite sports, food likes and dislikes, health and illness and courtesy formulas. Topics of personal interest that span home and school can also provide opportunity for promoting carry-over. These could include discussions of self, home, family, housekeeping, money, shopping, clothes, sizes, shapes, transport, distances, time and speed, volume and weight, television programs, plants, animals (including birds and fish), food, weather, environment, seasons and seasonal activities, occupations, sports, toys, and leisure activities, to mention but a few. Children who are old enough can be helped towards carry-over by participating as responsible beings in the planning of their own programs and home assignments. They can make recordings of their speech at school and play them back for their parents at home. They can, when taught in groups, create plays so that each character in the play can record a part, all characters using their best, well-practiced speech for the public presentation of the play. The admiration by both adults and younger children of successfully produced plays of this sort can be highly reinforcing. As noted above, the aspects of training that will be remembered best and used most in speech communication will be those things that are of direct interest and benefit to the children themselves. Children will communicate much more frequently if they find it fun and if it serves a real purpose.

recommended further reading

In addition to further chapters in this book, the reader's attention is drawn to the wide range of materials available from the Alexander Graham Bell Association for the Deaf, the publishers of the present text. The following texts relating to spoken language communication in hearing-impaired children are also recommended: Ling (1984a), a book containing contributions by Beebe, Clezy, Cole and Paterson, and Pollack, with a commentary by the writer about four exemplary early intervention programs that promote spoken language development; Cole and Gregory (1986), a monograph on various aspects of auditory learning; Ling and Ling (1971) a thesaurus suggesting basic vocabulary and language; Ling and Ling (1978), an introductory text on verbal learning; Reed (1984), an introductory and very readable text that presents a predominantly British perspective on the education of hearing-impaired children; and Wood, Wood, Griffith, and Howarth (1986), also a text of English origin, that provides a first rate analysis of teaching and learning communication skills among hearing-impaired children of school age. Two publications relevant to verbal learning and curricula for school-age children are Kretschmer (1985) and Bunch (1987). Wilbur (1987) provides a comprehensive description of sign language communication and Ling (1984b) has edited a book on early intervention through total communication.

The reader's attention is also directed to Vaughan (1976), a book by mothers about their children's acquisition of spoken language. Readings that are relevant to intervention in communication development among normally hearing children include Blank, Rose, and Berlin (1978), a book that demonstrates the importance of communication to learning; Bullowa (1979), a text that concentrates on communication before speech; Fey (1986), a very readable and well-referenced book that emphasizes parental roles in language acquisition; Luterman (1987), an important text that provides insights on how families are affected by a child's hearing impairment; and McLean and Snyder McLean (1978), a thought-provoking text on promoting the acquisition of spoken language through adult-child interaction. For detailed and comprehensive books on language acquisition by normally hearing children, the reader is referred to the second editions of the introductory text by Owens (1988) and the text edited by Fletcher and Garman (1986). See References, pp. 433 ff.

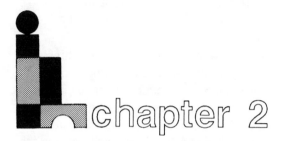

chapter 2

the dimensions
of speech

the dimensions of sounds

Speech sounds are very special because their principal use is to convey meaning. Like all other sounds, they have three dimensions: *intensity*, *duration*, and *frequency*. Each dimension can be measured objectively; that is by means of instruments. Each can also be judged subjectively; that is, by saying how loud, how long, or what pitch a sound appears to have to a listener.

loudness and intensity

Any given sound seems softer to a person far away from its source than to a person close to its source, and to most individuals who are hearing impaired than to people who have normal hearing. We perceive the strength of a sound as its *loudness*. Only if we measure its strength with instruments can we talk objectively about its *intensity*. Intensity is measured in decibels. The decibel (abbreviated dB) is based on a logarithmic scale. On this scale, a sound having a level 10 dB greater than another actually has 10 times the intensity; a level 20 dB greater has 100 times the intensity; a level 30 dB greater has 1000 times the intensity, and so on. The use of this scale has two advantages: it permits the representation of a huge range of intensities in simple figures, and it closely reflects how we hear. (In the middle of a normally hearing person's frequency range, sounds of 30 and 40 dB appear to be about twice as loud as those at 15 and 20 dB.)

The levels at which we hear are measured in dB above threshold, the intensity at which a sound can just be detected by young people with normal hearing. A gentle breeze blowing through the leaves in a tree under which one is sitting would create a noise consisting of various sounds at hearing levels (HL) of about 10 to 20 dB . A quiet whisper from about two yards away would be at about a 30 dB hearing level, and the loudest sounds in quiet speech at the same distance would occur at hearing levels of about 60 dB. Loud shouts from that distance would reach hearing levels of about 90 dB, and the noise from a chain saw could reach its user's ears at levels of up to 120 dB above a normal listener's thresholds. Sounds that are above this level can cause some discomfort or pain.

Relating decibels to hearing levels (HL) above normal listeners' thresholds is a useful convention. The decibel scale can be related to various reference levels, as we shall see in the next chapter; but in this chapter the decibel levels used will be as they appear on conventional audiogram forms, namely dB HL.

pitch and frequency

When sounds are judged to be high or low by a listener they are said to have a certain pitch. By convention, when sounds are said to have a certain frequency, one knows that they have been measured with instruments, and that the results in Hertz (Hz) can be specified. This distinction is made because, just as the loudness of a sound may be judged differently by different people, so can a given sound of known frequency appear to be higher or lower in pitch. The concept of frequency is very important in all aspects of speech and hearing. To clarify it, let us consider how different frequencies can be created.

When an object vibrates, some part of it moves backwards and forwards in space at a particular rate. If the object was in water, we would see the ripples caused by such vibration. When the object is in the air, similar waves are also created. The distance between waves or ripples is known as their wavelength. If air waves are neither too fast nor too slow, and are powerful enough to move a normally hearing person's eardrum, that person will perceive them as sound. The number of waves that arrive at the ear each second is known as the frequency of that sound. The slower and longer the waves, the lower their frequency; and the faster and shorter the waves, the higher their frequency.

An example of frequency as airwaves per second can be provided in relation to common experience. Almost everyone has heard a fly buzzing as it tries to escape from a closed space. When a big fly, trapped in a space, moves its wings up and down 260 times a second (and some flies do), it will create a sound with a frequency of 260 Hz. Middle C on a well-tuned piano vibrates at about this frequency (actually 261.62 Hz), and this sound is about as low as most people can whistle. A smaller fly more desperately trying to escape might move its wings twice as fast; that is, 520 times a second. It would then produce a sound an octave higher; that is, a sound of 520 Hz.

The term *octave* is more familiar to musicians than to others, but everyone has experienced what octaves actually are. Female voices are, on average, about an octave higher than male voices. If a man and a woman, both using the low range of their voices, sing a song in tune together, their voices will be an octave apart. The pitch of the sound /s/ is about an octave higher than that of the sound sh. Say these two sounds, and listen to the pitch difference between them. Try singing from the lowest note to the highest note you can comfortably reach. The range that most people with untrained voices can sing covers about two octaves. Technically, if an object vibrates (oscillates) twice as fast as another, it will produce a sound that is exactly an octave higher. Clinical audiometers are designed to produce test tones that are an octave apart. The term is explained here because it will be used both in this and in later chapters. The term *octave band* will be also be used. This simply means the range of sounds contained within an octave.

duration

The duration of different sounds helps us to identify them. Vowels tend to be longer than consonants. Sometimes the identification of a particular sound requires us to make a gap in the stream of speech; for example, just before we produce a plosive sound like /p/, /t/, or /k/ in the middle of a word. Sometimes the lengthening of a vowel before the final consonant tells us which of two sounds that consonant is supposed to be. For example, whisper the words *cap* and *cab*, and see how much longer the vowel has to be before the /b/. Most speech sounds, gaps in the speech stream, and differences in vowel length are quite brief, so we measure them in milliseconds (ms); that is, thousandths of a second.

why describe speech acoustics?

In this chapter on the production of spoken language, speech patterns (the acoustic properties of utterances), are described in terms of their intensity, frequency, and duration. Two aspects of every speech pattern are of interest: the segmental aspect that has to do with the properties of vowels and consonants, and the suprasegmental aspect that has to do with prosody, the tune and rhythm that underlies an utterance. This information on the acoustic properties of speech is relevant to several aspects of work with hearing-impaired children. First, it helps us to specify how sounds are made, and why particular speech patterns are distorted if children mispronounce them. This provides us with a foundation for speech development and speech teaching. Second, it helps us to know what sounds children with different types and degrees of hearing impairment can be expected to detect, discriminate, and identify through aided hearing - a subject that is followed up in Chapters 3 and 4. Third, it helps us know what possibilities there are for helping children who have no useful residual hearing to receive different aspects of spoken language through the use of other sensory aids, such as tactile devices or cochlear implants - a topic discussed in detail in Chapter 5.

Readers will be helped to understand the information provided in this chapter if they set out to experiment with the various speech patterns as they are discussed. Alone, or with friends they can discover both the way sounds change and the different sounds that can be produced as they adjust their speech organs. This is a fun way to discover what the lungs, larynx, pharynx, velum, tongue lips and/or jaw, separately and jointly, contribute to the production of the various acoustic patterns that make up spoken language. Such activity with sounds and with sentences will also help readers to identify the wide range of acceptable variations in speech that can be used without restricting intelligibility. Such knowledge and experience is essential if one is to listen to a hearing-impaired child's speech, identify any problems present in it, and set out in a rational manner to improve it.

breath and voice

The sounds of speech are produced by forcing breath from the lungs, through the vocal tract, and out to the air that separates talker and listener. The flow of breath, and the way it is influenced by the speech organs, create the fluctuations in air pressure, and the particular resonances that we perceive as different sounds. The length and the shape of the vocal tract change throughout childhood and puberty, until its adult dimensions are reached. It is usually larger in adult males than in adult females, and larger in adult females than in children. A diagram of the vocal tract is shown as Figure 2-1.

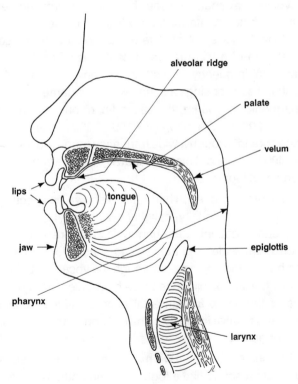

figure 2-1. **A diagram of the vocal tract showing the principal organs involved in speech.**

The larynx is the first in the series of speech organs met by the breath as it is expelled from the lungs. This is the organ containing the vocal cords (sometimes known as the vocal folds). A whisper is produced when the vocal folds are held slightly apart and the pressure of breath rushing through the space between them causes turbulence. (This space is called the glottis.) Voiced sounds are produced when, as breath is expelled, the vocal folds are held together so that they vibrate, opening and closing rapidly. The way the vocal folds are used to create voice is much the same as the way the lips can be used to produce a "raspberry." If the vocal cords are large, long and brought loosely together, a low voice will result. If they are smaller, made shorter, and held together more tightly, then a higher pitched voice will be heard. While the mass of the vocal cords depends on the size of the larynx, we can adjust their length and tension. Such adjustments allow us to sing and to speak with intonation.

Voices may sound as if they have, at any given moment, just a single "pitch" -the fundamental frequency (F_0) that carries the tune of a person's voice. In fact, this is not so. The voiced sounds produced by the larynx are made up of a wide range of harmonics. The first harmonic is the fundamental frequency. The other harmonics are multiples of this note. Thus, if one says or sings a sound with a fundamental frequency (that is first harmonic) of 100 Hz, the second harmonic of that sound will fall at $2 \times 100 = 200$ Hz, the third at $3 \times 100 = 300$ Hz, and so on. Harmonics of voice spread through a wide frequency range, but become quite weak above 4000 Hz or so. This is illustrated in the narrow band spectrogram presented as Figure 2-2.

The *intensity* of each harmonic is shown on spectrograms such as this as dark (high intensity) or light (low intensity) markings. The *duration* of the sound containing the harmonics is represented as length along the horizontal scale, and the *frequency* as height on the vertical scale. As the breath and voice pass through the vocal tract, the structures that lie above the larynx influence these harmonics in ways that help to give voices of the same fundamental pitch a different character. It is the number and relative intensity of the harmonics that give voices a different timbre, or quality.

Blowing over a bottle will make the air inside it resonate - sound out - and create a sound like a foghorn (if the bottle is big and the aperture is small), or like a whistle (if the bottle is small and the aperture is large). A complex cavity, such as the vocal tract, also resonates when puffs of air from the larynx set the air it contains in motion. The vocal tract is a complex shape, so several harmonics in various parts of the speech spectrum become louder than others when different sounds are being produced. This is why some of the harmonics in Figure 2-2 are darker (stronger) than others.

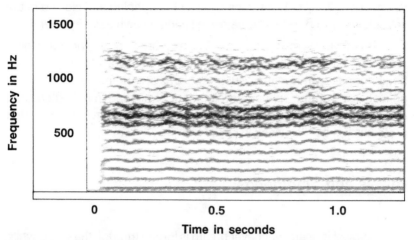

figure 2-2. **A narrow-band spectrogram showing the harmonics of voice. Time is represented on the horizontal axis, frequency on the vertical axis, and intensity by shading. The more intense the sounds, the darker the mark levels. On this spectrogram, the harmonics, multiples of the fundamental frequency, can be seen as a series of parallel horizontal bars. Vocal tract resonances make some harmonics stronger than others.**

The most important speech organ in the vocal tract is the tongue. It is mainly the position and the configuration of the tongue that make one vowel different from another; and it is the contact of the tongue with the teeth or palate that allows most consonants to be made. The pharyngeal walls that surround the space at the back of the tongue, the velum (soft palate) above the back of the tongue, the hard palate above the front of the tongue, the lips, teeth, and jaw, all help to shape the vocal tract, and all contribute to the particular quality of a speaker's voice.

The nose may also be considered part of the vocal tract because some consonants, appropriately called the nasals, (/m/, /n/, and ng in English), are made by directing the breath stream through the nose. This is done by lowering the velum and relaxing the pharyngeal walls to create an opening to the nose from the throat, called the velo-pharyngeal port. Some vowels may take on a nasal quality if this space is not closed during their production and some consonants, such as fricatives (/s/, /f/, th, /v/, sh, etc.), will be produced weakly, if at all. This is because they require a strong oral breath stream (air-flow through the mouth) which cannot be produced if the breath is allowed to escape through the nose. When we breathe through the nose, the velo-pharyngeal port is open. When we yawn, or swallow, it closes. One can feel the opening and closing of the velo-pharyngeal port by alternately initiating a yawn and saying /m/.

Breath and voice are the most basic components of speech. If there is a fault with the breath stream, the quality of both voice and speech will be abnormal. Unfortunately, such problems are often allowed to occur unnecessarily in the speech development of hearing-impaired children and to persist into their adult lives. The prevention and treatment of such problems will be discussed in Chapter 9.

vowels and diphthongs

A vowel is heard whenever breath is forced through the larynx while the mouth is open. If the vocal cords are close together and vibrating, the vowel will be voiced; and if the vocal cords are held slightly apart the vowel will be whispered. As the pulses of air from a voiced vowel, or the rush of air from a whispered vowel leave the larynx, they activate the air in the cavities of the mouth and make them resonate. The same effect occurs when we blow across the top of closed tubes, such as bottles. They begin to sound out at a high, medium or low pitch according to their size and shape. Those with large cavities and small apertures have a low pitch, and those with small cavities and large apertures have a high pitch. The mouth can be regarded as a tube that can be formed to make cavities and apertures of various shapes and sizes. Such shaping is done principally by means of movements of the tongue, lips and jaw. Different vowels are made, then, when the mouth assumes one configuration as compared with another, because different resonances are produced by these different configurations.

The broad peaks of resonance that occur as the breath stream passes through the vocal tract are called formants. Each configuration of the vocal tract gives rise to several of them. The first two (counting from low to high) are the most important. Any sort of energy that causes the air in the vocal tract to resonate will produce formants. Thus, they occur when the vocal cords vibrate to produce voicing, they are created when one whispers, they result when a vibrator is held against the face or throat, and one can hear them if one lightly taps the throat or the cheeks with one's fingers, or even if puffs of air are blown into the mouth from outside. It is the presence of formants of different frequencies that give each of the vowels, spoken or whispered, the acoustic characteristics that permit us to identify them. Let us look at the different configurations of the vocal tract that produce the formants of three vowels that can serve as reference points for all others - oo, ah, and ee.

If the tongue is high in the back of the mouth and the lips are rounded, we will produce an oo vowel. If the tongue is low in the middle of the mouth, the jaw is lowered, and the lips are neutrally spread, we produce an ah vowel. If the tongue is high at the front of the mouth and the lips spread, we produce an ee vowel. All other vowels are made by adjusting the tongue to intermediate positions and configurations. When we produce vowels with voice, they are heard categorically; that is, we hear the vowel as such, but not its component formants. This is not the case when we use a forced whisper. With loudly whispered vowels, we can hear not only the vowels as such, but, if we listen carefully, we can also hear the pitch of their formants. The positions of the tongue for the three vowels mentioned above and the frequencies of their formants are illustrated in Figure 2-3.

The spectrograms in Figure 2-3 show the widely different formants associated with each vowel. They also show that the lower formants tend to be stronger (have a greater intensity) than those that are higher in frequency. The two that are lowest in frequency carry information about many aspects of speech. These are labelled as Formant 1 (F_1) and Formant 2 (F_2) respectively. The relative frequencies of the formants (low, middle or high) are similar for each vowel, although they may differ from person to person. The approximate center frequencies of F_1 and F_2 for the three vowels oo, ah, and ee as spoken by the writer are as follows:

oo	F_1 = 300 Hz;	F_2 =	800 Hz
ah	F_1 = 700 Hz;	F_2 =	1,250 Hz
ee	F_1 = 300 Hz;	F_2 =	2,400 Hz

To have a concept of where these formants fall in the frequency range, one may think of the lowest formants of these vowels (300 Hz) as being pitched just above the middle C on a piano - at about the same frequency one obtains by blowing across the top of a medium-sized bottle. The highest frequency (2,400 Hz) is at about the middle of the range within which most people can whistle. The second formant (F_2) is the most important of all in the identification of vowels.

Diphthongs consist of two vowels sounded together to make one phonetic unit. To produce the diphthong in the word *eye*, the tongue has to move quickly and smoothly from approximately the ah to the ee position. The diphthong in the word *how* is similarly produced by moving the tongue from near the ah to near the oo position.

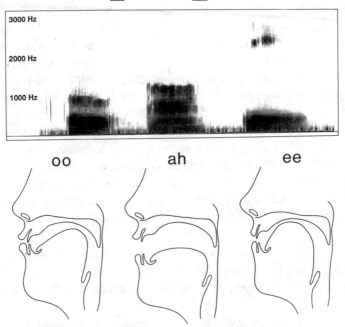

figure 2-3. A diagram depicting the approximate tongue configurations for production of the three vowels ah, oo, and ee, and (above) broad-band spectrograms showing the formants of these vowels as produced by the writer. Because broad-band spectrograms sample frequency bands that are twice as wide as those in narrow-band spectrograms (as in Figure 2-2), they highlight formants rather than harmonics.

There is a reasonably simple way of calculating the approximate formant frequency values of all English vowels. First, remember the values of oo, ah, and ee. Second, arrange the vowels in order of ascending F_2 values. This can be done by using the sentence *Who would know more of art must learn, and then take his ease* to construct a chart, such as shown in Figure 2-4. Third, draw a vertical line on this graph from the word that contains the vowel in question to intersect the lines of the graph. Looking from the points of intersection to the scale at the left, one can read off the approximate center frequencies of the first two formants of that vowel. The vocal tracts of females and young children tend to be smaller and shorter than those of an adult male, such as the writer, so the center frequencies of their formants could be as much as from 20-40 percent higher, depending on their size (see Figure 2-4).

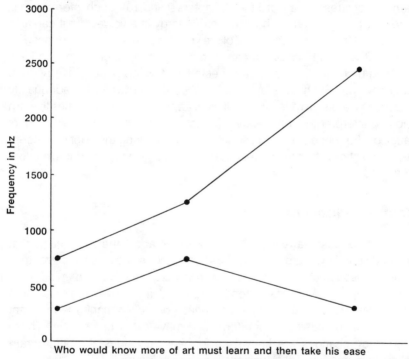

figure 2-4. A chart showing the approximate center frequencies of the first and second formants of the three vowels oo, ah, and ee, as spoken by the writer. The points at which a vertical line drawn from any word would intersect the two lines in the diagram permit one to read off the approximate F_1 and F_2 center frequency values of the intermediate vowels.

It is important to know where the formant frequencies of the various vowels lie because, as we shall see in the next chapter, this information allows one to predict fairly closely what sounds will be audible to children with different aided hearing levels. Note, by reference to Figure 2-4, that unless hearing is present beyond 1000 Hz (the center frequency of an audiogram), some vowels may sound like others because F_2 of most vowels will not be audible, and F_1 of several vowels are alike in frequency.

Vowels are important in speech for several reasons. They differentiate words that would otherwise sound alike - for example, booed, bowed, bored, bard, bud, bird, bad, bed, bade, bid, and bead. But vowels do more than differentiate between words. They also help to carry the prosody of a sentence - the rate and rhythm of speaking, the intonation pattern, and the amount of stress on a word (see Chapters 9 and 10). Such information is present throughout the whole range of energy in a vowel, but it can also be derived from one component of the vowel, such as the first formant (F_1). This fact is important, for it means that many of those children who have hearing up to 1000 Hz can be expected to develop good prosody (tune and rhythm). Such development requires that children are adequately aided, as well as provided with sufficient appropriate opportunities to learn how to interpret low frequency information through using their residual audition. Further discussions about vowels - ensuring their optimal reception, and stimulating their effective production - are provided in Chapters 3 and 10.

formant transitions

Vowels also carry important information about the consonants that precede or follow them. This fact has been recognized since ancient times when consonants (con-sonants = with vowels) were first named as such. As the major speech organs (tongue, lips, and jaw) move from or towards the necessary positions for the production of a consonant, the resonant frequencies of the vocal tract (formants) move either up or down. These frequency changes are known as formant transitions. A spectrogram showing some formant transitions is shown in Figure 2-5.

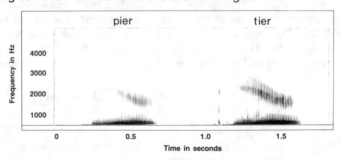

figure 2-5.   A broad-band spectrogram showing CV and VC transitions - the interaction of vowels and consonants. The transitions (rapid changes in formant frequency) shown are those created by saying the words *pier* and *tier*.

To understand clearly how formant transitions are created, take a bottle and fill it from a fast dripping tap of water. As the water moves up towards the top of the bottle, the drips make the air left in the bottle resonate. The resonant pitch of the air left in the bottle becomes higher and higher as the bottle fills. You have just created, in slow motion, a formant transition with water in the bottle, much as you make formant transitions in speech when you move your tongue up towards the front of your mouth to make a /t/ consonant in words, such as *hat* and *hot*.

Speech intelligibility is strongly affected by the presence or absence of formant transitions. If the tongue is moving in the right direction, and at the right speed, the formant transitions will be produced as they should be. Say the two words *hop* and *hot* without sounding out the final consonants. Stop the vowel with the lips for the /p/ and with the tongue for the /t/, and you will still hear each word quite distinctly. The way your tongue and jaw moved to stop the vowel created the formant transitions that are sufficient to specify the consonants. As the vowel came before the consonant in this example, you created a vowel-to-consonant (VC) transition. When a consonant comes before a vowel, a consonant-to-vowel (CV) transition occurs. The rate and direction of formant transitions can partly - or in some cases wholly - specify which consonants are present in words.

When hearing-impaired speakers talk very slowly, prolong their vowels, or fail to move their tongues as they should, appropriate formant transitions will not be produced. Thus, if you ask hearing-impaired individuals to say *hop* and *hot*, and you cannot hear the difference unless they explode the /p/ and /t/ (you must listen, not speechread), then you know that their tongue movements are the source of the problem. One can, of course, prevent or correct this problem (see Chapter 10).

Transitions that support the identification of different speech sounds as they change from one vowel context to another are considered to be variant cues. Such cues can easily be heard by contrasting the whispered words *cake* and *cook*. The /k/ sounds at the beginning of each word are quite different in pitch.

The second formants of the vowels carry most information about adjacent consonants. As shown in Figure 2-4, the frequency range of the second formants is from about 750 to 2500 Hz. The greater the amount of hearing over this frequency range, the more consonants individuals are likely to be able to identify through the perception of formant transitions. Children with no hearing above 1000 Hz. are likely to be able to identify only a few consonants in this manner when they occur in the context of back vowels like oo and aw that have low frequency F_2 components. This fact provides a helpful teaching strategy: to enhance the characteristics of consonants for profoundly hearing-impaired children with no audition beyond 1000 Hz, evoke them in the context of back vowels.

Some hearing-impaired individuals, particularly those with relatively little hearing and limited auditory experience, may find it difficult to identify consonants through the auditory perception of formant transitions. Their ability to perceive small changes in frequency through aided hearing might be inadequate. Even multi-channel tactile devices and cochlear implants convey degraded information on formant transitions (see Chapter 5). Fortunately, as discussed below, there are multiple cues to the identification of consonants, and if the variant cues associated with formant transitions are not available to a listener, then invariant cues, such as nasal murmurs, fricative turbulence and plosive bursts may suffice. Speech sounds that cannot be identified through hearing or other sensory aids may still be recognized with the help of speechreading - the process of gathering information by watching the lips.

types of consonants

Consonants are most realistically seen as different ways of releasing, arresting, or interrupting vowels in running speech. They may be classified according to their manner of production (how they are made), their place of production (where they are made - at the front, middle or back of the mouth), and whether they are produced with or without voicing. In this section, the manner, place, and voicing differences among consonants will be described, and basic information about the acoustic properties of the consonants presented. Some of the implications of this information for speech production among hearing-impaired children will also be discussed.

manner of consonant production.

Consonants can be made in numerous different ways. Each different manner of producing sound (through the nose, through the mouth, by pops, hisses, or gradual and sudden stops) can be a meaningful way of creating words so that one is distinct from another. Consonants that close off the vocal tract completely and "explode" as they release a vowel, like /p/ and /b/, are called *stops* or *plosives*. Those that are made through the nose, like /m/ and /n/, are called *nasals*. The consonants /l/ and /r/ that make the breath stream pass by the sides of the tongue are known as *laterals*, while those that cause the breath stream to become turbulent, like /s/ and /f/, are called *fricatives*. The consonants that begin the words *we* and *you* are called *semi-vowels*, and are among the least used of sounds. The consonant spelled ch as in cheese, is an *affricate*. The strategies that can be used to help hearing-impaired children acquire manner distinctions are treated in Chapter 11.

place of consonant production.

Consonants may be made at different points in the vocal tract, as shown in Figure 2-6. Those that are made with both lips, such as /p/ or /b/, are called *bilabials*; with the lips and teeth, such as /f/ or /v/, *labio-dentals*; and with the tongue and teeth, such as th, *lingua- dentals*. The most frequently occurring consonants are those made with the tongue in contact with, or near the alveolar ridge, the ridge just behind the upper teeth. These sounds, which include /s/, /l/, /n/, /t/, and /d/, are called *lingua-alveolar* consonants. Those made by forcing air over or around the sides of the tongue near the palate are called *lingua- palatal* consonants. They include sh as in shoe, ch as in cheese, and /r/ as in red. Consonants that are made by the tongue touching the roof of the mouth near the soft palate (the velum) are termed *lingua- velar* sounds, and they include the /k/, /g/, and ng. The sound /h/ is made by forcing air through the glottis, and is, therefore, called a *glottal* consonant. The further away from the lips consonants are produced, the less frequently they tend to occur in everyday speech.

Because the speech sounds in a normal utterance are coarticulated (are an inseparable part of the stream of speech), vowels will influence the production of adjacent consonants, and *vice versa*. Verify this by saying the two words *she* and *shoe*, and listening carefully to the sh sound in each word. The sh in the first word will higher in pitch than the sh in the second. This is because the lips are spread and the tongue is forward in preparation for the vowel ee, as in *she*, but the lips are rounded and the tongue is taken further back in the mouth in preparation for producing the vowel oo, as in *shoe*.

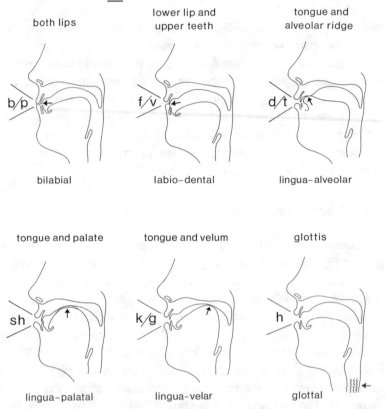

figure 2-6. **The vocal tract in relation to place of consonant production. The shape of the lips and the tongue, as well as the point of contact or close approximation of the various organs (specified in each diagram), will vary considerably according to vowel context. The speech organs approximate and leave these positions dynamically as the various consonants release, interrupt and arrest the various vowels.**

The same effect can be heard with other consonants. Say *key* and then *too*. The /k/ is the higher pitched of the two sounds. Now reverse the syllables: say *tea* and then *coo*. The /t/ will now be heard as the higher pitched of the two consonants. Such experiments indicate that there are at least as many ways of producing consonants as there are vowels that precede or follow them. This is one reason why it is impossible to chart the exact location of a consonant on a graph, such as an audiogram.

Each consonant would occupy a range rather than a location on such a graph. These normal modifications of sounds that occur as a result of coarticulation (being produced next to others in running speech) will only become part of a hearing-impaired child's speech, if sounds are developed and practised in utterances of at least several syllables.

Following vowels, consonants that are produced at the very front of the mouth will lower all formants. Alveolar consonants, such as /t/, /d/, and /n/, lower the first formants (F_1) of preceding vowels, but make their second formant (F_2) transitions point towards a locus of about 1800 Hz. The velar consonants such as /k/, /g/, and ng when following a vowel, lower first formant (F_1) transitions but make most of the second formant (F_2) transitions point to a locus of just over 3000 Hz. When these consonants precede rather than follow the vowel the transitions move away from the locus towards the vowel formant position. These influences due to coarticulation are illustrated in the spectrograms shown as Figure 2-5 (p.36). If place distinctions are not emerging in the speech of hearing-impaired children whose audiograms show responses in the range 2000 - 3000 Hz, question whether they are receiving sufficient amplification over that frequency range.

Adjustments made as we speak that allow sounds in a sequence to fit snugly together as described in the previous paragraph may be made several syllables ahead by a practiced speaker. The process of planning such adjustments is known as *feedforward*. Feedforward is not carried out consciously by normal speakers. It can be developed in hearing-impaired children only by ensuring that utterance length is not restricted. Natural coarticulation will only occur if feedforward is operating. This, in turn, requires that utterances reflect the expression of ideas in units of several words in length. Feedforward and coarticulation will be inhibited if speech sounds and words are produced in isolation.

Coarticulation, then, affects the frequency of consonants in highly consistent ways. For this reason, it serves to provide listeners with predictable ways to identify, as well as to produce, normal speech patterns. Normal speech is a stream of coarticulated sounds rather than a series of isolated elements. *To produce speech sounds so that they move towards and away from each other in a natural manner within each utterance is just as important as the production of the particular speech patterns themselves.*

The pursuit of natural sounding, well coarticulated (rather than well articulated) speech demands that the practice of having hearing-impaired children produce and rehearse consonants in isolation be abandoned. Developing sounds without reference to phonetic context is to teach an unvarying production that will come to impede both perception and pronunciation in everyday speech. While one may elicit continuants (sounds that one can continue to produce for a few seconds), such as /n/, or /s/ in isolation, one must immediately encourage their use in a variety of syllables, words, and phrases thus ensuring that their pronunciation varies naturally according to context as it does in everyday speech. Strategies for developing place distinctions in speech production are discussed in Chapters 12 and 13.

voiced and unvoiced consonants.

Many of the consonants in English are members of voiced and voiceless pairs. For example, /b/ and /p/ are such a pair, as are /z/ and /s/. When we say sets of two words containing these consonants, for example *bear* and *pear*, or *buzz* and *bus*, the difference between members of these pairs is that of consonant voicing. When a voiced consonant releases a vowel, vocal cord vibration begins as the consonant is produced. When an unvoiced consonant releases a vowel, vocal cord vibration does not begin until after the consonant has been released. Words are said so quickly that the difference between vocal cord onset in pairs of words like *bear* and *pear* have to be measured in thousandths of a second. In fact, just over 20 ms is a common voice onset time (VOT) difference. When a voiced consonant stops a vowel as it does in the word *cub*, the vowel is lengthened, and runs into the final consonant, but when an unvoiced consonant is found in that position, as in the word *cup*, the vowel is shortened, and no voice runs over into the final sound. But the voiced-voiceless distinction can be made even when we whisper, and no voice is present at all. This is done by lengthening the vowel and shortening the consonant if the final sound is voiced, and the reverse if it is unvoiced. Test this out by whispering the words *hiss* and *his* (Strategies for the development of voiced-voiceless distinctions are suggested in Chapter 14).

consonant blends.

Two or more consonants that are adjacent in a word or in running speech are called consonant blends, or clusters. Initial blends are those that occur at the beginning of a word (as in blend). Medial or intervocalic blends appear between vowels in the middle of words (as in rented). Final blends are commonly found in many English words, such as hold, camp, and round, but most final blends are made through adding plural, possessive, or tense markers to existing words (as in cats, Bob's, and spilt). Consonant blends also occur between words in running speech because spoken language consists of an integrated stream of sounds rather than a series of distinct elements. There are several examples in the preceding sentence, including "consonant blends," "running speech," "spoken language," "integrated stream" and "sounds rather." There are also multiple blends that contain more than two adjacent consonants as in the word *sounds*.

For the purpose of teaching consonant blends, it is helpful to think of them as being either sequentially or concurrently articulated. In sequential blends, the first consonant has to be completed before the next can be formed. The initial blend in the word *slow* provides an example. In contrast, with concurrent blends, both consonants are formed before the first is completed. Thus, in the word *blow*, the tongue is already in position for the /l/ before the /b/ is released. If it is not, then intrusive voicing occurs between the two consonants. This fault makes a word such as *blow* have two syllables instead of one, turning it into something nearer *below* than *blow*. Such a fault upsets the rhythm of speech, and makes it less intelligible. In some concurrently produced blends, such as the /tr/ blend in the word *trail*, each element of the blend is modified to such an extent that the resulting word may sound as if it could be spelled *chrail*. We certainly do not hear the two consonants as they occur in the words *tail* and *rail*.

Hearing-impaired children, like those with normal hearing, must become aware of the way consonants are blended and words put together in a stream if they are to speak and understand speech adequately. Thus, "The boys' truck", "The boy's truck", and "The boy struck", contain the same between-word (interlexical) blends, and are all are said in much the same way, though they mean different things. Speakers can sometimes differentiate such passages by using prosodic cues, such as a change in voice pitch to mark word boundaries, but when a speaker does not do this, the listener must differentiate them according to the context in which they are spoken. The most important context in this regard is how such a passage relates to the other parts of the message that precede or follow it.

Consonant blends are more commonly met than simple consonants - those that appear singly before, between, or after vowels - and they are much more difficult to produce. Just because a child has developed speech sufficiently well to produce simple consonants in vowel contexts, one cannot assume that he or she can produce words or running speech that demand consonant blending.

Many initial and intervocalic blends are formed with consonants that are difficult for some children to master - and for some clinicians and educators to teach. They include /r/ and /s/. Examples of such blends occur in the words *brown*, *try*, *slow* and *stop*. As mentioned above, a large proportion of final blends involve the /s/. Interlexical blends can be formed from the combination of any of the consonants. Sometimes, the mispronunciations of words that young children know occur because the child has not yet mastered the blends that are created by abutting words. Only the constant use of spoken language in meaningful communication is likely to afford children with enough practice to achieve mastery of blends in words, and fluency in the process of blending sounds in adjoining words. These skills are an essential part of using words in a normal stream of speech. Strategies for the effective development of blends in the speech of hearing-impaired children are suggested in Chapter 14.

speech production and hearing impairment

In order to assist hearing-impaired children to develop pleasant and highly intelligible speech, the facts presented in this chapter must be borne in mind. It is particularly important to remember that all sounds - vowels or consonants - change in frequency, intensity, and duration, according to the context in which they are produced; that there is no such thing, for example, as a /t/ in isolation - only a range of /t/ sounds, each of which fits with the vowels and consonants that precede or follow it. The ways consonants change with context can be both heard and felt by whispering syllables or words. Say words such as *tea* and *too*, and *cow* and *key*, and pay particular attention to the tactile and kinesthetic sensations in the mouth that are produced as you say them. The tactile sensations arise through both the tongue and the palate as the two touch and remain in contact. The kinesthetic patterns are felt as the tongue moves from one place in the mouth to another. These are the sorts of sensations that hearing-impaired children must use to the greatest possible extent in developing feedback skills.

The way that each sound feels as speech is produced is very important in developing the spoken language of children who have no sense of audition, and on this account cannot use hearing to detect the sound waves created by their own speech. Such children must learn to rely, even more than normally hearing talkers do, on articulatory feedback instead of auditory feedback as they learn. Children who lose hearing after they have learned to talk, for example as a result of meningitis, can learn to maintain their already acquired speech skills if they are helped to establish how speech *feels* rather than how it used to *sound* to them. Just as each speech pattern of English sounds different to a normal listener, so does each speech pattern feel different to a normal speaker.

In the past, numerous studies have been undertaken on the speech patterns produced by hearing-impaired children. In essence, they show that every aspect of speech development can suffer as a result of hearing impairment. The findings of studies carried out in the past are, of course, no guide as to what one should expect from exemplary teaching programs today. Rather, they reflect how speech was acquired by children who were educated some time before modern knowledge about speech and language acquisition, and modern sensory aids were available. Teachers and clinicians simply could not work as effectively before hearing aids came into widespread use, and before other sensory aids were invented. Present-day and future studies should show fewer faults, and a smaller range of faults, than used to be commonly found. Studies of hearing-impaired children's speech from now on should reflect the enormous benefits to speech that can result from using appropriate hearing aids or other technological devices, and also show the benefits to be gained from providing children with experience of spoken language from very early infancy.

Some hearing-impaired children and adults in the future may exhibit many, if not all, of the faults of speech reported in the literature, but in such cases the cause will be attributable more to impoverished teaching than to their auditory deficits. Children with no problems other than hearing impairment can learn to speak intelligibly, many normally, if they are provided with right sort of opportunities and conditions.

Procedures for eliciting speech patterns from hearing-impaired children and integrating them into their spoken language are described in Chapters 8 - 13. In the next three chapters we shall consider the other side of the communication coin - speech reception - and how it complements speech production in the acquisition of spoken language.

suggestions for further reading

Comprehensive texts that provide in-depth information on normal speech production include those edited by Minifie, Hixon and Williams (1973) and MacNeilage (1983). An introductory treatment of speech acoustics is provided by Boothroyd (1986). The acoustic aspects of speech production by normally hearing and hearing-impaired speakers have been addressed in Ling (1976), and in Ross and Giolas (1978). Advanced texts on specific aspects of speech production such as respiratory function (Hixon and collaborators, 1987), and laryngeal function (Baer, Sasaki and Harris, 1987) are also available.

The abnormalities commonly found in the speech of hearing-impaired children have been the subject of numerous texts including Calvert and Silverman (1983), Hochberg, Levitt and Osberger (1983), Lauter (1985), and Markides (1983). The relative levels of speech intelligibility achieved by hearing-impaired children taught in oral and total communication programs have been reported in Schildroth and Karchmer (1986). Journals such as The Volta Review (see Perigoe and Ling, 1986) and the Journal of Speech and Hearing Research (see Forner and Hixon, 1977) carry many articles reporting research on various aspects of speech production in hearing-impaired children. See References, pp. 433 ff.

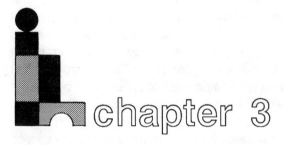

chapter 3

speech reception (1): the auditory channel

the senses in speech reception

Hearing-impaired persons must be able to perceive the various components of the speech signal if they are to communicate through the use of spoken language. There are three senses that permit some form of speech reception: audition, vision, and touch. Most people, even those with normal hearing, use all three modalities. Those who have normal hearing primarily use audition to receive speech, but they can also see the movements of talkers' faces as they are spoken to, and they can feel their own speech organs moving and touching different parts of the mouth as they themselves are speaking. Most of those with hearing impairment can, given appropriate hearing aids, be helped to hear something (usually a great deal) of the speech signal and to make optimum use of all three senses in speech communication. Few children have too little hearing to benefit from hearing aids. Usually, they are among those who have suffered a loss of hearing from a disease, such as meningitis, after having been born with normal audition. Most children who are, or become, totally or near-to-

47

tally deaf can, however, learn and/or maintain spoken language through the use of vision, cochlear implants, tactile devices, or natural touch.

Speech reception by hearing-impaired children is a complex topic. The intent here is to present sufficient information about it to ensure that readers know how speech can best be presented to individual hearing-impaired children in order to promote their optimal development of spoken language. The topic will be explored in three chapters. This chapter begins with a simple account of the auditory system and how it works, continues with a discussion of the causes and measurement of hearing impairment, and then explains how audiograms relate to the acoustic components of speech. The Five-Sound Test is introduced as an example of how significant components of speech can be used to determine whether sounds in each part of the speech frequency range are audible to aided and unaided listeners. The next chapter relates to hearing aids and the use of aided hearing. As there is more to speech reception than meets the ear, Chapter 5 will describe how other senses and devices can provide a supplement or an alternative to the auditory presentation of speech.

the auditory system

As shown in Figure 3-1, the first part of the auditory system to be encountered by sound coming from an external source is the *outer ear*, which consists of two components: the external ear (the pinna) and the ear canal (the auditory meatus). The external ear serves to funnel acoustic energy into the ear canal. Sounds that pass through the ear canal reach the sensory system which lies deep inside the skull, by way of the *middle ear*. The middle ear consists of a small space (the middle ear cleft) that extends from the eardrum (tympanum) to the *inner ear*. The eardrum serves to convert sound waves into mechanical energy (vibrations). The middle ear space is bridged by three tiny bones (ossicles) called the hammer (malleus), anvil (incus), and stirrup (stapes), and these carry the vibrations produced by sound from the eardrum across the middle ear cleft to the inner ear.

A small tube (the Eustachian tube) leads from the back of the throat to the middle ear cleft. It serves to balance the air pressure present in the middle ear with that of the outside air so that the eardrum can move freely.

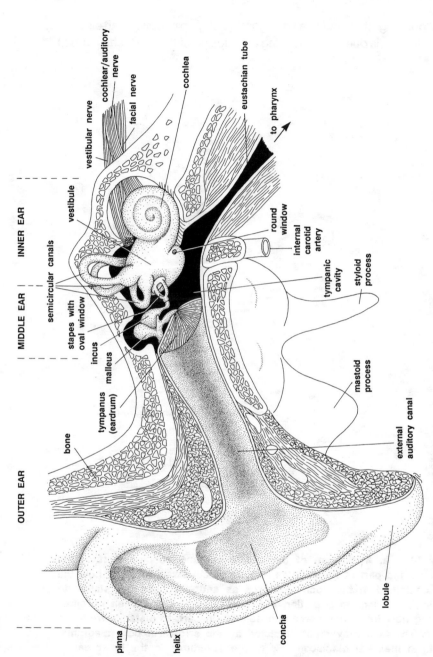

OUTER EAR

MIDDLE EAR

INNER EAR

pinna

helix

concha

lobule

external auditory canal

mastoid process

bone

tympanus (eardrum)

malleus

incus

stapes with oval window

semicircular canals

vestibule

styloid process

tympanic cavity

internal carotid artery

round window

to pharynx

eustachian tube

cochlea

facial nerve

cochlear/auditory nerve

vestibular nerve

figure 3-1. A diagram showing the main components of the human auditory system.

(The "popping" that occurs as one goes quickly up or down in an elevator or an airplane is due to the opening and closing of the Eustachian tube.)

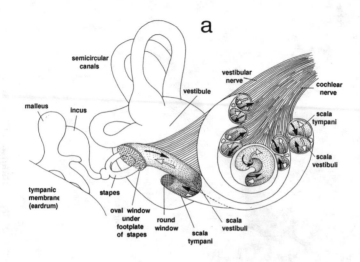

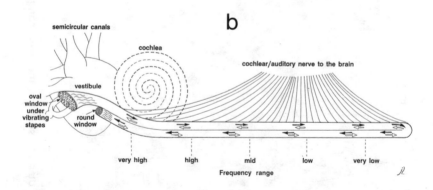

figure 3-2.   a. A diagram of the middle ear and cochlea. Part of the vestibule and part of the cochlea have been cut away, to show how the fluid contained in the cochlea moves as sound causes the stapes to vibrate. b. A diagram depicting the cochlea as if it has been unrolled, showing how frequency perception relates, in part, to distance from the stapes. The fluid movement, depicted by the arrows in both diagrams, results in maximal displacements of the structures in the inner ear at different points along the length of the cochlea, depending on the rate at which the stapes vibrates. Such displacement results in patterns of receptor cell stimulation that permit analysis of a sound's frequency.

The *inner ear* (cochlea) converts sound vibrations into nerve impulses that travel by way of several synapses along the *auditory nerve* to the auditory centers (the auditory cortex) of the brain (see Figure 3-2a). The cochlea is encased in bone and occupies a space shaped like the inside of a small snail shell. The inside of the cochlea contains fluids supporting the receptors that convert the variety of vibrations (mechanical energy) into nerve impulses (electrical signals) that provide the raw material for auditory comprehension. As the stapes vibrates, it acts like a pump to create waves in the fluid contained in the cochlea. The round window in the cochlea permits this fluid to move, and to create patterns of maximum tissue displacement at points along the cochlea that differ according to the frequency of the sounds. High-frequency sounds (rapid vibrations) create patterns that stimulate the receptor cells at the end of the cochlea nearest to where the stirrup bone connects. Other receptor cells respond to the different patterns of tissue displacement created by sounds of lower and lower frequency as the turns of the cochlear become smaller and smaller. This arrangement permits the analysis of incoming sounds to begin in the cochlea (see Figure 3-2b).

the outer and middle ear

The purpose of the outer and the middle ear is to *conduct* the sound waves from the outside world to the cochlea. Impairments that occur in the outer or middle ear are therefore considered to be *conductive* in origin.

Hearing impairments originating in the outer or middle ear can be *unilateral* (affecting one side) or *bilateral* (affecting both sides). Conductive hearing impairments can be detected quite simply by audiometry. Most can also be detected by tympanometry, a procedure carried out with a device that creates different air pressures in the ear canal to determine if the eardrum moves normally.

Conductive hearing impairment can affect a large proportion of children during their school years. In Western countries, up to 10 percent of children of elementary school age can be affected at any given time. Episodes of conductive deafness are usually short lived among such children. Much higher proportions of native populations all over the world tend to suffer hearing loss. At any given time, some 85 percent of Eskimo, North American Indian, Australian Aboriginal and similar populations may suffer hearing loss that is due primarily to middle ear disease.

Most of the serious problems that arise in the outer or middle ear, and lead to hearing impairment, can be overcome through medical or surgical treatment. Objects obstructing the ear canal can be removed; children born without external ears or ear canals can have them created by surgery when their heads are fully developed; perforations of the eardrum can be helped to heal; diseases that cause inflammation of the middle ear (otitis media) that often results in very painful earache can be treated with drugs, and/or helped by the insertion of ventilation tubes; allergies causing blockage of the Eustachian tubes will usually respond to medication; and the ossicles (little bones) that bridge the middle ear cleft can be mobilized or replaced if they do not function properly.

Conductive hearing impairment is not a great barrier to the acquisition of spoken language provided it is recognized and treated appropriately. At worst, it results in moderate hearing impairment. Because conductive impairment attenuates sounds over the whole frequency range to much the same extent, hearing aids are usually very effective in overcoming its effects. When conductive hearing impairments are not recognized, when they are allowed to persist, or when they cause hearing levels to fluctuate, language learning in early infancy, and academic progress in school can be seriously impeded by them.

the inner ear

The purpose of the cochlea is to translate sound vibrations that we cannot feel into *sensory* information for *neural* transmission (transmission along the nerve) to the brain. Impairments that occur in the cochlea and/or auditory nerve are therefore considered to be *sensori-neural* in origin. Although just one ear can be affected by a disease, such as mumps, sensori- neural hearing impairments are usually bilateral. They can stem from a variety of causes. In the main, they are due to genetic disorders, viral infections suffered by the mother during pregnancy, injuries or difficulties experienced at birth, viral infections in childhood, toxic substances, aging, or to damage caused by excessive noise. The list is not exhaustive. Sensori-neural hearing impairments affect about one child in a thousand at birth. Impairments that originate in the cochlea are mainly due to malformation or destruction of the receptor cells.

Although mild forms of hearing impairment involving the cochlea and the auditory nerve do occur among children, severe or profound disorders are more commonly met. A trend towards milder impairments has been reported, but some infections in childhood, such as meningitis, can still result in a total loss of hearing. When hearing is lost due to sensori-neural impairments it cannot, as a rule, be restored by either medical or surgical treatment. The treatment for fluid leaking from the cochlea (perhaps as a result of head injury) and the provision of a cochlear implant (see Chapter 5) may possibly be regarded as exceptions.

Problems affecting the auditory nerve are relatively uncommon. If surgery is required for an auditory nerve disorder - to remove an acoustic neuroma, for example - there is little chance that any sense of hearing will be preserved on the affected side.

The most common treatment for children with sensori-neural hearing impairment, then, is audiological and educational rather than medical or surgical. The most usual form of audiological treatment is the provision of hearing aids that are selected to meet the specific needs of the recipient. Educational treatment is most usually concerned with ensuring that hearing impairment interferes as little as possible with a child's overall development. To this end, parents and other family members, as well as the children and their peers, are generally encouraged to become involved in auditory management programs.

central auditory processing

Up to now, the outer, the middle, and the inner ear have been discussed. These structures comprise the peripheral (outer part of the) hearing mechanism. They are responsible for the conversion of information about our acoustic environment to nerve impulses for transmission to the brain. Central processing mechanisms are required to interpret such information. Relatively little is known about the central auditory processing of spoken language. A brief review of the levels of auditory processing that are intrinsic to the interpretation of spoken language will serve both to illustrate the complexity of the system, and to provide a foundation for the understanding of how hearing-impaired listeners may compensate for their auditory deficits.

In order for the comprehension of spoken language to take place, selective attention must first be given to the speech stream, and some sort of sensory storage must come into play, because words and sentences do not arrive instantly. The sounds that go together to make words, and the words themselves, may not be perceived as whole units, so they must be analyzed and retained until the listener, using previously acquired knowledge about phonemic features, phonological rules, motor speech cues, situational cues, linguistic context cues, and suprasegmental patterns, arrives at a decision about what has been said. Once some words are recognized they must be re-coded, rehearsed, and stored again while more words are arriving at the ear. When the message is complete, it may be very meaningful to the listener and, on this account, remembered. If the message is not significant it will be quickly forgotten.

There are at least four stages through which speech patterns are processed. We may label them *detection, discrimination, identification,* and *comprehension.* Most simple hearing tests measure detection. When hearing is tested using a choice between two items, discrimination is involved. When a test requires that any word or other test item be recognized, either from a closed set (a limited number of items) or an open set (an unlimited number of items), then identification must take place. There can be no "pure" tests of auditory comprehension, because the understanding of a message goes beyond the spoken *form* of a message to conceptualization relating to its *content.* Auditory tests in which words are used inevitably involve central auditory processes, and their results will be influenced by the listener's language background. For example, a French speaker tested with English words, or an English speaker tested with French words, could well appear to have a hearing impairment. Children can also appear to have either a peripheral or a central auditory problem when tested with words selected from an adult's vocabulary, or with sentences having linguistic structures that are unfamiliar to them.

All levels of central auditory processing must be affected if serious hearing impairment results from damage to the outer, middle, or inner ear (the peripheral hearing mechanism), because listeners have to develop special ways of dealing with spoken messages when their hearing impairments degrade the speech signal. Spoken language is inherently redundant; specific features of both its form and its content can be derived from more than one of its components so that, when part of the message is missing, the whole can still be interpreted. The process (often referred to as "closure") is closely akin to understanding the content of a note read from a partly obliterated page. For hearing-impaired listeners to achieve comprehension of degraded auditory signals, they have to rely a great deal on interpreting the whole message when words may be partially or wholly missing. Usually they can be helped in this process by the addition of other sensory information to the auditory signal. Vision and touch can be used for this purpose, as discussed in the next chapter, and as indicated in the theoretical model presented as Figure 3-3.

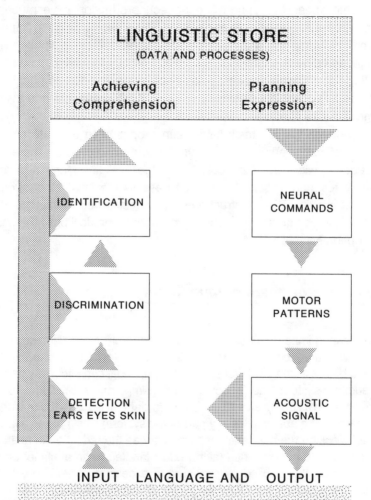

figure 3-3. A model showing the four major levels of processing that are involved in speech reception and speech production, the cognitive-linguistic store being common to both. The descending arrows on the left indicate that an ongoing, active search for meaning originates from the highest levels of linguistic processing. Feedback is shown to be a significant aspect of speech production.

Figure 3-3 is based on evidence (to be more fully discussed in the next chapter) that visual or tactile information is compatible with, and can assist at, all four levels of auditory processing: detection, discrimination, identification, and comprehension. In addition, it shows that the linguistic store required for comprehension is also needed for planning expression; that speech reception and speech production have much in common. The linguistic store as depicted here is not the passive recipient of verbal information. It actively directs the production of spoken language, and directs attention to incoming verbal information, as well as holding data relating to all aspects of spoken language - its phonemic features, its vocabulary, its syntax, its semantic components, and a wide range of verbal concepts.

Although various tests have been proposed to evaluate certain aspects of central auditory processing in adults and children, there has not been a widespread acceptance of their validity. Many new and different tests are required in order to assess the integrity of such a complex system. The construction of such tests, their evaluation, and their widespread acceptance await a stronger theoretical base than has so far been established.

the effects of hearing impairment

Hearing impairment can range in degree from a condition so slight that it can barely be noticed to total loss of auditory function. It can be caused before, during, or after a child is born, and it can affect any part of the auditory system. The causes of hearing impairment, briefly reviewed below, can be as complex as a genetic disorder that leads to the malfunction, or even the absence, of any part of the system; as simple as a lump of wax blocking the ear canal; as temporary as the reduction in hearing that sometimes occurs when taking off or landing in an airplane; or as permanent as that caused by exposure to excessive noise. (Consistent exposure to sound at high levels even over short periods of time [minutes] can permanently damage hearing. This is why airline workers have to wear ear muffs when working near running jet engines.)

If sufficiently severe, and if it is not treated effectively, hearing impairment can have numerous effects on both children and adults. Except for earache, usually the result of acute middle ear infection, hearing impairment is not associated with physical pain. Nor can it be seen. It can, however, have far-reaching effects, much as a stone, dropped into water, will cause an ever-widening circle of ripples. Its *primary effect* is to filter sound in such a way that the auditory detection of speech is either partially or totally excluded.

The most important *secondary effect* of hearing impairment is to restrict both verbal and non-verbal aspects of functioning, particularly the acquisition and/or use of spoken language in communication.

The *tertiary effects* of hearing impairment are as significant as they are varied. Restricted communication due to deafness affects not only easily observable facets of human functioning, such as language use, educational achievements, and social interaction, but much more subtle aspects of personality. These adverse effects can eventually extend into every aspect of a hearing-impaired person's life. Thus, when hearing impairment restricts a child's language development and communication, it will also prevent optimal educational attainment. A child leaving school with less than adequate academic skills, is likely to experience, among other things, restricted employment options, limited income, and circumscribed leisure activities.

Hearing impairment tends to impair a person's ability to localize sound. This particular effect is not a matter of major significance, although it can adversely influence the learning of spoken language.

When hearing impairment is experienced by older children or adults, its effects tend to be less severe than those experienced by young children with a similar degree of impairment. This is not to make light of hearing problems that are suddenly or gradually experienced after early childhood, but rather to point out some essential differences. Older children and adults who suffer hearing impairment can usually manage much more efficiently than children who become hearing-impaired at an early age because they have the linguistic experience and social skills that permit them to fill in missing information, much as a skilled reader can complete a partially obliterated written message.

Given the importance of the impact that hearing impairment in childhood has on the acquisition of spoken language, it is usual to differentiate between two groups of children; those who become hearing-impaired *pre-lingually* (before language is acquired), and those who suffer hearing loss *post-lingually* (after language skills are established). Different strategies are required to develop and maintain their spoken language skills. Similarly, the types of educational settings required by children in the two groups, and the most efficient procedures for developing their academic skills will also differ.

Finally, the effects of hearing impairment are not limited to the afflicted individuals. Such effects extend to their families and to society at large. It should not, perhaps, be surprising that hearing impairment has such pervasive outcomes. Most of what we know of the world external to us is learned through either hearing or vision. The languages that most people know are normally acquired through the ear.

the measurement of hearing

audiometry

The simplest way to measure a person's hearing, and one that has been universally adopted, is to present a tone of a given frequency (say 1000 Hz) and then vary its intensity until a listener can just detect it. This intensity level, called a threshold of hearing, is then recorded, and the procedure repeated in turn at both higher and lower frequencies until hearing levels have been determined for a wide range of sounds. The instrument used to measure hearing in this way is called an *audiometer*. Audiometers are usually calibrated in five dB steps. Differences of less than this amount are not regarded as clinically significant. Using such an instrument to test hearing is a process known as *audiometry*.

All clinical audiometers produce pure tones; that is, tones having only one component of a given frequency, and the most common audiometric test is carried out using headphones to deliver such tones to the ears. Since the sound presented in this way travels through the air in the ear canal, such evaluations are termed *air conduction* tests. For these conventional sorts of hearing tests, audiologists switch the tones on and off, while those being tested indicate when they can hear the tones being presented, usually by raising a hand. The sort of audiometry in which a child is required to respond by turning, moving a toy, saying "yes," or raising a hand (as adults usually do) to let the audiologist know when a tone is detected is known as *behavioral* testing.

Some audiometers are not built to produce stimuli at the extremes of either the frequency or the intensity range of speech. For example, some do not provide a 125 Hz tone, even though the fundamental of a male voice may be half that frequency, and many do not have output levels beyond 110 dB, even though many hearing aids amplify speech to greater levels of intensity. Hearing beyond the limits of such audiometers, particularly in the octave bands centered on 1000 and 2000 Hz, can be very useful indeed to a profoundly hearing-impaired child in the process of verbal learning.

When responses are obtained to low frequency sounds (125, 250, and 500 Hz) at intensities of 115 dB or more, the individual being tested may be feeling rather than hearing them. Indeed, if extremely high intensity sounds yield thresholds that do not extend up to and beyond 1000 Hz, the likelihood is that they are vibro-tactile rather than auditory, and that the individual with such restricted thresholds would be able to respond at similar intensity levels if the earphones were placed on the hand rather than over the ears. Closely related to this phenomenon is the wearing of hearing aids by individuals who have no hearing, but who obtain information on the spoken word from the vibro-tactile sensations that the hearing aid produces in the ear canal.

The extent of any hearing impairment, as established through the completion of an audiometric test, is calculated by comparing the individual's thresholds with those of normally hearing listeners. This is accomplished quite simply, because the reference level (0 dB hearing level) on clinical audiometers, and on the audiogram form shown as Figure 3-4, is known as audiometric zero - and audiometric zero is the average level at which young adults with no history of ear problems can just detect sounds at the specified frequencies.

To determine whether the hearing impairment originates in the outer or middle ear as compared to the inner ear, tones from the audiometer can be delivered by a vibrator placed behind the ear on the mastoid bone rather than through headphones. This, predictably enough, is called *bone conduction* testing. Because sound transmitted through the mastoid bone to the cochlea will be heard quite clearly if the cochlea is unimpaired, it can be concluded that those who have better thresholds for bone conducted sound than for air-conducted sound have a defective outer or middle ear. When individuals have different air conduction and bone conduction thresholds, they are said to have an *air-bone gap*. If an air-bone gap exists, conductive hearing impairment is suspected. Many types of conductive problems can be verified using an *otoscope* to look down the ear canal or by *tympanometry*, a procedure that requires the use of an electronic device to change air pressure levels in the ear canal.

Not all audiometry is carried out in the manner described above. Some children are too young to respond reliably to this form of testing. When this is the case, the audiologist may use an audiometer to produce pure tones that warble and present them through loudspeakers rather than headphones. Tests in which sounds are presented through loudspeakers rather than headphones are called "sound field" tests. Sound field tests can also be carried out with narrow bands of noise rather than warble tones.

When children are too young to respond voluntarily to tests of hearing, they may be tested through the use of Visual Response Audiometry (VRA). To carry out this type of testing, auditory stimuli of known intensity and frequency are presented to the child through a loudspeaker. The child is placed on mother's lap or in a high chair, and then visually reinforced (rewarded) for turning towards the source of the sound. The audiologist provides the reinforcement by activating an electrically driven toy placed on or near the loudspeaker.

Children who are too young to respond even to VRA audiometry can still be tested. Indeed, hearing tests can be carried out on newborn babies by means of Electric Response Audiometry (ERA) and other forms of electro-physiological testing in which no overt response is required. Indeed, such tests can be (and usually are) carried out when the children being tested are sleeping or heavily sedated. Such audiometry is now in widespread clinical use. Simply stated, ERA involves the presentation of rapidly occurring sounds at known levels of intensity. The electrical activity related to these stimuli in various parts of the central auditory nervous system is detected by means of electrodes placed on the child's scalp. A computer is an intrinsic part of this system. It is used to average these electrical responses in order to separate them from noise. This permits the results to be read from a simple graph. Only for sounds that the child can hear will the graph show lines that have well-defined peaks and valleys.

audiograms

An audiogram is a graph on which a person's thresholds of hearing are recorded (see Figure 3-4). Intensity is represented on the vertical axis of the audiogram form as hearing levels specified in dB (decibels above normal thresholds of hearing), and frequency is shown along the horizontal axis in octave intervals (intervals that are twice the frequency of the previous interval, thus 125, 250, 500, 1000 Hz, and so on). Usually, the intensity scale begins at less than audiometric zero (for those who have particularly good hearing), and ends at about 120 dB (a normal dynamic range of hearing).

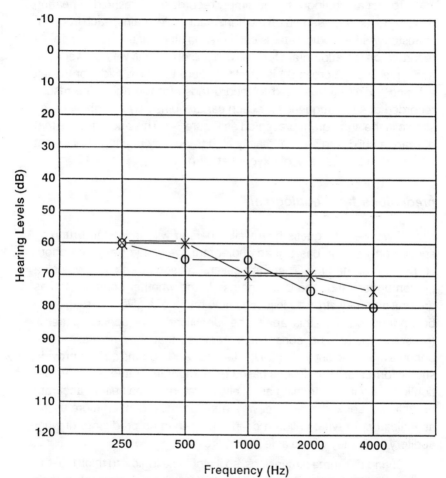

Frequency (Hz)

figure 3-4. A typical audiogram form. The zero reference line represents the average threshold levels of normal young adult listeners. The audiogram is that of a six-year-old boy who has not yet produced /s/. (See the case history of Brad towards the end of this chapter.)

Most forms for plotting an audiogram cover the frequency range from 125 Hz to 8000 Hz. All speech sounds have components within this range, although some speech sounds, such as the fundamental of a deep male voice, can be much lower, and others, such as the turbulent hiss of fricatives, much higher. For example, it is quite normal for a bass voice to be as low as 60 Hz, and an /s/ sound to have a significant amount of energy at well over 16,000 Hz.

To plot an audiogram, one simply records the threshold of hearing (hearing level) represented on the horizontal scale against each frequency tested. As the audiometer is calibrated in steps of five dB, the points recorded on the audiogram form always fall on, or half way between the horizontal lines. A cross (X) is used to record the thresholds for the left ear, and a circle (O) is used to record those for the right. The results recorded at each frequency for each ear are joined by straight lines, as shown in the audiogram presented as Figure 3-3. This audiogram is that of Brad, a child with severe, mainly high-frequency hearing impairment attributed to anoxia (lack of oxygen) at birth.

predictions from audiograms.

If we were to guess how well a person will understand running speech only on the basis of an audiogram, we would be wrong about 30 percent of the time. There are several reasons for this. How well a person understands the language used, and whether contextual cues are present, may strongly influence how much of a given message can be understood. But this apart, the identification of speech patterns (prosody, vowels and consonants) requires that their acoustic components are sufficiently clear to the listener. Audiograms cannot provide such information. Predictions based on audiograms rather than evaluation in the course of training are likely, therefore, to be neither accurate nor reliable. Looked at another way, audiograms are much more useful as indicators of what children cannot hear than as predictors of what auditory skills they will be able to acquire.

Sound has three dimensions, so it would be logical to think that the measurement of people's hearing should involve assessment of their ability to detect differences in the *intensity*, *frequency*, and *duration* of sounds. This can be done but, as explained above, routine audiometry involves only two of these three dimensions. Audiograms contain no information on how well the third dimension of sound - duration - can be perceived. Thus, children who have trouble in hearing the relative duration of sounds or the gaps between them, could have difficulty in following speech, but their audiograms would not indicate this problem.

Audiograms are typically based on thresholds for "steady state" pure tones - sounds that do not vary in intensity and frequency. But speech is quite unlike this. Speech patterns are both complex and constantly changing. There are, inevitably, great differences among children in their ability to resolve sounds that change rapidly in these dimensions. In addition, audiograms are records of the faintest sounds that can be heard by an individual, but nobody listens to speech at such low levels of intensity. Furthermore, audiograms cannot show how much auditory learning a child has experienced or what potential a child may have for auditory learning. Not surprisingly, then, two or more hearing-impaired children can have identical audiograms, and yet have very different listening skills - very different levels of ability to understand speech through hearing.

Hearing loss due to noise exposure is one of several types of auditory deficit that not only reduces hearing acuity, but also reduces a person's tolerance for sounds of high intensity. Sounds that are quiet to normally hearing listeners may not be audible to such individuals, but more intense sounds may appear to them to be too loud for comfort. This phenomenon, one that cannot be predicted from an audiogram, is known as loudness recruitment. In its most severe form, the presence of this problem may reduce the dynamic range of hearing so much that sounds go from "too quiet to hear" to "too loud to tolerate" when intensity levels are increased by just a few decibels. Loudness recruitment is rarely so extreme, but it can lead to difficulties in the selection and adjustment of hearing aids (see Chapter 4).

Certain predictions - about what children will not be able to hear - can, of course, be made with considerably more than 70 percent confidence from accurate audiograms. The sort of specific prediction that can be correctly made on the basis of Brad's audiogram presented as Figure 3-4 is that nothing will be audible in the conversational level speech addressed to this child from a distance of two yards when he is not wearing his hearing aids. One can also completely rely on certain general predictions, such as *persons with no hearing beyond 1000 Hz will not be able to hear unvoiced fricatives*. We know that this will be so because all significant energy in these sounds falls above that frequency. If children have audiograms that show no hearing above 1000 Hz and they can hear unvoiced fricatives, then either their audiograms are inaccurate or their hearing aids are distorting sounds very badly.

If any of these negative predictions are borne out by observation of a child in the course of an intervention program, then non-auditory strategies can be used to develop that child's spoken language. Such strategies are discussed in later chapters. Before employing alternative sense modalities, however, the hearing levels recorded on audiograms should be verified in the course of treatment, initially over some months. Predictions, such as those stated above, are, of course, only as reliable as the audiogram itself - and audiograms, particularly those derived from behavioral testing, may not be completely reliable for several reasons. Behavioral testing requires a child's complete cooperation and full attention. Some children are very difficult to test, and on this account their responses may be misleading. Just because their responses are recorded on an audiogram form does not guarantee that they are true hearing levels. This is a fact of life, not a criticism of audiologists or audiological tests as such.

audiograms and the acoustics of speech

As shown in the previous chapter, the speech patterns of English vary considerably in intensity, frequency and duration - all three dimensions of sound. It is the interaction of these three dimensions of sound that gives speech patterns their phonetic identities. There is no absolutely right way to produce speech sounds so, although there are differences between one talker and another, a wide range of dialects and accents can be understood.

To recapitulate the points made in Chapter 2 for the purposes of the present discussion, the most powerful sounds in speech are the central vowels - those made with the largest oral cavities and the widest opening of the mouth. The weakest sounds are those that restrict the breath flow maximally - the fricatives /f/, /s/, and unvoiced th. Those with the highest frequency are these same fricative sounds, all of which have components up to and beyond 15,000 Hz. The longest and lowest-pitched speech patterns are those associated with prosody - the fundamental voice frequency and components of rhythm, intonation, and stress that collectively are known as suprasegmentals. The vowels are longer than most consonants, and their lower and stronger (F_1) components fall below 1000 Hz. The higher (F_2 and F_3) components of vowels fall mainly between 1000 and 3500 Hz. The consonants are spread widely across the frequency range of speech, and vary greatly in duration and intensity. The shortest sounds in speech are the stops that occur at the end of syllables or words, such as up in the phrase *up there.*

The overall intensity of conversational speech normally varies within a range of about 30 dB from the quietest consonant (unvoiced th) to the loudest vowel (aw as in the word *bawl*). This amount of acoustic variation is known as the *dynamic range of speech.* Speech sounds within this dynamic range vary not just in relation to each other, but according to whether the words in which they occur are stressed or unstressed. For example, the two words *for* and *four* are pronounced similarly when said one by one. However, in a sentence, such as *I waited there for four hours,* the word *four* is likely to be stressed (emphasized). Stress in words results in more than just a change in intensity.

At a distance of about two yards (an average distance for conversation), the quietest sounds in everyday speech are about 30 dB greater than audiometric zero and the loudest, about 60 dB. Intensity is the most variable dimension of speech. In the absence of reflection and reverberation, sound increases in intensity by about 6 dB with every halving of distance, and decreases by the same amount with every doubling of distance, between the talker (or other source) and the listener. When a mother is talking to her hearing-impaired child at home and in the course of quiet play (as in the sketch presented as Figure 3-5) the acoustic conditions are at their most favorable. This is an important point and one that will be taken up again later on in relation to hearing aid use.

The overall frequency range of speech does not vary a great deal and, because the broad frequency characteristics of speech sounds are known, it is possible to relate certain aspects of speech quite closely to vertical bands drawn on an audiogram. By doing this one can relate speech reception to individual children's plotted hearing levels, and be better able to specify what sort of speech features may or may not be detected if they are fitted with appropriate hearing aids.

As suggested in the previous section on audiograms, it is possible to say that if there is no hearing in a certain frequency band one can predict that a certain range of sounds will not be heard. We can now add that if sound patterns of a certain frequency, as specified below, occur at levels 10 dB or so better than individuals' aided thresholds in that frequency range, those patterns will be *detected.* However, sensorineural hearing impairment may not only filter sounds, it may also distort them. If this is the case, then speech patterns as specified below may be detected, but those having components in that frequency range may not be *discriminated, identified,* or *comprehended* because of such distortion.

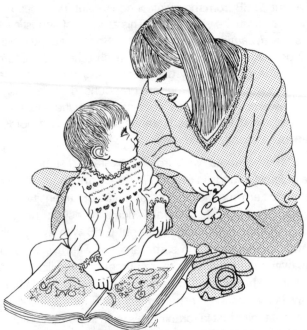

figure 3-5. A mother talking to her young hearing-impaired child under optimal learning conditions: through one-to-one interaction; by following the child's interests; and by ensuring the best possible listening opportunities (being on the child's level, at close quarters, and in the favorable acoustic environment provided by the home). Such strong visual focus is rarely necessary when useful residual hearing exists, and maximum use is made of it.

speech components and frequency bands

In the following paragraphs the components of speech that fall in various frequency bands will be specified. Each band will be centered on one of the octave intervals represented on an audiogram form (125, 250, 500, 1000 Hz, and so on), and extend by a half octave in each direction. Such octave bands are shown by the vertical bands of shading shown on the the audiogram form presented as Figure 3-6. The lighter (banana-shaped) area in Figure 3-6 depicts the approximate intensity of significant speech components as they occur in the writer's conversational speech at a distance of two yards. This area may be considered as the CLEAR zone - the zone in which conversational level elements in the acoustic range of speech occur. The approximate intensity levels of the vowels oo, ah, and ee, and the consonants sh and /s/ are shown in the frequency bands where most of their energy is to be found.

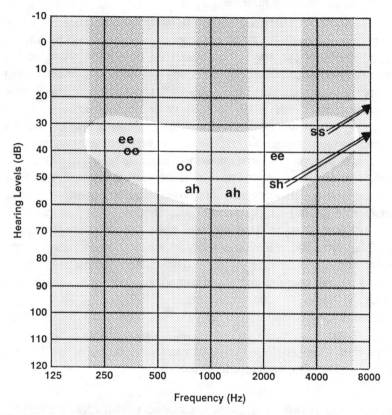

figure 3-6. An audiogram form showing octave bands centered on the audiometric frequencies (vertical bands of shading), and the CLEAR zone in which the Conversational Level Elements in the Acoustic Range of speech are to be found. The approximate center frequency and intensity of the formants of each sound used in The Five-Sound Test as produced by the writer at a distance of two yards are depicted in the CLEAR zone.

Many speech sounds share common properties. For example, /m/, /n/, and ng share nasality, all fricatives, such as /f/, /s/, and sh, share turbulent breath stream, and all plosives, such as /p/ and /b/, produce bursts as breath is released. By and large, such common components fall within the same, or within adjacent bands of frequency. This being so, one can think of speech as having relatively few significant acoustic component features, rather than many individual speech sounds. To think this way is to be concerned with the similarities among speech sounds rather than with their differences.

To assess whether *common components* of sounds are present or absent in a child's production or perception of speech can be a more economic way of carrying out an evaluation than by focusing on the presence or absence of the speech sounds (phonemes) themselves. For example, one can listen to a child's speech in order to determine whether particular components, such as nasality or fricative turbulence, are present or absent. Once the significant components of speech that are causing the individual some difficulty have been specified, one can then find ways to provide cues that make them easier to hear, see or feel. For example, all the nasal sounds have a low frequency murmur, and all the fricatives have a significant amount of high frequency energy. If a child is neither perceiving nor producing certain of these components, then one must first question whether these speech sounds are being appropriately amplified or if other sensory information is adequate over the frequency range in which they occur. The speech components (rather than the speech sounds) that are of primary importance in speech, and that fall within each frequency band, are listed in Figure 3-7. To stress the importance of vowel-to-consonant and consonant-to-vowel formant energy, formant transitions in this list will be specified as T_1, T_2, and T_3 components - they are found in the frequency range over which the first, second, and third formants move as we talk.

the intensity levels of significant speech components

The intensity levels of the components of speech listed in Figure 3-7 vary considerably from one frequency band to another. The several examples that follow serve to indicate how extensive these differences are, and how important it is to take them into account when providing amplification for hearing impaired individuals.

The octave band centered on 1000 Hz contains the central vowels, which are more intense, but no more important, than any other vowels (see Figure 3-7). They happen to be so because the mouth is more widely

125 Hz	F_0 of most adult male voices

250 Hz	Voicing cues
	F_0 of most female and child voices
	The low harmonics of adult male voices
	The nasal murmur (F_1 of /m/, /n/, and ng)
	F_1 of high back and high front vowels

500 Hz	Primary cues on manner of production, most consonants
	Harmonics of most voices
	F_1 and T_1 of most vowels
	Noise bursts of plosives in back vowel contexts
	T_1 of the semi-vowels
	F_1 of the laterals /l/ and /r/

1000 Hz	Additional cues on manner of consonant production
	The harmonics of most voices
	T_1 of the laterals /l/ and /r/
	F_2 of nasal consonants
	F_2 and T_2 of back and central vowels
	The noise bursts of most plosives
	T_2 of the semi-vowels

2000 Hz	Primary cues on place of consonant production
	Additional cues on manner of consonant production
	The harmonics of most voices
	F_2 and T_2 of front vowels
	The noise bursts of most plosives and affricates
	Turbulent noise of fricatives sh, /f/, and th
	T_2 and T_3 of /l/ and /r/

4000 Hz	Secondary cues on place of consonant production
	The upper range of harmonics, most voices
	F_3 and T_3 of most vowels
	The noise bursts of plosives and affricates
	Turbulent noise of voiced and unvoiced fricatives

8000 Hz	Turbulent noise of all fricatives and affricates

figure 3-7. A chart showing the components of speech that fall within the octave bands centered on the audiometric frequencies 125 to 8000 Hz.

opened for vowels like aw and ah than for other vowels like oo and ee. In producing the latter sounds, the shape of the vocal tract and the height of the tongue obstruct breath flow and thus reduce their intensity. Anyone who has tried to tape-record words containing these and other vowels at a consistent level is familiar with their differences in intensity. Also, the harmonics of voice decrease in intensity as they become higher in frequency. This, in turn, causes speech sounds to be weaker in the octave band centered on 2000 Hz than in the octave band centered on 500 Hz.

Several cues that lie within each frequency range also vary in intensity. For example, the nasal formants are quieter than the harmonics of voiced sounds that are present in the octave bands centered on 250 and 500 Hz. The second formants of the front vowels are less intense than the fricative turbulence associated with both the sh and ch sounds in the octave band centered on 2000 Hz. The fricative turbulence of /s/ in the octave band centered at 4000 Hz is stronger than that of the /f/, and of the unvoiced th that occurs in the same frequency range. Fricative turbulence associated with voiced affricates and voiced fricatives is also less intense, though no less significant, than that of their unvoiced counterparts. In short, the intensity levels of the significant components of speech do not correspond all that closely with the average intensity levels across the speech range.

As a first step in selecting amplification for severely and profoundly hearing-impaired children, the writer measured the levels of significant components in his own conversational speech at a distance of two yards. They occurred at levels that, when entered on an audiogram, created the banana-like shape shown as a shaded area across the audiogram form presented in Figure 3-6. This CLEAR zone does not correspond closely with the average intensity levels that occur in the various frequency bands across the long-term speech spectrum, because the components that are really important in speech discrimination and spoken language reception are less intense than the average levels of sounds at the high and low ends of the speech frequency range.

the five-sound test

It is useful to check on children's hearing before setting out to teach them, by using the information contained in Figure 3-6. The approximate center frequencies of the formants of the three vowels oo, ah, and ee, and centers of energy in the consonants sh and /s/ are shown at their approximate intensity levels in this figure. By saying these sounds at various distances, and asking children (with their eyes closed to prevent response to visual cues) to clap when each sound is heard (a detection test), or to repeat the sound when it is heard (an identification task), it is possible to check on how well the child's auditory system (hearing plus hearing aid) is working. The child shown in the sketch presented as Figure 3-8 is responding to the Five-Sound Test. Her teacher uses the test as the first activity of each school day.

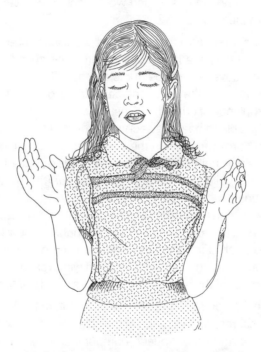

figure 3-8. A child responding to The Five-Sound Test by clapping each time one of the stimulus sounds is detected. The procedure was routinely used with this child prior to spoken language lessons, and results have ensured the detection of problems with the child's hearing or hearing aids whenever they have occurred.

The validity of the Five-Sound Test depends on the intensity of each sound in the test being presented at about the same level as that found in everyday conversational speech. If, for example, a child responds when the examiner makes the /s/ as loud as he can, one cannot conclude that the /s/ will be audible at the quieter levels that are typical of everyday conversation. Further, any speech sound can vary in everyday discourse by as much as 12 dB according to whether it is stressed or unstressed. A hearing-impaired person may, therefore, be able to hear stressed, but not unstressed sounds. To determine whether the /s/ or any other of the elements in the Five-Sound Test would be audible to the child in quiet conversation, one must, therefore, test by producing the sounds at the quieter levels met in such conversation. This can be achieved if the person who administers the test first rehearses sentences containing these speech sounds in unstressed words, and then tests with them at this pre-determined level.

The five sounds selected represent significant cues in each frequency range. If they are not audible, then other cues in each octave band as listed above will not be audible either. Thus if children cannot detect the /s/ sound, they will not be able to detect /f/ or the high frequency turbulence of other fricatives. If they cannot hear the sh sound, they will not be able to hear the second formant of the vowel ee and the transitions that provide cues on the consonants preceding or following the front vowels. If neither the oo nor the ee is audible to profoundly hearing-impaired children, then the nasal murmur (the lowest formant of all nasal sounds) that occurs around 300 Hz will not be heard either. Similar deductions can be made in relation to sounds in each frequency band. Teachers, clinicians, and caregivers should all know the distances over which each child in their care can hear each of these sounds, and ensure that they communicate with the child within earshot, the distance within which most of these sounds can at least be detected.

The principle underlying the selection of items in the Five-Sound Test is, then, that response to each of the selected sounds will signify the audibility of that and other speech components in each of the octave bands as outlined above. This principle is not always understood. For example, some talkers use the aw to replace the oo vowel in the test. But the aw vowel is the loudest speech sound and its first formant is much higher and louder than that of the oo. Its use will not, therefore, verify that sounds in the octave range centered on 250 Hz are audible. If the oo vowel as produced by a particular talker does not contain an F_1 components at about 300 Hz, then it should be replaced not by the aw vowel, but by the /m/, for its detection by severely hearing-impaired children will depend mainly, if not exclusively, on the presence of audition in the frequency range centered on 250 Hz. Indeed, it would be reasonable to add the /m/ as a matter of routine, and thus create a Six-Sound Test.

The Five-Sound Test is useful as a quick check on whether the child's hearing aids are functioning adequately or whether their performance has deteriorated since the hearing aid selection process was completed. For example, if a child wakes up with a cold, an allergy, or middle ear infection that was not present the previous day, responses to the Five-Sound Test are likely to be poorer than they were the previous morning. If the child has no symptoms suggesting any such sickness, the hearing aid rather than the child may have developed a problem. In either case, one may consider the child's listening system to be functioning at less than an optimal level.

In general, children having unaided hearing levels of, or better than, 80 dB at 250 Hz, 100 dB at 500 Hz, 110 dB at 1000 Hz, 115 dB at 2000 Hz, and 85 dB at 4000 Hz should, with appropriate hearing aids and earmolds, be able to detect and probably discriminate between and among most of the significant speech components listed as falling in each octave band described above. The use of the Five-Sound Test as part of the follow-up to hearing aid selection is strongly recommended (see Chapter 4). It was designed to be a simple and easy-to-administer test of detection. Its simplicity does not, however, negate its validity. Reference to Figure 3-3 will remind the reader that without audibility (detection of sounds), there can be no auditory discrimination, identification, or comprehension.

audition of speech components in spoken language

Using the information about speech and audiograms provided above, one can answer some of the questions that can be used to determine whether or not a hearing-impaired child is aided well enough to detect certain important aspects of speech. For example the following observations, musings, and questions might run through the head of a professional working in an auditory - verbal management program:

"This four-year-old, severely hearing-impaired girl is not making a nasal/non-nasal distinction when she talks. Anna substitutes /b/ for /m/, and /d/ for /n/, and is not yet producing an ng. She may not be able to hear the difference between nasal and other sounds. I wonder if the nasal murmur (falling at about 300 Hz) is audible to her? It should be if the aided threshold is better than 40 dB around 250 Hz! If it isn't, we'd better increase the gain in the low frequencies because she has enough unaided hearing (70 dB Hearing Levels) at 250 Hz to ensure an adequate response to all nasal sounds. If it is, then we'll make sure that the nasal/non-nasal distinction is an item for discrimination in Anna's auditory learning program. We mustn't allow this pattern of substitution to become habitual."

"Brad, this six year old severely hearing-impaired boy is not using an /s/ sound in his everyday speech. I wonder if he can hear it? If he has been taught to produce it through the use of hearing he should be able to generalize it to everyday speech - providing it's audible at a normal conversational distance of a couple of yards or so. Well, his audiogram (see Figure 3-4) shows that he has unaided hearing levels of 75 - 80 dB at 4000 Hz, but his aided thresholds at this frequency are at 45 dB. That would allow him to detect the /s/ through the use of hearing only when the teacher or clinician is as close as about eighteen inches. (Given a 6 dB increase in intensity with each halving of distance, an /s/ that has an intensity of about 35 dB [hearing level] at two yards, would have an intensity of 41 dB at one yard, and 46 dB at eighteen inches). There's not enough amplification to permit him to hear a conversational level /s/ further away than that. He may have the wrong sort of earmolds, an inappropriate hearing aid or both. Let's arrange to have the audiologist look into this. Many children with 75-80 dB unaided hearing levels wear hearing aids that provide 45 dB gain or more at 4000 Hz, and thus permit them to hear a conversational level /s/ at much greater distances. Why not this one?"

Observations and decisions, such as those sketched in the above examples, can be made on the basis of the information already presented. More such vignettes will be provided in later chapters.

raising voice levels

There is a general tendency to speak more loudly to hearing-impaired people than to others in the hope of making speech more intelligible to them. Shouting may help some, but it is usually of limited benefit. Raising voice levels increases the amount of low-frequency energy in an utterance (which is usually quite audible to hearing-impaired people) but does not increase the high-frequency energy (which is usually much less audible) to the same extent. Readers can verify this for themselves. First whisper then say quietly, "This is my sister." Then repeat it more loudly, and ultimately shout the same sentence, all the time listening very hard to the level of the /s/ in the utterance. While the vowels and voiced sounds increase a great deal, the /s/ will remain much closer to a constant level.

Because most hearing-impaired people have much better hearing for the low (as opposed to the high) frequencies, one can increase their hearing problems rather than overcome them by talking loudly. This is because an excess of low sounds can cause masking of the high-frequency consonants. It is much better to talk to hearing-impaired people quietly and at close quarters. Quiet speech increases the ratio of high-to-low frequency energy, and being close makes everything louder to the listener. It also raises the speech signal above the ambient noise more effectively than speaking loudly from a distance. In addition, being close (without being invasive) is socially much more desirable than raising one's voice, something that is often associated with anger. It is also more appropriate for people who have aided hearing, a topic to which we shall now turn.

recommended further reading

Sanders (1977) provides a wide-ranging and easy-to-read introduction to speech perception, and Lieberman (1972) provides an excellent account of the importance of prosodic features. Boothroyd (1982) presents a well structured introduction to hearing and the auditory management of hearing impairments in young children. Two texts on medical aspects of hearing impairment are recommended, one edited by Martin (1981), and the other by Pappas (1985). Introductory level information on hearing, sound, and the auditory system is available in Martin (1986). Further reading on audiological testing and management can be found in Bess (1988), and Pollack (1988). Genetic factors leading to speech and hearing problems are discussed in an excellent and comprehensive text by Jung (1989) and, in less depth, in a further text on audiology - the third edition of *Hearing in Children* by Northern and Downs (1984). See References pp. 433 ff.

chapter 4

speech reception (2): aided hearing

introduction

The previous chapters contain information on speech production, speech reception, the acoustics of speech, the human auditory system, and the effects of hearing impairments. That information is essential for the full understanding of the present chapter on aided hearing. This chapter includes a broad description of currently available hearing aids, a commentary on the basic procedures involved in selecting appropriate instruments for children, an explanation of aided audiograms, a description of the audiologist's role as a support person in a school environment, and some suggestions on how best to use aided hearing for the development of spoken language skills in hearing-impaired children.

The most important tools available in the management of almost all hearing-impaired children, are appropriately selected hearing aids. However, hearing aid selection is neither a simple nor an entirely scientific set of procedures. To provide children with the utmost information about speech, hearing aids must be selected and adjusted according to the type and extent of their hearing impairments, personal characteristics (e.g., age, stage of development, and size), as well as the characteristics of the environment in which they will be used. Ideally, hearing aids should provide sufficient amplification to enable the child to hear as many quiet sounds as possible without having so much output that loud sounds become too loud to tolerate. That is, they must place sounds within the child's dynamic range of hearing (the range between the quietest sound individuals can hear, and the loudest sound that they can hear comfortably). They must also have a suitable frequency range (so that the highest and the lowest pitched speech sounds that fall within the child's auditory range are adequately amplified). Last, but not least, they must reproduce sounds faithfully (so that the time, frequency, and intensity components of speech are not unduly distorted).

The more profoundly hearing-impaired the individual, the more difficult it is to select hearing aids that meet the ideals outlined above. Consequently, an audiologist may have to make compromises in order to achieve an optimal hearing aid fitting. Because people have different degrees and types of hearing impairments, different hearing aids with different adjustments are needed to meet these individual needs. Accordingly there can be no "best hearing aid on the market" — only a range of instruments, one or two of which are likely to be the most appropriate hearing aids for a particular child.

Very few hearing aids are likely to suit a child without adjustment — or some form of fine tuning. Most types of hearing aids currently available can be adjusted in several different ways. The volume control can be turned up or down so that there is enough overall gain (amplification) to render most speech sounds loud enough for improved listening. The on/off switch is sometimes part of the volume control. A small screw can usually be turned to emphasize high or low-frequency speech sounds according to individual needs. Individuals with a dynamic range of hearing that is smaller than the acoustic intensity range of speech, may need hearing aids that can be adjusted to provide some form of automatic gain control (AGC). This permits the intensity range of speech to be compressed, and on most hearing aids, the extent of such compression can also be adjusted by the turn of a screw. Such a feature in hearing aids may be an advantage to some, but not all hearing-impaired children. Compression of the intensity range of speech is itself a distortion and it may detract from the perception of important acoustic cues within spoken language by children with a wide dynamic range of hearing.

Currently available hearing aids, in spite of their sophistication, are not satisfactory in every way: they usually distort sounds to some extent; they are prone to feedback if used at high output levels; it is difficult to hear well with them in noise; they are quite easily damaged; and frequently break down, even when they receive required daily care. For these and many other reasons, audition through hearing aids does not compare with having normal hearing. Hearing aids are, however, indispensable to hearing- impaired individuals who wish to communicate with people in the world at large and for children who are learning speech communication skills. The next generation of hearing aids will be partly digital, and function in many ways like calculators or computers. They will provide even more adjustment options than present day instruments as well as automatically reduce background noise and feedback. Until recently, most digital hearing aids were too large to be worn behind the ear, but digital hearing aids of this type are now available and controlled trials with various types of digital hearing aids have already been carried out. However, further research is needed before it will be possible to specify what advantages digital hearing aids might ultimately have for children with different hearing impairments.

Some of the main difficulties in current hearing aid selection processes are discussed in the following paragraphs. The discussion indicates that a considerable amount of art as well as science must be employed by audiologists, because precision in all aspects of the selection process is not yet within their grasp. Hearing aid selection may always have to involve some judgements involving trial and error. This should not perturb parents and professionals unduly, because speech itself cannot be defined all that precisely, either. None of the problems associated with hearing aid selection has prevented the advantageous use of hearing aids by many children.

about hearing aids.

Three main sorts of hearing aids are manufactured to meet the variety of needs that exist among hearing-impaired individuals: head-worn, body-worn, and special-purpose instruments. Children most commonly use the type worn behind the ear. Other sorts of head-worn hearing aids include those housed in eyeglass frames, and those made to fit entirely in the ear canal. Hearing aids designed to be worn on the body were in general use before head-worn hearing aids became available. Many people, including young children, continue to use this type of hearing aid. Special-purpose hearing aids include few truly personal instruments. Most special-purpose hearing aids are used in educational settings and are shared by several children. These include hearing aids that use infra-red waves to transmit the talker's voice, speech-training aids, and group-hearing aids — so-called "hard-wire" systems that have their components (microphones, amplifiers and headphones or other receivers) connected by external cables. The FM (radio) unit is an exception among special-purpose hearing aids because many children use it as often away from as within educational settings.

Both head-worn and body-worn hearing aids can be purchased with or without a telephone coil. Switching from the microphone (M position) to the telephone coil (T position) on the hearing aid, can enable listeners to hear telephone conversations much more clearly. This is because the speech signal is then received through induction. Induction occurs when a magnetic flux crosses a coil in such a way that it generates an electrical current. The telephone receiver creates a magnetic flux that is caused as a talker's voice is transmitted through it. This flux, when it crosses the coil in the hearing aid, causes the same sort of speech-generated current to flow in (and be amplified by) the hearing aid. The telephone coil in a hearing aid can also permit speech reception through induction from a loop of wire that encircles a room or a chair, or from one that is worn by a child as a means of linking a radio receiver to personal hearing aids.

earmolds

Personal hearing aids, whether they are body-worn or head-worn are coupled to the ear by means of earmolds. To be comfortable and effective, earmolds must fit the wearer's ears perfectly. Since the size and shape of individuals' ears vary considerably, earmolds have to be created from an impression carefully taken of each ear. Earmolds are manufactured in a plastic material, such as lucite. A hole of suitable size (the bore) is drilled through the earmold to direct the sound from the hearing aid into the ear canal. Pliable, soft earmolds are most appropriate for children, because they are easier than hard plastic ones to put in the ear, usually provide a better acoustic seal (prevent the leakage of sound), and are less likely to cause damage if the ear happens to be struck or bumped during play. Various earmolds, to be discussed in more detail below, are shown in Figure 4-1.

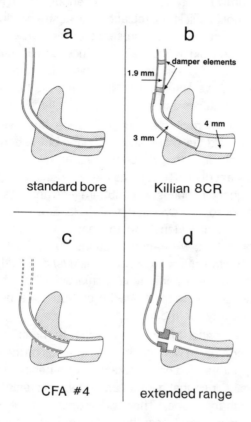

figure 4-1   Various types of earmolds. Each one affects the transmission of sound in unique and fairly predictable ways (see text).

An earmold can cause acoustic feedback (a whistling noise) if it does not fit sufficiently well. Such feedback is caused when loud sounds leaking from around the earmold enter the microphone of the hearing aid and are re-amplified. Most people have heard the acoustic feedback that often occurs in public address systems when a microphone has been placed near the loudspeakers or the system has been turned to a high level, causing it to howl. Acoustic feedback can also be caused by sound leaking through over-thin tubing leading from a hearing aid to an earmold. Not all annoying sounds associated with hearing aids are caused by acoustic feedback. Electrical feedback, arising from faulty circuitry in the hearing aid, can cause a variety of similar noises to occur. Children's ears grow rapidly during certain periods. When earmolds are outgrown, they should quickly be replaced, because a hearing aid cannot amplify speech effectively in the presence of feedback. Lowering the volume of a hearing aid will certainly reduce or eliminate feedback caused by an earmold that has been outgrown or for some other reason fits badly. However, overcoming feedback in this way is to be avoided because it usually reduces amplification to an ineffective level.

An earmold is more than a coupling device. It is a very important part of the hearing aid. Its shape and the shape of the bore profoundly affect the quality of sound that will be heard. Earmolds that have tubing and bore of constant diameter, such as the one depicted in Figure 4-1a, transmit low-frequency sounds well, but are less and less effective for the transmission of sounds over about 1500 Hz. Earmolds with a flared, horn-shaped bore that widens into the ear canal, such as the one depicted in Figure 4-1b, will transmit sounds quite effectively up to at least 8000 Hz. The transmission of sounds like /s/ and /f/, that contain a great deal of high-frequency energy, is optimal when both the tubing and the bore of the earmold widen from the earhook of a behind-the-ear hearing aid all the way into the ear canal.

It is a simple matter for anyone to listen to the effect that a long narrow tube, as compared with a widening bore, has on the transmission of sound. First, put the two hands together, one behind the other, and bend the fingers over so that a long narrow tube is created. Say a long /ssssssss/ through this "tube." Then widen open out the hands so the path through them is narrow near the mouth and becomes increasingly wider. Say the same sound through this hand configuration. Now alternate the two hand configurations, all the while saying /sssssss/, and note how the sound changes character. When said through the tube-like configuration the higher components of the /s/ are lost. Talk through the two hand configurations, and hear how different speech sounds under the two conditions.

Earmolds must be kept clean and free of wax, not only for hygienic, but also for acoustic reasons. A small accumulation of wax in the tip of any earmold will cause a reverse horn effect, one that will lower the intensity of high-frequency components considerably. Indeed, wax in the tip of the earmold is a common reason for a child being unable to hear sounds, such as sh and /s/, when the same child could hear them over considerable distances on a previous test.

Children with hearing levels of over 100 dB at 2000 Hz are often helped by CFA #4 earmolds (see Figure 4-1c), which can improve the transmission of sounds at and beyond 2000 Hz by as much as 15 dB, as compared to an earmold with a standard bore. CFA# 4 earmolds usually provide better transmission of speech sounds than the Killion 8CR in the range 2000 Hz plus or minus a half octave, but they are not as effective as 8CR earmolds above 5000 Hz. Transmission of sounds in the 2000 to 3000 Hz range is very important for the reception of cues that signal many important speech components, including cues on place of consonant production (see Figure 3-7). Young children who need better transmission in the high-frequency range than earmolds with a standard bore provide, may have ear canals that are too small to accept earmolds with a flared bore. In such cases it is often possible to create earmolds that provide high-frequency emphasis through the use of other earmold designs. The extended range type of earmold (see Figure 4-1d) is constructed with a small resonance chamber at the point where the tubing enters the earmold. Depending on the dimensions of this chamber, different parts of the high-frequency range can be selectively emphasized.

An earmold is only one component of a hearing aid system to be considered in arranging for sounds in a certain frequency range to transmitted at relatively higher (or lower) levels of intensity. Hearing aids that amplify sounds more effectively in one frequency range than another can also be selected to help meet individual children's needs. Modern hearing aids can also be adjusted, by the turn of a screw, to provide extra amplification of either high-frequency or low-frequency speech components.

It helps in the selection of appropriate hearing aids if the child comes to the selection process already in possession of appropriate earmolds. With a reliable audiogram in hand, and using the type of information present in the above paragraphs, the type of earmold that will most effectively transmit the range of sounds that a child requires can be fairly accurately specified. A few examples will suffice to illustrate this point.

Jackie's audiogram shows thresholds of 80 dB at 250 Hz, 95 dB at 500 Hz, and 115 dB at 1000 Hz, with no further responses beyond this frequency at the limits of the audiometer (120 dB). The objective in this case would be to ensure that Jackie could be aided in such a way that she could hear speech components over the frequency range of her residual hearing (up to and including 1000 Hz). A standard bore earmold (Figure 4-1a) would be most effective because it adequately transmits the low-frequency range. Earmolds designed to transmit high-frequency sounds (Figure 4-1b,c, and d) would be of no help and, indeed, could be disadvantageous, because the unnecessary transmission of high-frequency components beyond the frequency range of Jackie's audition might well cause feedback that could be avoided with standard molds.

Kim's audiogram shows thresholds of 80 dB at 250 Hz, 90 dB at 500 Hz, 105 dB at 1000 Hz, and 115 dB at 2000 Hz with no further responses at the limits of the audiometer (120 dB). The objective in this case would be to ensure the audibility not only of the low-frequency speech components, but of those falling in the octave band centered on 2000 Hz. An earmold with a standard bore does transmit sounds around 2000 Hz, but not very effectively. Earmolds with a horn configuration are most effective for the transmission of sounds at higher frequencies. The most effective type of earmold for Kim would, therefore, be either a CFA #4, or an extended frequency range mold tuned to enhance transmission in the frequency range centered on 2000 Hz (see Figure 4-1c and d).

Laurie's audiogram is relatively flat, with hearing levels of about 85 dB from 250 to 4000 Hz. The goal here is to ensure that she will be enabled to detect sounds at all frequencies within her range of hearing, including those, such as the /s/ and other fricatives, that occur in and above the octave range centered on 4000 Hz. Earmolds having a standard bore (Figure 4-1a) would not transmit sounds at this frequency effectively. An earmold with a horn configuration, however, would enable her to detect such high-frequency energy, providing that the hearing aid selected for her provided sufficient amplification in this frequency range, and also providing that her ear canals were sufficiently large to accept an earmold with a flared, horn-shaped bore. However, Laurie's ear canals are too small to accept such earmolds. An earmold of alternative design, having the extended range configuration (Figure 4-1d) could, however, still permit the transmission of all sounds from around 250 Hz up to and including those around 4000 Hz. Of course, an earmold cannot assist in the transmission of sounds unless the hearing aid amplifies and reproduces them satisfactorily, and many hearing aids are deficient in this respect. Both the hearing aids and the earmolds will influence the outcome of hearing aid selection procedures. Just as there is no one type of earmold, so is there no one type of hearing aid (or combination of earmolds and hearing aids) that is optimally suitable for all children. There are dozens of different types of earmolds and hearing aids available, each capable of modifying the acoustic signal. Audiologists therefore have to make the best of the numerous choices open to them in meeting their amplification goals for individual children. They may have different goals, and also follow different procedures from those stated or implied in this chapter. Like all responsible professionals, audiologists should be able to give good reasons for following their chosen procedures and making particular recommendations relating to auditory management.

head-worn instruments

Head-worn hearing aids can provide as much gain as any other type of hearing aid, but unless the earmolds used with head-worn aids fit very well indeed, they may produce a great deal of feedback and very little usable power. Head-worn hearing aids are prone to feedback because the microphone and the earmold are close together. This is true of hearing aids that fit in the ear canal as well as those worn behind the ear. Head-worn aids are cosmetically favored over body-worn hearing aids by most people, but they also have several other advantages over body-worn instruments. Because they are not worn on or under clothing, they do not amplify the sound caused by the instrument rubbing on material, and they may permit some children to localize the sound. In-the-ear hearing aids are not suitable for most children. They are built into the individual's earmolds, and children therefore tend suffer feedback as they outgrow them. The head-worn hearing aids of choice for most children are those worn behind the ear. Their advantage in relation to the transmission of high-frequency sounds through earmolds having a flared (horn shaped) bore has been mentioned above. Damper elements that will smooth out unwanted peaks of resonance can also be readily fitted in the earhook or in the tubing leading to the earmold in such hearing aids (see Figure 4-1b).

body-worn instruments

Body-worn instruments are often recommended for young children whose ears are not sufficiently strong to support behind-the-ear models, whose ears are small, or whose ear canals cannot readily accept ear-molds. Body-worn hearing aids can be more durable than head-worn hearing aids if they are carefully fitted in a suitable harness. Under these circumstances they are less likely to be damaged by food or drink, and less likely to be lost. Body-worn hearing aids are certainly less prone to feedback than head-worn hearing aids due to the distance between input and output (microphone and earmold). Some very profoundly hearing-impaired adults prefer them on this account. However, the direct coupling of the earmold to the external receiver rather than through the use of tubing leaves less freedom to promote the transmission of high-frequency sounds. Without tubing to help, a sufficiently long bore of increasing diameter cannot be formed. If worn loosely against clothing, body-worn aids will create a rubbing sound that will tend to mask all unvoiced fricatives and most plosive bursts.

special purpose instruments

A variety of special hearing aids, primarily designed for use in schools is also available. By far the most important of these, and the only type that will be discussed here, is the FM (frequency modulated radio) unit. Several manufacturers produce such units. Their purpose is to permit children to hear talkers (usually the teacher) effectively from a distance. An FM unit consists of a radio microphone that is worn by the teacher (or other caregiver), and a small receiving unit worn by the child that can usually be coupled by some means to the child's personal hearing aids. Self-contained FM units that do not couple to personal hearing aids, but have receivers and earmolds like those of body-worn instruments, are also available. Some teachers working with classes of children find these more reliable and prefer them on this account. The reduction of intensity with distance that normally occurs between talker and listener is avoided through the use of FM units. They also provide a better signal-to-noise ratio (speech minus noise measured in dB) be-cause the teacher's microphone, being close to her mouth, allows her speech to enter the system at levels well above those of the ambient noises in the room. The child, for these reasons, can receive much clearer speech patterns than would be possible with a personal aid at the same distance from the teacher. In short, an FM unit effectively brings the teacher's speech as close to the child as her mouth is to the microphone.

FM units are particularly appropriate for hearing-impaired children attending regular schools or classes. They can also be very useful to parents or professionals when they are taking their children out to a zoo, or to participate in an outdoor sport. They also permit children to hear caregiver's commentaries on things that they are attending to even when they are otherwise out of reach. Some children who can detect only low-frequency sounds at high-intensity levels can gain auditory experience effectively only through the consistent use of FM hearing aids. Others with a similarly limited range of audiometric responses rely on FM units to provide them with helpful vibro-tactile sensations related to speech as they use the high-sound-pressure levels delivered to the ear canal to feel rather than hear what is said to them. (Multi-channel electro- or vibro- tactile devices would probably be more efficient for such children.)

FM units can, like all other types of instruments, be used inappropriately. A child may be carefully and optimally fitted with personal hearing aids and then be expected to wear an FM unit coupled to them during school hours. Providing the FM unit does not change the output characteristics of the individual hearing aids too much, such use of it can be an advantageous. However, before FM units are used as a matter of course with children, they should be evaluated to determine just what sort of signal they will produce for the child. It is possible for a child to hear less well with an FM unit than with personal hearing aids. Louder is not necessarily clearer. Thus the FM system to be used with a particular child should be selected and evaluated with the same level of care as that exercised in selecting that child's personal hearing aids.

hearing aid selection

In this chapter, it will be assumed that all children suffering from binaural sensori-neural hearing impairment will normally receive two hearing aids — one for each ear. The superiority of binaural over monaural amplification for all but a small minority of children is no longer in question. Both ears should participate in the auditory processing of speech. Binaural fitting will therefore be assumed in this chapter. It will also be assumed, in view of the difficulty of the task, that the selection of appropriate hearing aids will be made only by qualified (and preferably experienced) audiologists. Experience is advantageous because it is much harder to fit hearing aids to children than to adults. While adults can respond verbally and very clearly in response to tests involving speech, young children can not. Moreover, adults, with their well-estab-lished language skills, can function effectively with hearing aids that would be quite inadequate for children who have yet to learn their language.

Hearing aids have to be selected on audiologists' knowledge in four areas:

1. the physical and electro-acoustic characteristics of the hearing aids;

2. the acoustics of speech as outlined in Chapters 2 and 3;

3. the methods for determining hearing levels and supra-threshold characteristics of person to be fitted; and

4. how to verify whether the hearing aid selected on the basis of such information does, indeed, provide optimal amplification over the desired frequency range and, if not, how to adjust the instru-ment so that it does).

These tasks are neither simple nor straightforward, and audiologists' evaluation and control of these aspects of hearing aid selection can, at best, be approximate. Each of the four aspects will be discussed separately in the following paragraphs.

characteristics of hearing aids

Detailed knowledge of the physical and electro-acoustic charac-teristics of specific hearing aids must be part of the extensive range of background information that audiologists must bring to the hearing aid selection task. Since many new models are introduced annually, they must continually update that knowledge. They must know, before they see a child, the range of instruments available, their size (many children's ears are too small to support some behind-the-ear models), how much gain (amplification) they will provide, the upper limit of their power (i.e. their saturation- sound-pressure levels), their frequency range, the extent to which gain, power output, and frequency response can be adjusted, their ruggedness (because young children can easily damage them), their compatibility with FM systems used in the child's local school, availability of local servicing, whether the supplier will loan hearing aids in the case of breakdown, their cost, and so on.

Manufacturers provide audiologists with data sheets that specify the electro-acoustic characteristics of each type of hearing aid they make. Computer aided selection of hearing aids according to such manufacturers' specifications has been developed and can greatly assist audiologists in the hearing aid selection process. However, as individual hearing aids of any given type vary to some extent, the actual performance of each has to be individually checked in the selection process. This task has been simplified by the various computerized devices that have now become commercially available for measuring the electro-acoustic characteristics of hearing aids. But knowing what the hearing aid will provide is not enough. The ear canals of the children and the earmolds with which hearing aids are coupled to their ears can cause sound pressure levels at the eardrum to be quite different from those predicted on the basis of electro- acoustic testing of the hearing aids. To overcome this problem, many audiologists now determine exactly how much amplification is actually being provided *in the ear canal* by inserting a small tube leading to a microphone past the earmold. With the help of a computerized system that analyzes the output from this probe-tube microphone, information about in-the-ear sound pressures at various frequencies can be immediately obtained. Computerized probe-tube microphone systems that provide the means to measure in-the-ear hearing aid performance are very helpful because, in addition to their usefulness in the selection process, they can be used to determine the exact nature of faults that may develop in hearing aids.

speech acoustics

The major purpose of fitting hearing aids is to permit hearing-impaired individuals to hear speech. True, hearing-impaired musicians and music lovers may wear hearing aids to help them to create and enjoy other forms of sound, but most people with auditory problems want help with speech communication. Audiologists must be utterly familiar with the acoustics of speech and how hearing aids can modify the transmission of its components. Without a thorough knowledge of speech acoustics, audiologists could only try one hearing aid after another and see whether, by chance, one happened to provide more than the average amount of help. Alternatively, they could select hearing aids for individuals according to a formula — a procedure akin to painting pictures by numbers. Audiologists who are familiar with the acoustic properties of speech can select or change the performance characteristics of hearing aids logically, and often quite precisely, to suit the needs of individuals, and thus provide them with optimal amplification. This section is designed to outline the sort of thinking that relates knowledge of speech acoustics to hearing aid selection for children.

In selecting hearing aids, audiologists have traditionally used a variety of procedures principally based on theories derived from clinical practice. They have, that is, determined what tends to suit different types of hearing impairment best by observing what happens when they try different types of available amplification. Such theories obviously reflect the limitations of available instruments. Theories derived through reference to speech acoustics are currently gaining acceptance. This is a substantial advance, for it opens doors of enquiry beyond the boundaries of pragmatic study. Some such theories suggest that an average of the intensity levels representing the long term speech spectrum (the average amount of energy at each frequency generated by many utterances produced by many speakers) should be used to determine how much amplification should be provided at each frequency. The notion here is that the greater the intensity of speech, the smaller the amount of amplification that will be required for its detection by the hearing-impaired listener.

There is fairly close agreement among speech scientists about the shape and the overall intensity of the long-term speech spectrum. However, there is not yet close agreement among audiologists about how the amplification of speech in the various frequency bands should be modified to suit the needs of different hearing-impaired listeners. The amount of amplification provided in each frequency, if based on an unadjusted average speech spectrum, would not critically influence speech intelligibility for adult listeners who have a wide dynamic range of hearing (e.g., those who have mild to moderate hearing loss and tolerance for high intensity sounds). However, for children with a more restricted dynamic range of hearing, the use of an unadjusted average would yield less-than-ideal results, because the intensity of the significant acoustic elements in speech (those that have to be detected in order to *learn* spoken language) does not correlate that closely with the overall average intensity of speech. One's concern should be less with average overall levels of speech in various frequency bands than with the levels of crucial speech components within these bands (a concept introduced in Chapter 3).

Predicting needs on the basis of average speech spectrum levels tends to lead to under-amplification in the lower and higher ends of the frequency range, particularly for profoundly hearing-impaired children. For example, one crucial speech cue in the octave band 250 Hz, plus and minus a half octave (see Figure 3-5) is the presence or absence of the nasal murmur. The audibility of this cue is essential if children with no hearing beyond 1500-2000 Hz are to avoid the problems they commonly experience with nasalization and denasalization in their spoken language. However, it is one of the quieter components of speech in this frequency range, and well below the level of the average speech spectrum. The most common error among hearing-impaired children who are deprived of this speech cue (the nasal murmur) is that its absence leads to confusions between /m/ and /b/ as well as /n/ and /d/. The reason for this can be seen by referring to the spectrograms presented as Figure 4-2. Covering the frequencies in and below the octave band centered at 250 Hz will make the /m/ *look* like a /b/ on a spectrogram, just as providing too little amplification at 250 Hz will make it *sound* like a /b/ to many hearing-impaired children.

The low-frequency range is often reduced substantially in the selection of hearing aids for adults, largely because considerable amounts of ambient noise met in certain work and social environments have low-frequency spectra that, amplified, can mask higher frequency sounds. While perceived quality of the speech signal may be reduced by the loss of this frequency range, adults are compensated for the limitation by the relief from masking they experience and can tolerate well because they can deduce, from their knowledge of language, what they would have heard if it were not for their hearing impairment. It cannot be assumed, however, that children can benefit from any limitations in range that are acceptable, or even advantageous, to adults. The task for adults is to comprehend a language they already know, regardless of the influence of the various acoustic environments in which they have to communicate. Instruments that are unnecessarily limited in some way should not be imposed on children who have yet to learn their mother tongue in situations that can, more often than not, be acoustically controlled.

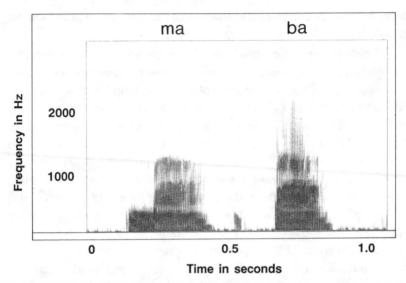

figure 4-2 Broad-band spectrograms of the syllables ma and ba. Cover the area just below 500 Hz and note that, if the frequencies in the range 250 Hz plus or minus a half-octave are eliminated, differences in the remainder of the sounds are difficult to see. Similarly, if amplification in this frequency band is insufficient, differences in the remainder of the sounds could be difficult for severely and profoundly hearing-impaired children to discriminate. Because too little amplification would render the nasal murmur inaudible to them, they would probably be unable to distinguish between nasal and non-nasal sounds.

Over-reduction of low-frequency sounds can not only eliminate the most important cue to nasality (the nasal murmur), it can also eliminate the audibility of the first formants (F_1) of the high back and high front vowels oo and ee. This may not be very important to hearing-impaired adults, particularly if they can hear the higher formants of these vowels. However, if it renders F_1 of the high front vowels inaudible (as it may do to a severely or profoundly hearing-impaired child), it may also eliminate the suprasegmental patterns (the prosodic features of speech). It will certainly eliminate them for children who have no hearing beyond 1000 Hz. Articulation index studies (studies that show how much information is carried by the different frequency bands) demonstrate that loss of the low frequencies affects word discrimination by adults to a relatively small extent. However, the adverse effects of such loss on the suprasegmental structure of utterances, and the reduction in perception of meaning that results at sentence and discourse levels, are of immense importance to children who are in the process of developing language.

A similar example of under-amplification that can occur at the high end of the speech frequency range by using the average speech spectrum as a guide to desirable levels of gain (amplification), can be provided in the octave band centered on 4000 Hz. All fricatives (such as /f/, /s/, and th) are cued by turbulent air stream energy in this frequency range. Voiceless fricatives (such as /f/ and /s/) have high-frequency components of much greater intensity than voiced fricatives, such as /v/ and /z/, and hence cues to the presence of the latter will not be rendered audible to many children unless more amplification than that suggested by the average speech spectrum is provided. The confusions that occur when these cues are not available to hearing impaired children are, predictably, often with the nasal consonants. For example, /z/ and /n/ are readily confused in the absence of high-frequency cues because the voicing component of the /z/ in the absence of the fricative cue resembles the nasal murmur. Speechreading cannot help hearing-impaired children in this instance because the sounds /z/ and /n/ cannot be discriminated visually. The reader is referred to the earlier discussion on speech acoustics in Chapter 3, from which further examples, and particularly important ones relating to transitional cues in speech, may be derived.

Any theory of hearing aid selection based on speech acoustics is further complicated by the amount of variability in the intensity levels of the speech signal that occurs with distance. The approximate intensity levels of conversational speech at a distance of two yards were described in the previous chapter. Such distances and levels may be valid for many adult-to-adult and adult-to-older child conversations, but they will not hold good for parent-infant interactions; and, of course, the distance between children's mouths and the microphones of their hearing aids will not vary as much as between mother and child; nor will they usually exceed a few inches. Each time distance is halved between talker and listener, the intensity of the speech sounds will increase by approximately 6 dB. This means that a change in distance between a talker and a listener from two feet to three inches (a change that may readily be observed as mothers care for and communicate with their children) will result in speech intensity differences of approximately 18 dB. If one adds to this figure the 30 dB dynamic range of sound in speech, and about half that again in recognition of voice intensity changes associated with normal vocal stress patterns in motherese (the way mothers tend to talk to their children), then one begins to understand the problems of coping with the expected dynamic range of speech that must be handled by both the hearing aid and the defective ear. Adequate theories for hearing aid selection must accommodate such variability.

Future audiological management theories must also incorporate an additional unknown — one that exists in relation to the different intensity levels of their own and other's voices as they are experienced by those who wear hearing aids. Since the microphones of children's head-worn hearing aids are at a few inches from their own lips, and may be at a distance of several yards from another talker's, intensity differences of well over 20 dB between their own and others' voices usually exist. If children are to hear their own voices and monitor their own speech, they must adjust to living with such differences. How such adjustment can best be promoted remains to be determined.

In spite of the insightful application of knowledge relating to speech acoustics, current hearing aid selection procedures may meet with only qualified success for other reasons discussed below.

hearing levels and supra-threshold characteristics

Both the quantity and quality of supra-threshold hearing (audition of sounds above the threshold of detection) are important in the management of hearing impaired children. How much hearing remains to a child will, in the main, determine what sort of hearing aid should be selected. Whether the hearing that remains will permit sufficiently fine discrimination of complex sounds that vary in intensity, frequency, and time will largely determine how well speech will be heard. Quantity and quality of hearing tend to be closely related: those with the greatest dynamic range of hearing usually hear speech with the least amount of distortion.

All hearing-impaired individuals have a limited dynamic range of hearing. Alice, for example, has thresholds of detection (hearing levels) averaging 60 dB and loudness discomfort levels (LDLs) averaging 105 dB. Her dynamic range of hearing is 105-60 = 45 dB. Ben, on the other hand, has exactly the same pure tone audiogram as Alice (60 dB), but his LDLs average 120 dB. His dynamic range of hearing is 120 - 60 = 60 dB. It is, therefore, much easier to find and adjust a hearing aid for Ben than it is for Alice.

As stated in Chapter 3, children's hearing levels now can be determined from an early age by objective, electro-physiological tests of hearing. But to calculate the available dynamic range of hearing one must also establish loudness discomfort levels (LDLs). These have to be determined by guesswork supplemented by observation of the child's gross responses to different sounds of high intensity.

There is no agreed stimulus for the establishment of discomfort levels, but observation of responses to narrow band noises is a commonly used procedure. If the procedure has not been sufficiently sensitive, and the output of the hearing aid selected is too great for a child's comfort, the presentation, at close range, of sounds with a wide frequency range and sudden onset (like the sound produced by tapping a tambourine) will usually elicit flinching or some other form of response signalling distress. If the procedure has led to defining the LDL at too low an intensity, then too small an estimation of the child's dynamic range will be made. Estimations of LDL that are either too great or too small can have adverse effects that merit further discussion.

There is risk that some residual hearing may be lost if there is long-term exposure to hearing aids that have extremely high levels of output. The risk is small, because children will more frequently resist wearing the hearing aids than tolerate sounds that are uncomfortably or dangerously loud to them, but it is certainly there. When children refuse to wear their hearing aids it is usually because they are too powerful, not powerful enough, not helpful in assisting them extract meaning from what is said (see later sections in this Chapter), or because the earmolds cause irritation. Signs of distress arising from over-amplification are most likely to appear within a few days either when a child is wearing hearing aids for the first time, or when new hearing aids have been selected. Attention to the possibility of output levels that are too high must, therefore, be given for two important reasons: the risk of rejection of the hearing aid, and possible damage to residual hearing.

The possibility that output levels are not sufficiently high should also receive careful attention. Unless children with hearing aids use as much of their dynamic range of residual hearing as possible, their auditory reception of speech will not be optimal. They will be likely to miss certain speech components if the output from the hearing aid is unnecessarily limited.

The definition of each child's dynamic range for intensity (within which listening will be a comfortable experience) is, therefore, crucial in the overall selection process. The greater the dynamic (as well as the frequency) range of speech available to hearing-impaired children the easier it is for them to develop spoken language skills, assuming that the hearing aids selected allow for the full utilization of this potential.

The quality of a young child's supra-threshold hearing is notoriously difficult to establish. This is mainly because such children tend to have a relatively limited attention span, and also tend to be less able than adults to describe what it is that they can hear. When children are first fitted with hearing aids, the quality of their hearing is, therefore, best established through observation of their responses in the course of auditory-verbal training. In short, the best way to find out how well hearing-impaired infants can learn to discriminate between sounds, identify and use words, and comprehend spoken language is not through audiological tests, but through using auditory-verbal procedures to develop their spoken language. Later on, when children have sufficient verbal skills, the quality of their supra-threshold hearing can be tested using more complex means of evaluation including speech tests of hearing.

the validation of the selection process

Tests to determine the validity of the hearing aid selection process have to be carried out in various ways on several occasions; when the hearing aid is first worn, on a day-by-day basis once it is habitually worn, and then during regular follow-up sessions. When the hearing aid is first worn, systems in which a tube leading to a microphone is inserted past the earmold into the ear canal (probe tube systems) can be used to indicate whether the hearing aid and its coupling to the ear are as predicted from the selection procedures. On a day-by-day basis, observation can be used to whether an infant responds (often by quieting or stilling) to speech, and whether there are any signs of intolerance to a range of acoustic stimuli.

Once the hearing aids are in constant use (and this should be only a matter of a week or so at the most), the Five-Sound Test (described in Chapter 3) can be used, day-by-day, to determine the distances over which older children can hear sounds in each frequency range. This test is a face valid measure of a child's ability to detect sounds. Auditory detection must be ensured if higher level auditory processing is to occur. Also, children who have been fitted with appropriate hearing aids should be regarded as having auditory systems that extend not from the ear to the brainstem, but from the microphone of the hearing aid to the auditory cortex. If a child's ability changes, then either the hearing aid or the child's hearing must have changed, and the audiologist should be asked to determine why.

The integrity of each child's auditory system must be, indeed can only be, maintained through regular audiological follow-up. Such follow-up should include electro-acoustic checks on the hearing aids (for their performance may deteriorate quite rapidly), as well as the usual battery of audiological tests. In addition, the audiologist should determine whether anticipated changes in children's customary auditory responses and patterns of vocalization have begun to emerge. They should begin to occur as soon as they have been using the hearing aids for some weeks and have had the opportunity to hear meaningful spoken language often enough and clearly enough. Consistent, measurable, and rapid progress in the acquisition of spoken language skills are important measures of an effective hearing aid selection procedure. Among normally hearing children between one and four years of age, such progress can be observed day after day. It is not too much to expect on a week-by-week basis from children enrolled in appropriate aural habilitation programs.

Three types of measures should then be used to determine whether the hearing aid selection procedure has validity: immediate clinical assessment; day-by-day observation of auditory responses, preferably using a consistent set of stimuli, such as those included in the Five-Sound Test; and regularly scheduled follow-up tests that evaluate the hearing aids, the child's hearing, and the child's progress in learning spoken language skills. Follow-up tests sometimes indicate that the hearing aid has deteriorated through use. They may also show that the thresholds of young children are actually better than when the hearing aid was selected because their responses to behavioral tests were initially unreliable. They may, alternatively, show a change for the worse because there has been an actual loss of hearing. Because any of these changes could come about quite quickly, follow-up tests should be scheduled at intervals of three months or less. Less frequent follow-ups may be scheduled once the child has acquired sufficient spoken language to be able to report unusual difficulties in hearing reliably.

Children eighteen-months-old and older are able to indicate difficulties with hearing aids after only a few months of auditory experience if that experience has permitted them to derive meaning through listening. Only if the hearing aids are making sounds and speech more meaningful to them do children have any reason to be concerned about whether they are in good working order or not. Children who do not in some way inform caregivers when they are having a problem with one or both of their hearing aids have not learned to derive meaning through audition. Children who obtain significant benefit from a hearing aid (derive meaning from sound) want to wear their hearing aids at all times. Some prefer to go to bed with at least one hearing aid on. This behavior is very much in contrast to that of children who either prefer not to wear their hearing aids or who wear their hearing aids turned off or turned down so far that they cannot hear. Caregivers, both professionals and parents, must recognize that their part in the developing children's attitudes towards amplification is of the utmost importance. Caregivers' positive or negative feelings towards hearing aids and/or the acquisition of spoken language are quickly perceived.

To summarize, then, a child's failure to report problems with hearing aids, to wear them, or have the volume adjusted appropriately suggests one or more of several possibilities; namely, that:

- the child is not sufficiently mature to report problems;
- spoken language has little significance (meaning) for the child;
- caregivers have a negative attitude towards hearing aids;
- caregivers have a negative attitude towards spoken language;
- the auditory-verbal experience the child receives is inadequate;
- inappropriate hearing aids have been selected;
- the child has no useful residual hearing, and should be using a different type of sensory aid (a tactile device or a cochlear implant).

audiologists as support personnel

Clinical audiologists are experts in more than the non-medical aspects of hearing, hearing impairment, and hearing aid selection. In addition to these central aspects of audiology, they also act as support personnel for the parents and other professionals concerned with the spoken language development of hearing-impaired children. Accordingly, their task is to assure, inform, assist, and generally collaborate with the parents and other professionals concerned with the long-term treatment of their clients. To do their job effectively, they must ensure that their work ends up helping hearing-impaired individuals to function optimally when communicating through speech. To this end, they must be concerned not only with the selection of hearing aids, but with the quality of the spoken language acquisition programs that the infants and children they test might follow. Optimal outcome of audiological practice cannot be achieved within the walls of a clinic or the hours of a normal working day.

aided audiograms

There are various ways in which hearing test results can be reported and different charts that can be used to show the outcome of hearing aid selection. The regular audiogram can be used, and this procedure is traditional. It will be used here to illustrate what happened to a seven-year-old boy called Alan.

aiding Alan

Alan was seen by the writer following audiological testing in another center. His parents brought an audiogram with them. It showed his loudness discomfort level (LDL), his unaided thresholds, and the levels of his aided sound field responses (A−A). These were plotted on the audiogram form shown as Figure 4-3a. It can be seen that Alan is able to respond to less intense sounds at all frequencies when wearing, as compared with not wearing, his hearing aids. But is this amount of gain clinically significant? Can the outcome of the selection procedure used with Alan help him acquire spoken language skills? Is this hearing aid fitting optimal for him? The answers to these questions are a resounding NO. The selection procedures discussed above would have shown that Alan's hearing aids were providing less than optimal auditory help. Indeed, they would have demonstrated that the only sounds that Alan could hear in conversational level speech at a distance of two yards, while wearing the hearing aids that had been selected for him, were a few central vowels.

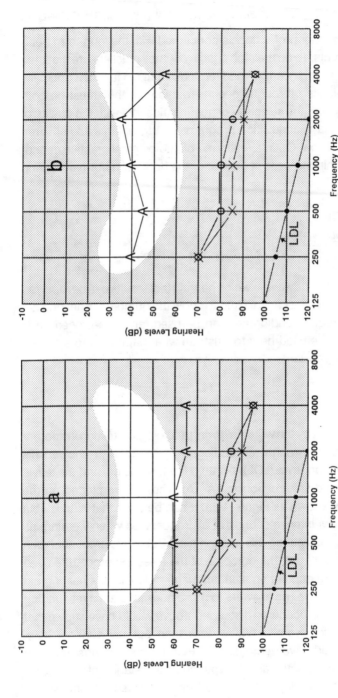

figure 4-3. a. Alan's aided (A—A) and unaided (O—O and X—X) thresholds in relation to the CLEAR zone (the approximate zone in which the conversational level elements of speech are present in the acoustic range normally created by a speaker at a distance of two yards). Only one response appears within this zone - the one at 1000 Hz. This permits Alan to hear only one of the elements of The Five-Sound Test, namely the vowel ah. b. The improvement in Alan's aided thresholds following adjustment of the hearing aid and the fitting of new earmolds. Only the /s/ and other sounds in the octave band centered on 4000 Hz cannot be amplified sufficiently, and remain inaudible to him.

Reference to Figure 4-3a indicates the extent to which Alan's hearing aids fall short of permitting him to detect sounds across the speech frequency range. The only aided response (A) that falls within the CLEAR zone — the zone surrounding the stimuli used in the Five-Sound Test, is the one obtained at 1000 Hz. (This zone is so called because, to be detected through audition, its Conversational Level Elements must fall within this range for Auditory Reception. The position of Alan's aided audiogram in relation to this zone depicts the extent to which significant speech components spoken in a conversational level voice at a distance of two yards were detectable by him using the hearing aid as initially selected. His aided audiogram overlapped with this zone at only one frequency, namely 1000 Hz. This limited range of detection could provide Alan very little significant information about speech. Not surprisingly, the Five-Sound Test confirmed that only the ah vowel was the only item audible to him.

Children with much greater hearing impairments than Alan can be expected to detect much more of speech than he was receiving when he was first seen. In theory, children with Alan's degree of hearing impairment should be able to detect all but the high-frequency sounds of speech. Accordingly, steps were taken to correct this situation. Alan's audiologist agreed to work with the writer with a view to improving his amplification. She pointed out that his behind-the-ear hearing aids could be adjusted to provide better amplification for the lower, but not for the higher frequencies. At the turn of a screw, the hearing aid adjustments were made, and immediately Alan was able to respond to sounds in the octave bands centered on 250 and 500 Hz. This enabled him to detect all vowels, the nasal murmur, and the relative intensity, frequency, and duration of all voiced sounds. However, his inability to detect sounds in the octave band centered on 2000 Hz remained a matter of some concern. His earmolds had a standard bore — a configuration that is not ideal for high-frequency transmission. New earmold impressions were taken, and CFA#4 type molds that would provide better sound transmission at 2000 Hz and above were ordered. These permitted Alan to respond to the sound sh produced at a conversational level over a distance of more than three yards, and to discriminate between syllables, such as /rarara/ and /lalala/. Following the adjustments to the hearing aids and the provision of new earmolds, Alan's aided audiogram was as shown in Figure 4-3b.

Although the improved low-frequency response resulted in a gain of 30 dB at 250 Hz, there was no risk of upward spread of masking — a situation in which low-frequency speech sounds limit the perception of higher frequency sounds — because the gain in the higher frequencies was increased to comparable levels. Had the aided audiogram been sloping downwards by a significant amount such masking might well have occurred. The octave band centered on 4000 Hz could not be brought into the CLEAR zone. Alan's hearing impairment in this frequency range was simply too great for this to be achieved with any available hearing aid. The adjustment of the hearing aid as in Figure 4-3b did not cause sounds to exceed Alan's loudness discomfort level (LDL), which is depicted on both of his audiograms.

The difference in Alan's performance, due to improved amplification, was noticeable within days. He attended more readily to speech addressed to him and he made fewer mistakes in speech reception. For example, he no longer confused "how are you" with "how old are you," and he made fewer speechreading errors. Within weeks, he was producing the /b/ and /m/ appropriately, and was making other nasal/non-nasal distinctions. Within a few months, he had acquired and spontaneously began using the sh and ch sounds, and was producing speech with more natural intonation and clearer rhythmic patterns.

Alan's case is, unfortunately, not an isolated one. Three very similar cases were brought to the writer's attention in different cities within the course of a few months of his first seeing Alan with a view to recommending suitable speech goals and strategies for accomplishing them. When hearing aid adjustments had been made, and Alan had begun to benefit from them, it became clear that he did not, in fact, require formal speech teaching. He rapidly acquired new sounds simply through having sufficient, better quality auditory experience. Not all audiologists are in a position to assess the results of their hearing aid selection procedures, particularly on a day-by-day basis or over the course of an extensive educational program. Such a limitation may lead to overly-cautious fitting procedures, such as were initially adopted with Alan. The low-frequency response of his hearing aid was deliberately reduced to avoid amplifying environmental noise and to prevent upward spread of masking. But such caution was unnecessary because Alan was not exposed to intense noise, and the hearing aid was not providing enough amplification for the detection of either low or high-frequency sounds in any case. If treatment programs do not have an audiologist on staff who is able to monitor a child's auditory progress, then parents or other professionals must do it. Everyone concerned with the development of hearing-impaired children's spoken language must be able to ascertain that their children are hearing optimally every day of their lives. They must be prepared to question if their children's responses do not appear to be optimal, to recognize malfunctioning aids, to check the adequacy of earmolds, to carry out everyday checks on hearing aids, and to have them fixed when they go wrong (as they almost certainly will).

Audiograms constructed by using other conventions may be a little more complex, but they can also more accurately represent what actually happens in real life. The type of aided audiogram presented to describe Alan's history is, in a way, somewhat misleading; amplification does not, in fact, change the child's hearing levels. It simply increases the intensity of sounds. The next type of aided audiogram described will illustrate this.

aiding Barbara

Barbara is a five-year-old child whose parents brought her to the writer for a consultation because she was not producing fricatives. Barbara's unaided hearing levels in both the left ear (X – X) and the right ear (O – O) averaged about 85 dB over the frequency range 250 to 4000 Hz (see Figure 4-4a).

The CLEAR zone depicted in previously presented Figures has, as inspection of this Figure shows, been shifted down on this audiogram form, and has assumed a somewhat distorted shape. In this sort of aided audiogram, the shape and position of the CLEAR zone will depend on the amount of amplification provided at each frequency. In Figure 4-4a, the shape of the CLEAR zone reflects the amount of gain provided by Barbara's hearing aids at each frequency. (It no longer represents the approximate intensity range of the five sounds as measured at a distance of two yards. It shows the approximate intensity range of these elements as they are spoken at that distance *and then amplified by the child's hearing aids*.) Figure 4-4a also shows that the octave frequency range centered on 4000 Hz is not amplified sufficiently to permit Barbara to detect the /s/ in normal conversation addressed to her from six feet away. The Five-Sound Test confirmed that Barbara's hearing aids did not permit her to detect the /s/. She could, as one would expect from this aided audiogram, detect all three vowels and the sh.

Barbara's hearing aids were already adjusted to provide as much high-frequency energy as they could produce. We therefore looked for the sort of earmolds that would provide better transmission in this frequency range. Killion 8CR type earmolds were selected. When they. were fitted, more high frequencies became available. The improvement in Barbara's amplification fact is reflected in the adjacent aided audiogram shown as Figure 4-4b. This shows that Barbara's responses at 4000 Hz are now contained within the CLEAR zone. A repeat of the Five-Sound Test showed that Barbara could detect a conversational level /s/ at two yards as soon as the new earmold was fitted. She began to use the /s/ in plurals and possessives, and other fricatives in her communicative speech a few months later. Now, at age eight, she has normal spoken language. The time spent in selecting an appropriate earmold was a small price to pay for Barbara's acquisition of the /s/ — one of most heavily used morphemes in English. It also prevented the need for any formal teaching of speech.

Recently, other types of intensity vs. frequency charts have come into more common use. Such charts are presented in Figure 4-5. This Figure will be used to show Carleen's hearing impairment, and to demonstrate how the gain provided by the hearing aid she had received was modified to meet her needs.

aiding Carleen

Carleen is a four-year-old girl who had developed a high pitched, rather nasal voice. Her unaided audiogram is shown in Figure 4-5a. This chart is unlike the previous ones in three respects. First, it is presented the other way up — with loudness discomfort level at the top, and normal thresholds of detection at the bottom. Second, these thresholds (the average of normally hearing young adults) have been obtained in a sound field rather than through headphones. Third, responses are not charted in relation to audiometric zero, but in dB sound pressure level (SPL) relative to 20 microPascals (fPa), because this way of presenting audiometric data is consistent with the way that manufacturers present their specifications of hearing aid performance. Accordingly, such a chart can be used to incorporate, and directly compare, three types of data required for hearing aid selection; namely hearing test results showing the individual's dynamic range of residual audition, the amplified or

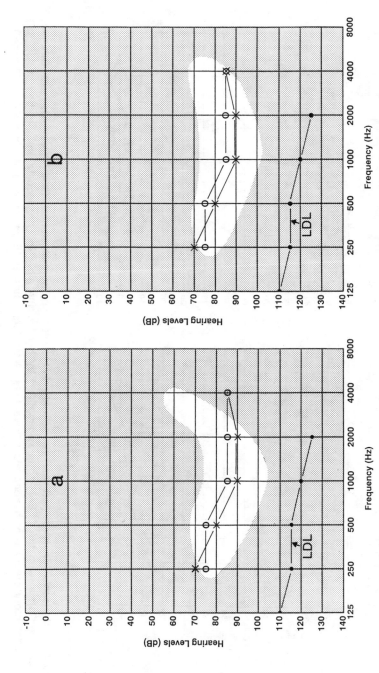

figure 4-4. Audiograms showing Barbara's hearing levels and the effects of amplification on the intensity levels of speech she received: a. Barbara's thresholds in relation to how speech components in the CLEAR zone were amplified by her hearing aids. b. The satisfactory outcome of appropriate earmold selection: all significant components of speech have been rendered detectable.

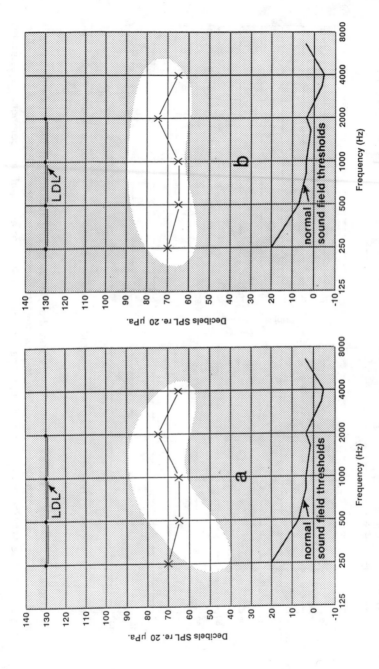

figure 4-5. Carleen's unaided (left ear) thresholds in relation to normal sound field thresholds (dB SPL re. 20 microPascals): a. with the CLEAR zone as amplified by her hearing aid. (Note inadequate amplification at 250 Hz.) b. The satisfactory outcome of hearing aid adjustments. (Note thresholds at all frequencies are in the CLEAR zone.)

unamplified dynamic range of speech, and the frequency vs. intensity characteristics of a hearing aid.

Carleen's hearing levels as represented on a conventional audiogram would appear as a straight line falling from 50 dB at 250 Hz to 70 dB at 4000 Hz. In Figure 4-5, however, her hearing levels appear as a crooked line because they are plotted above normal sound field thresholds. Normal sound field thresholds vary because, as stated in Chapter 2, the human ear is not equally sensitive to sounds at all frequencies.

The CLEAR zone representing the intensity of conversational level elements in the acoustic range of speech, as produced at a distance of two yards and then amplified by Carleen's hearing aids, is also shown in Figure 4-5a. Carleen's responses in relation to this CLEAR zone indicates that she can detect sounds in all frequency bands except those in the octave band centered on 250 Hz. She was able to respond to the oo vowel in the Five-Sound Test, but only at distances of less than a yard. On this account she was tested with the /m/ to determine whether the loss of this frequency range when at a distance from the talker was important to her. She failed to detect the sound at distances greater than two feet. The reduced frequency range was, therefore, considered to be a problem, because Carleen had developed speech that was both high-pitched and nasal. In order to provide her with stronger supraseg-mental and nasal cues, an internal (screw) adjustment was made to her hearing aids, and she was tested again. The results are shown in Figure 4-5b. A repeat of the Five-Sound Test confirmed that she was able, following the adjustment, to detect all three vowels and both consonants at a distance of over two yards. Following a few months of therapy in a parent-infant program that provided abundant informal learning oppor-tunities and some unisensory teaching, Carleen modified her speech in the desired manner and now, some years later, has normal speech and a very pleasant voice quality.

Audiograms charted in sound pressure levels (SPL) make it easy for audiologists to work with modern computerized equipment. True, referring a child's responses to SPL rather than audiometric zero may appear strange at first, but direct comparisons of different measures on the same graph reduces possible errors. For example, a child with average thresholds of 90 dB (HL) has average thresholds of about 96 dB(SPL). So, a hearing aid with an output of 120 dB(SPL) would not be providing the child with 120-90 = 30 dB gain, but 120- 96 = 24 dB gain. Using the 20 fPa baseline makes it easier for the audiologist to visualize just what hearing aids will do for an individual. If the audiologist is using a computerized probe-tube microphone system (see Figure 4-2) as part of the selection and fitting procedure, there is also an added advantage: the audiologist can test and adjust the performance of the hearing aid as it is being selected — a procedure adopted in aiding Dawn.

aiding Dawn

Dawn is a four-year old child with similar levels of hearing impairment in both ears. Her left ear thresholds (X—X) are depicted in dB SPL in Figure 4-6. (In order not to clutter the audiogram forms with unnecessary data, only her left ear thresholds will be used in presenting her case.) This Figure shows Dawn unable to hear any conversational level speech elements unless she is wearing hearing aids because her unaided thresholds across the whole speech frequency range all lie outside the CLEAR zone. Dawn has used a body-worn instrument since she was seven months old. She has acquired very natural language, and speaks in a pleasant voice — the outcomes of having been enrolled in an excellent auditory-oral parent-infant program. She is now to be fitted with behind-the-ear hearing aids. The purpose of presenting Dawn's case is not to show yet another case of inadequate hearing aid selection, but to explain how appropriate hearing aids can be selected through the use of *in the ear* measures using a computerized probe-tube system. Dawn has had new CFA#4 type earmolds made so that her new hearing aids can be selected with them in place.

First, the average intensity of the speech elements (the line in the CLEAR zone), and Dawn's thresholds (X—X), as shown in Figure 4-6a, are entered into the computer. *Second*, the probe-tube is carefully placed in her left ear canal with its tip close to the eardrum, and the earmold inserted. *Third*, one of the preselected hearing aids is placed over her left ear, connected to the earmold, and switched on. *Fourth*, a continuous 60 dB SPL tone that ranges from the lowest to the highest frequencies in the speech range is then fed into the hearing aid. Immediately, a line showing how much this tone has been amplified by the hearing aid shows up on the computer screen. As depicted in Figure 4-6a, the screen now shows three lines: the average level of speech in the CLEAR zone; Dawn's thresholds just as they are presented in Figure 4-6 (in dB SPL); and the output of the hearing aid (H—H) as measured in Dawn's ear canal. *Fifth*,

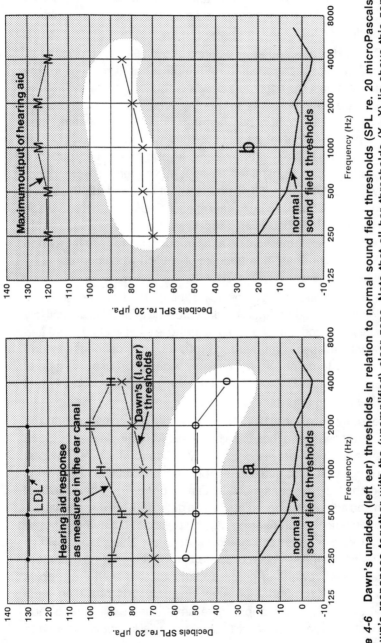

figure 4-6 Dawn's unaided (left ear) thresholds in relation to normal sound field thresholds (SPL re. 20 microPascals):
a. Dawn's responses together with the (unamplified) clear zone. Note that all her thresholds (X—X) lie above this zone and that she can, therefore, hear nothing of conversational level speech at a distance of two yards without her hearing aids. The response of the hearing aids selected for her (H—H) lies between her thresholds and her loudness discomfort level (LDL). b. The levels to which the CLEAR zone has been amplified by the hearing aid selected in relation to Dawn's thresholds, and the maximum output of the hearing aid (M—M).

the suitability of the particular hearing aid is considered. Comparison of Dawn's thresholds (X—X) and the hearing aid's output (H—H) shows that the gain provided by the hearing aid exceeds Dawn's thresholds at all frequencies.

Following the procedures as outlined above takes several minutes. The procedures are then repeated on the other ear. It remains for the audiologist to adjust the maximum power output of the hearing aids so that the sounds they reproduces do not exceed Dawn's loudness discomfort level (LDL). When her hearing aids were adjusted, their maximum power output at each frequency was below her LDL, as depicted (M—M) in Figure 4-6(b). The amount of in-the-ear gain provided by this hearing aid as transmitted through this earmold can be determined by subtracting input (60 dB) from output (as charted). By adding the amount of gain provided by the aid at each frequency to the average intensity of the CLEAR zone it can be seen, as also shown in Figure 4-6b, that there is sufficient amplification at all frequencies to permit Dawn to detect all of the significant components of speech when addressed by talkers at a distance within two yards.

Because traditional ways of doing things tend to persist, more conventional aided audiograms with data presented in dB HL are unlikely to be entirely replaced with charts, such as those used in Figures 4-5 and 4-6. However, because computerized probe tube microphone measurements are likely to come into increasingly widespread use, the type of audiograms shown in Figure 4-6 will probably be more commonly met in the future than at present.

The examples given in this section have all featured the speedy and satisfactory adjustment of hearing aids by relatively simple means. Such adjustments are not unrealistic for many children. Making the widest possible range of sounds detectable is but a basic requirement, however. For some children, this is as much as can be done. For others, optimal selection and adjustment based not just on detection, but discrimination, identification, and comprehension may be possible; but at the expense of much more extensive testing and observation. There are individual children for whom the selection of appropriate hearing aids is a far more arduous and less rewarding process than indicated by the examples used above. Only through a constant drive towards providing each individual child with more appropriate amplification will parents and professionals help children realize their full potential for spoken language development

the use of aided hearing

Making the most of a hearing-impaired child's residual hearing involves not merely obtaining the most appropriate hearing aids, but using them to the greatest advantage. Several things can combine to reduce the quality of a speech signal arriving at a child's ear. These include the hearing aids themselves, background (ambient) noise, reflected sound, and reverberation. Hearing aids are not high-fidelity instruments. They therefore cause some distortion of sound. Noise in the background can originate from a radio, television, heating or cooling systems, movements of objects or other people in the room, street noises coming in through the windows, and so on. Sound can be reflected from hard surfaces just as light is reflected from a mirror. When reflected sound becomes mixed with the original speech signal, the clarity of the speech that is ultimately heard will be reduced. The more hard surfaces there are in a room, the more likely it is that sounds will reflect from several of them almost simultaneously and thus make the problem worse. When sound bounces back and forth between and among several hard surfaces, reverberation is said to occur. Any or all of these sources of noise degrade the speech signal. Speech should be as much as 30 dB above competing noises if hearing-impaired children are to receive speech under the most advantageous conditions. This 30 dB signal-to-noise ratio is less important to normally hearing individuals. It is very common for hearing aid wearers to report that their greatest difficulties in hearing are due to noisy backgrounds. When adults who know their language and all of the conventions underlying discourse report this, imagine what a serious problem it poses for children who have yet to learn their speech communication skills.

It is possible to overcome the effects of noise on speech in several ways. First, one must make sure that the hearing aids themselves are not producing it. Caregivers (parents, teachers or clinicians) can check this by listening to the hearing aids through an earmold of their own or through a specially designed stethoscope. Such a check should be made frequently. Second, one must ensure that there is as little background noise as possible in the rooms where most spoken language communication takes place. Radios and televisions should not compete with the spoken language being addressed to the child. It may not be possible to exclude all noises, but drapes, carpets, cushions, and soft furnishings will help absorb unwanted sound as well as prevent its reflection and reverberation. A thick cloth on a table, for example, will be advantageous in reducing the noise that is created as children play with bricks or other hard toys. Third, and perhaps the most important, caregivers should be close to the child when they speak. This will ensure that whatever is said will be louder to the child than any noises in the background except those that are very loud. Such an advantageous signal-to-noise ratio can be obtained through this simple procedure because the level of speech can increase by as much as 6 dB with every halving of distance between talker and listener. The importance of providing the child with clearly spoken language that is well above the levels of background noise cannot be over-emphasized.

auditory training or auditory learning?

Many auditory training procedures still in use in some special schools for the hearing-impaired were originated before the Second World War. They were mainly designed for teaching scheduled lessons to groups of children through the use of hard-wired amplification systems — hearing aids that were neither wearable nor portable. In contrast, procedures to promote auditory learning are more recent and have been developed through experience with personal hearing aids as they were gradually miniaturized — made small enough to be worn habitually all day and every day. Some of the concepts that have been applied in auditory training over the years will be briefly described below, and then compared with modern day concepts that underlie auditory learning. Rather than having to acquire auditory skills through specific training procedures at carefully scheduled lesson times, children can now unconsciously learn at least a significant proportion of such skills by dint of being exposed all day and every day to sounds in the environment.

Traditional auditory training programs began with discrimination between non-verbal sounds, such as bells, drums, and whistles, and then moved on to discrimination between speech sounds and words. They were based on the notion that one should proceed from gross to fine differences. Since auditory responses cannot be directly observed, speech or motor responses were demanded as immediate evidence of hearing. Such training, therefore, tended to exclude the more complex types of verbal communication that the children would need outside the training sessions. Most training of this sort was also undertaken with classes of children who had widely differing abilities rather than with individuals.

There is no evidence to support the notion that children learn spoken language skills any better for having first been exposed to non-verbal sounds. Nor is there any evidence that children should acquire auditory skills through discrimination and identification training on a limited range of stimuli graded according to their apparent difficulty on a gross-to-fine continuum beginning with non-verbal sounds. Non-verbal sounds are of much longer duration than speech sounds, and do not usually relate closely to any of the dimensions that are important in speech. By the time a bell has been struck and allowed to ring long enough to be recognized as a bell, for example, one could say a whole sentence, such as *My mummy has a bell on her bike*.

Certainly, there is a place in a child's auditory repertoire for non-verbal sounds. Encouraging a child to listen for — and recognize — meaningful environmental sounds can be an interesting and stimulating activity. It can also encourage children to attend more closely to all aspects of their acoustic environments. Music can also attract children's attention, and be used in dancing and games. Many hearing-impaired children enjoy learning musical instruments. Music consists mostly of notes that fall well below 1000 Hz, and, remember, middle C on the piano (just over 260 Hz) is near the low-frequency end of the audiometric scale. Music is, therefore, mainly within the residual hearing range of the majority of hearing-impaired children who, in spite of traditional neglect of voice production, can learn to sing. Tape recorded stories with script, music, environmental sound effects, and different talkers (including the children themselves) are much more fun than a story consisting only of speech produced by one talker.

Most hearing-impaired children who are optimally aided will experience environmental sounds in the context of their everyday lives. For such children they will, through the context in which they are heard, become a meaningful part of their auditory development. For the few children who have so little hearing that they are unaware of many everyday environmental sounds, there is much to recommend including such sounds in a formal auditory training program. Survival may depend on a child recognizing a car horn and the siren of a police car or ambulance. However, carry-over to real life situations must be an objective of such a program. While such carry-over is possible, the generalization of auditory recognition of sounds to the auditory reception of speech is unlikely. Formal auditory training that has focused on the development of discrimination and identification of environmental sounds has not been shown to yield gains in children's ability to comprehend or use spoken language, yet such gains are the only logical goal for devoting significant amounts of time to this sort of training.

Children are most likely to learn spoken language skills through direct exposure to a great deal of spoken language in situations that allow the child to deduce the meaning of what is said. The concept underlying auditory learning as compared with auditory training is that the acoustic information presented to the child must be optimally audible (detectable), and aimed at developing comprehension. Teaching auditory discrimination and auditory identification skills can be part of an auditory learning program, but attention should be given to these skills only when the child's responses indicate that such attention is necessary — for example, teaching a child to discriminate between nasal and non-nasal sounds or to identify an /m/ sound as such would be undertaken only when it became evident that the child was unable to do this in the course of everyday communication.

Most modern educational programs now focus on auditory learning through real-life experience more extensively than on formal auditory training. This is a healthy development because formal auditory training can only be successful if it relates closely to children's speech, spoken language development, cognitive levels, and everyday life experiences. It is inappropriate, for example, to spend time teaching a child to make auditory figure-ground (speech in relation to noise) discriminations in class, if that child can, through wearing optimal amplification at home as well as in school, learn to make such discriminations spontaneously. This is not to say that discrimination training should be completely rejected; simply that it should not be a primary focus of any program. It should be provided as and when children demonstrate the need for it through their failure to make appropriate auditory discriminations in the development of their everyday listening skills. Formal training in auditory figure-ground discriminations is justified for children who have not learned them spontaneously. As a further example, consider a child who has not spontaneously learned to attend to acoustic feedback on a speech production task, such as judging whether he is producing an /b/ or an /m/. The child can be taught to make this auditory discrimination in a formal manner. However, the outcome of the work cannot be considered as successful until the child comes to use the skill thus acquired in the course of speech communication outside class. Further discussion of formal teaching and informal learning of spoken language will be found in Chapter 7.

In this section, auditory skills have been considered as leading to comprehension when they relate to the interpretation of auditory experiences in the context of meaningful, real-life situations; when the focus of the training is not on teaching the children to hear, but rather on giving them reason to learn to listen. Listening has been presented as occurring only when children seek to extract meaning from the acoustic events that surround them all day and every day. This is true whether the meaning is derived from auditory information alone, or auditory information supplemented by other cues. It is through comprehension, not discrimination or identification exercises, that we integrate new, incoming information with the material previously stored in memory and direct our attention (our search) for further information and deeper meaning. In short, skills in comprehension and speech reception work to enhance each other (are mutually reinforcing). This fact applies whether the child is using acoustic hearing aids, more than one sort of sensory information, or a different sort of sensory aid.

This chapter has been concerned exclusively with the use of hearing. There are many hearing-impaired children who, in the hands of informed caregivers, and with the consistent use of appropriate personal hearing aids from early infancy, require nothing more in the way of special help to acquire excellent spoken language than the opportunity to hear plenty of it under acoustic conditions that optimize its quality, and in social settings that clearly provide it with meaning. In general, children with no additional handicaps and hearing levels of less than 60 to 70 dB can be expected to develop natural language under such conditions. Such children may, however, generally require FM units and support services during their school years to maintain their language growth and ensure their academic development in face of the difficulties caused by hearing impairment in regular school settings. Children with hearing levels that average more than about 70 dB usually need other forms of help in addition to hearing aids and informed caregivers if they are to acquire spoken language effectively and efficiently. Among these other forms of help are more structured teaching. Some children with hearing impairment greater than about 95 dB may need more than one sort of sensory input and, where appropriate, the use of a new type of electronic device. Information on the different types of electronic devices that can be used to provide supplementary or alternative cues for improving the reception of spoken language will be presented in the next chapter.

suggestions for further reading

Boothroyd (1982) provides a good introduction to aided hearing as well as to the auditory management of hearing impairments in young children. Vaughan (1976) is an excellent book about the contributions that *learning to listen* can make to children's spoken language development. Written by parents for parents, this is a gem that should be read by all concerned with aided hearing. More conventional and comprehensive texts on auditory management of hearing-impaired children are those edited by Beasley (1984), Jerger (1984), and Ross and Giolas (1978). A comprehensive treatment on facilitating classroom listening among hearing-impaired children has been provided by Berg (1987). The many ways in which telephones can be used by hearing-impaired individuals have been described by Erber (1985), and the use of various types of general and special purpose hearing aids has been discussed by Ling and Ling (1978). General information on aided hearing can be found in Pollack (1988), which contains an excellent chapter on amplification for young hearing impaired children by Seewald and Ross. Many issues relating to amplification are also treated in Bess and Mc-Connell (1981). Further recommended texts on audiology are Bess (1988), and the third edition of *Hearing in Children* by Northern and Downs (1984). Specific discussion of earmold design in relation to the acoustic effects on the transmission of sounds has been provided by Killion (1981) and Lybarger (1985). A monograph edited by Cole and Gregory (1986) entitled *Auditory Learning* also provides coverage of hearing aids and their selection as well as discussions of various procedures that have been found to optimize auditory learning. See References pp. 433 ff.

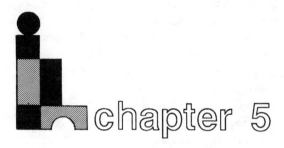

chapter 5

speech reception (3): supplementary and alternative channels.

supplementary information on speech

There are three senses through which we can gather information about the acoustic events that surround us: hearing, vision, and touch. When aided hearing provides inadequate sensory information for the comprehension of spoken language, vision and touch can be used as supplementary or alternative channels. This chapter provides a discussion of the ways in which vision and touch can be used to enhance speech reception and speech production. Speechreading, and the various devices that have been produced to augment its use with hearing-impaired children are examined, and intervention and evaluation strategies that one might adopt to ensure optimal selection and use of such devices are suggested. This chapter is the last of three concerned with speech reception. Subsequent chapters will be concerned with spoken language and speech production.

The visual cues provided by speechreading (see below) are a natural, and usually effective, supplement to hearing. This is mainly because the cues that speechreading provides, such as those on place of consonant production (see Figure 2-6), can usefully augment a message that is heard only in part. Speechreading cues are fragmentary. By themselves they convey incomplete information on speech. When vision is used as the primary modality, therefore, it has to be supplemented by cues provided through another sensory pathway, or by verbal or nonverbal context cues of some sort. Individuals who are familiar with the language and the topic under discussion, are at a great advantage as speechreaders because they can use their knowledge of the world to predict the course of a conversation.

Tactile cues relating to speech are of three types: those that talkers produce in the vocal tract as they articulate; those that can be obtained using the fingers to feel the effects of producing sounds; and those that can be provided through some sort of electronic device. All three types of cues can be used to assist in teaching severely and profoundly hearing-impaired children to produce sounds that they cannot detect through hearing. Most older children or adults who suffer a severe loss of hearing can continue to talk normally, partly because they are able to use the tactile and kinesthetic cues of the sort generated within the vocal tract during speech. Some deaf-blind people can understand the speech of others through placing their fingers on the faces of talkers. There are two types of electronic devices that can be used to assist speech reception through touch; one vibro-tactile, and the other electro-tactile (see below). Both allow touch, normally a close sense, to be used as a distance sense. So far, neither type of device has proved to be more than an aid to speechreading. The sense of touch, except as a source of supplementary cues for speechreaders, appears to have marked limitations as a pathway for the perception of spoken language.

Only in recent years have electronic devices for utilizing each of the senses been produced. Those discussed in this chapter include cochlear implants, visual aids and tactile devices. Cochlear implants have been generally available since the early 1980s. Visual aids and tactile devices have been used in schools or clinics for the purpose of providing special training relating to spoken language for many years. Tactile devices that are small enough to be worn, however, have only recently become available.

Several things make it difficult to compensate for hearing impairment through any device or procedure. These difficulties relate to the very complex nature of the speech signal, the widely different types and degrees of hearing impairment, and the fact that the alternative sensory systems available to human beings (the eyes and skin) are not as amenable to receiving speech signals as the normal ear. Most devices for helping those who cannot benefit sufficiently from hearing aids have, therefore, been designed to function as aids to speechreading. Research is required to determine how to make optimal use of the procedures and devices that are currently available, particularly with hearing-impaired children. While some devices and procedures, like hearing aids and speechreading, are compatible and mutually reinforcing, others are not, or may not, be so.

seeing speech

Speakers move their tongues, lips, and jaws when they talk. The art of understanding speakers by means of watching these movements, as well as their facial expressions, and even body postures, is known as speechreading. It was in recognition of the fact that much more than the lips are observed in everyday communication that the term "speechreading" became generally preferred to "lipreading." The visible components of speech can, however, specify but a small part of a spoken message. Some sounds are made without any visible cues, while other groups of sounds have the same visual patterns and are therefore frequently confused with one another.

The nature of information provided by the visible aspects of speech has been well defined, but some of the characteristics that differentiate good and poor speechreaders have yet to be discovered. Those who speechread well usually have a good knowledge of spoken language, make use of both verbal and non-verbal contexts to provide cues on the intent of the message, and are able to synthesize the partial patterns perceived into a meaningful whole. Others, who are equally intelligent, have similar visual acuity, and are just as well grounded in their native language, find speechreading skills notoriously difficult, if not impossible, to master. Most children are able to acquire effective spoken language skills through speechreading, if need be, providing that the limited amount of information that it can transmit is sufficiently supplemented by sensory aids, linguistic cues, knowledge of the topic, pertinent situations, and the prevailing social or educational context.

the information content in visual speech reception

The fragmentary nature of the information provided by speechreading has been mentioned above. Most readers, by introspection and experimentation (for example looking in a mirror), will be able to confirm the validity of the following notes on the visible features of speech.

Vocalization:
Neither speech-breathing patterns nor vocalization are visible.

Suprasegmental patterns:
Intensity, duration, and frequency of voice are not visible.

Vowels and diphthongs:
Lip shapes and jaw heights are visible, while tongue positions usually are not. Adjacent vowels are easily confused.

Consonants by manner:
Very few cues on manner are visible, hence sounds produced in the same place are often confused.

Consonants by place:
Bilabial, labio-dental, alveolar, and velar consonants are visually discriminable.

Consonants by voicing:
Cues on voiced-voiceless distinction are invisible, thus all cognate pairs (two sounds distinguished only by the presence or absence of voice) are frequently confused.

Word-initial and word-final blends:
Initial blends with elements having different places of production are the most easily differentiated, but none can be identified with certainty. Most word-final blends move to end in /t/, /d/, /s/, or /z/, the past tense, or the plural. The movement to one or the other is usually visible, but the sounds themselves, all alveolar consonants, are not discriminable.

speechreading and the acquisition of spoken language

Speechreading provides very little information on prosody (the tunes and rhythms of speech). Thus it does not help a child learn how to use breath effectively in relation to the demands of an utterance, nor does it help a child to master the skills involved in controlling the intensity, duration, and vocal frequency of sounds. A child must, therefore, be enabled to acquire and use these components of spoken language in some other way. They cannot be neglected because prosody (the suprasegmental aspects of speech) carries information on the type of sentence structure that is being used, highlights the new versus the old (previously given) information in an utterance, and leads the listener to focus on the crucial elements in sentences that are provided by linguistic stress. Further, it is voice quality that provides information about the mood, as well as the personal and social characteristics of the speaker. Speechreaders need this sort of information, and it can only be provided through hearing aids, cochlear implants, or tactile devices - instruments that use other sense modalities (also see Chapter 9).

Another major drawback associated with speechreading in early infancy is that contact with children who rely on vision can be completely lost when they are out of sight. Those with sufficient hearing can, in contrast, be kept in contact through voice over considerable distances. Hearing aids (and other sensory aids to be discussed below) are a great help in maintaining contact between caregivers and children.

Yet another drawback is that, through speechreading, infants cannot be provided with a commentary on objects, events and activities when they are directing their attention towards them. They must look to their caregivers for comments and discussion before or after rather than *during* events and activities. Talking to children about objects, events, and activities while they command their attention makes it easier for the children to perceive relationships between what they are doing (or what is being done) and what is being said. It therefore promotes much clearer comprehension of caregiver's utterances than talking about something that is to become, or already has become, part of children's past (even recent past) experience. Certainly, instant snapshots of an activity can help recapture some objects and events but, even then, the immediacy of the spoken word is lost, and delayed commentary can be awkward as well as confusing for children (see Chapter 7 for further discussion of this point).

Speechreading vowels poses many problems for severely and profoundly hearing-impaired children who are learning to talk. Pairs of words, such as *sheep* and *ship*, and *bad* and *bed* look alike. Indeed, all adjacent vowels tend to be visually confused. Children who acquire speech mainly through vision also tend to imitate only the lip and jaw movements associated with vowels because the tongue's normal movements towards particular vowels and the tongue's configurations during vowel production are hidden by the lips and the teeth. Those who base their vowel production on such inadequate information inevitably neutralize high front and high back vowels. By moving their tongues only slightly, if at all, from a central position they restrict the frequency range of their vowel formants and, as a result, the production of the formant transitions that are so important in the auditory identification of the consonants (see Chapter 2). The effects of such inappropriate tongue involvement have profoundly negative effects on speech intelligibility.

Consonants differing in manner, but produced in the same place in the vocal tract, are not readily differentiated through speechreading. Examples of those that appear alike are the stops and nasals, such as /b/ and /m/; the fricative sh and affricate ch; the fricative /s/ and the stop /t/; and the semi-vowel /w/ and the liquid /r/ in the context of back vowels. The /h/ is completely invisible because it assumes the exact shape of the vowels that follow it. In contrast, consonants that have the same manner of production, but differ in place of production are quite readily differentiated. For example, /b/, /d/, and /g/ do not look alike. However, these can all be confused with their voiceless cognates, namely the plosives /p/, /t/, and /k/. The visibility of word-initial and word-final blends can be deduced by the reader from knowledge of the relative visibility of the consonants from which they are constructed. For children who are in the process of learning spoken language, visual confusions among the consonants cause problems of speech sound perception and production, vocabulary acquisition, and all other aspects of language.

When the various speech sounds are produced in syllables, experienced speechreaders using vision alone can, on average, identify about 30 to 40 percent of them. This level of performance indicates the extent of the difficulties hearing-impaired children would have in the acquisition of spoken language if nothing more than speechreading were available to them. While those who already have language, well developed social skills, and awareness of contextual cues of all sorts may be able to make sense of what is said when about 60 to 70 percent of the utterance is missing, children without such advantages cannot derive clarity of comprehension from such an impoverished signal.

testing speechreading skills

Several tests of speechreading skills have been developed and numerous studies attempting to define the factors that lead to superior speechreading performance have been undertaken. As in many audiological test batteries, the basic language units in most tests of speechreading are syllables, words, and sentences and, in recent years, narrative aspects of discourse that are presented through tracking procedures. (These procedures involve a person reading a sequence of small chunks from a book or other text to the hearing-impaired person and finding out how long it takes for that person to be able to repeat back the chunks correctly.) It is always difficult to ensure the validity of many of these tests because, if they are administered live, there is room for non-standard procedures; and if they are filmed or videotaped, then they are presented "pan faced" with none of the facial and body posture cues that occur in real-life communicative situations (and so become lipreading rather than speechreading tests), and are two-rather than three-dimensional. Although recorded tests may take a child's language levels into account, they are often unrelated to the interests and communicative contexts of an individual child's life - factors that are known to influence speechreading performance strongly.

The search for the factors that underlie speechreading skill has not been exhaustive. For example, speechreading has been measured in relation to static measures of visual acuity. Yet speechreading requires, not observation of static speech postures, but dynamic tracking of complex movements. No attempt has yet been made to examine speechreading skills in relation to some of the dynamic tests of visual function that have been developed and are used to measure visual perception in relation to performance with balls in sports. Speechreading currently occupies a fairly large and diverse number of research workers, many of whom have developed an interest in the topic due to the continued creation of devices designed to support it. Advances that may pave the way to improved testing and training strategies are being made possible through the development of materials that are recorded on video disks and presented interactively under computer control.

developing speechreading skills

For those who have insufficient hearing to permit effective auditory speech reception, speechreading becomes an important supplementary or alternative communication channel. Those who need it must, therefore, be enabled to make the most of it. Many different training programs have been proposed for developing speechreading skills. Those for adults range from the essentially analytic, in which participants are taught to recognize the various positions the speech organs assume when making a sound - a procedure that focuses on postures rather than movements, to those that focus on the synthesis and presentation of spoken language forms that one would meet in a variety of personal and social contexts. There are adherents to both forms of training and, of course, to those that include something of each. The writer, who has experimented with all types of programs with numerous adults and children, has come strongly to favor emphasis on strategies that incorporate the dynamics of the speech stream, and emphasize communicative interchange in situations that as nearly as possible replicate real-life experiences.

Strategies that focus on learning rather than on teaching are much the most suitable for children, because development in the visual aspects of communication is greatly enhanced if children find speechreading meaningful and relevant to their personal interests, activities, and goals. Traditionally, however, there has been much more concentration on strategies that emphasize analysis rather than synthesis of the information provided by speechreading. Analytic programs are typically those in which mirrors are used in the course of teaching to provide models and feedback about lip positions and lip movements in relation to specific speech patterns. The actual value of using mirrors in training speechreading is suspect because they are not normally required to elicit approximations to either static or dynamically changing lip configurations, even in young children. Moreover, because many aspects of speech are not visible, practice with mirrors tends to lend speechreading an emphasis that can detract from the use of residual audition, whether it is used as a leading sense or as a supplement. The question "Mirror, mirror on the wall, can you help us much at all?" has been experimentally studied and the answer, in a word, appears to be "No."

It is certainly possible to train individuals to improve on specific visual discrimination tasks through analytic training, but however extensive it may be, analytic training is difficult for children to generalize (carry-over) into everyday situations. Some professionals commonly use a strategy that is designed to lead to carry-over of visual, or any other sort of sensory training ; namely, the rehearsal of discriminations first within a closed set (a task with but a few items for paired comparisons), such as the animals *cat*, *dog*, and *pig*, then rehearsal of identifications within increasingly open sets (tasks involving more and more items), such as all domestic animals and, finally, open sets that could include all forms of life.

Many professionals working with young and very young hearing-impaired children do not set out to teach them to speechread. Rather, they concentrate on establishing communication in relation to events that interest the children, and encourage their participation in situations designed to promote language learning. This way, the children, in deriving meaning from the interaction, acquire whatever speechreading skills they need as they acquire language.

Teaching strategies for speechreading, as for anything else should be adopted to optimize children's progress in accordance with their needs at any given time. No one method, collection of methods, or view on a procedure can possibly be valid for all children at all times. Children's language and their means of perceiving it are closely linked (see Chapter 7 for further discussion on this).

In spite of its problems, speechreading is, and always will be, an important aspect of speech reception for most hearing-impaired individuals. Not all children can acquire speech primarily through audition, and even those who can will sometimes find themselves having to function under conditions that are not conducive to listening. Recognition of the weaknesses of speechreading should not, therefore, lead teachers or other caregivers to reject it, but rather encourage them to seek its development in the most effective ways open to them. Children for whom speechreading is the primary avenue of speech reception should be helped to learn the skills involved through its association with every aspect of their lives at home and in school. Exaggeration of mouth movements should be avoided, particularly for such children. While exaggeration may help a child speechread a particular person, it often leads to an over reliance on that person as an interpreter. Most people whom children will meet in everyday life will not speak with ultra-visible lip and jaw movements and accompany what they say with expressions that can be seen only on extremely mobile faces.

speechreading as a supplement

Most of the information in speechreading is based on place identification (where the sound is produced in the vocal tract). This is not surprising, because perceiving spatial relationships is what the eye does best. This is important, for it is the various spatial relations that are created as the vocal tract moves to create the sounds that give rise to the frequency (spectral) content of speech. With the possible exception of multi-channel cochlear implants and multi-channel tactile devices, no device or procedure provides information related so clearly (albeit indirectly) to the spectral qualities of the vowels and consonants as well as speechreading does. This is speechreading's great strength as a supplement to low-frequency residual hearing, for even greatly impoverished audition, as well as most single-channel devices, can provide reasonably good time and intensity information (see below).

Speechreading is a useful supplement to residual hearing. The ways in which it can supplement residual hearing, and thus provide a reasonably complete pattern for speech reception, are shown in Table 5-1. In this table, the presence of cues in the auditory and visual modalities are indicated in relation to each of seven aspects of speech: Vocalization (breath and voice); intensity, duration and vocal frequency (IDF - the three components of suprasegmental patterns); vowels and diphthongs (V + D); consonants by manner of production (CxM); consonants by manner and place of production (CxP); consonants by manner, place and voicing (CxV); and initial and final clusters of consonants (Blends). When sufficient information can be received through the particular modality by most individuals, the appropriate cell is completed with the letter Y, when such information cannot be received the cell is completed with the letter N. When only partial information is likely to be received, a small letter "p" is placed next to the letter "Y" in the cell, thus Y_p. Through reference to Table 5-1 it is possible to ascertain whether particular speech patterns can best be developed through residual audition, vision, or a combination of the two. The usefulness of Table 5-1 can be extended by adding further rows to indicate the amount of information that a given child might be expected to receive from his or her cochlear implant or tactile device.

The fullest possible development of young children's skills in using residual audition, cochlear implants, or tactile devices may not be achieved if one or other of them and speechreading are consistently used together. This is pointed out because, while speechreading plus audition generally yields better performance than either alone, there is some evidence that higher levels of combined modality performance can be obtained if one modality alone is made part of each hearing-impaired child's daily experience. Indeed, giving part of each lesson over to developing auditory skills through the deliberate suppression of speechreading skills is a basic procedure among those who espouse an auditory-verbal philosophy. Those who follow this procedure may recognize speechreading to be an essential supplement for most hearing-impaired children under many real-life conditions, but consider that the maximum use of residual hearing and maximum auditory-visual performance can result only when such focus is given to audition alone.

	Voice	IDF	V+D	CxM	CxP	CxV	Blends
RESIDUAL AUDITION (<1000 Hz.)	Y	YYYp	Y	Yp	N	Y	Yp
NORMAL VISION	N	NNN	Yp	N	Y	N	Yp
RESIDUAL AUDITION AND VISION	Y	YYYp	Y	Yp	Y	Y	Yp

table 5-1 **The components of speech that can be detected wholly (Y), in part (Yp), or not at all (N) through useful residual audition that extends up to but not beyond 1000 Hz, normal vision, and the two together. Note that residual audition and vision together yield most of the available information on speech.**

supplements to speechreading

Linguistic competence, social experience, situational context (such as knowing what is being talked about and being conversant with the topic under discussion), verbal cues, non-verbal cues (such as facial expression and body posture), and sensory cues of one sort or another have all been mentioned above as providing significant supplements to speechreading. The most efficient speechreaders are those who can supplement the visual information available with additional input through another sense modality.

When speechreading is supplemented by information presented to either the ear or skin, scores on performance tasks through the joint use of the two modalities are usually considerably better than the sum of scores achieved on the same task through the two modalities separately. Thus, for example, it is not uncommon for children who score about 35 percent on a test of word recognition through speechreading and 15 percent on the same task through audition to obtain a score of over 75 percent when verbal materials are presented through speechreading and audition together. Such improvement in bimodal over unimodal performance tends to occur regardless of which of the three sense modalities are tested separately and then combined.

The greatest gains in performance are achieved when the information provided through another sense modality is not simply redundant, but complementary, to the visible aspects of speech. Good examples of complementary cues are those received through other senses that signal the presence of speech components that cannot be speechread, such as prosody, the nasal murmur, manner distinctions, and so on. This is not to say that all signals provided through another sense modality should be complementary. Redundancy provided through cues that have features in common with those available through speechreading can also assist individuals by bolstering their confidence about the nature of the visual signal. Certainly, speechreading cues are sufficiently meager to need as much augmentation as can be provided. It is not, therefore, surprising that the advantages of cochlear implants and tactile aids are shown most clearly when they are used to complement speechreading. Indeed, one thrust of modern research on speechreading is to determine more precisely the types of sensory information that most effectively augment speechreading performance.

With the creation of new devices, some deliberately designed as speechreading aids, it is important to pursue further research on the extent to which separate and intensive training of vision and another modality served by a device, such as a cochlear implant or a tactile aid, can substantially change levels of bimodal performance.

So far, we have discussed possibilities and limitations associated with speechreading as an alternative to hearing, as a supplement to hearing and as a procedure that can itself be supplemented through the provision of cues in other sense modalities. It should be clear that, with children who have but moderate-to-severe hearing impairments, speechreading usually serves as a supplement to hearing. With children who are totally or near-totally deaf, the reverse is true: speechreading becomes their primary means of receiving spoken language. Those who are fortunate enough to have even a minimal amount of residual hearing can use it to supplement the visual information on which they mainly depend. It is individuals with even worse hearing - those who obtain vibro-tactile sensations in the ear when they use a hearing aid - that are prime candidates for cochlear implants or tactile devices, for such instruments can usually supplement speechreading more effectively than vibratory sensations in the ear canal. An alternative to electronic devices does, however, exist for this small minority of children. It is a visual supplement to speechreading called Cued Speech.

Cued Speech

Cued Speech was invented by Cornett (1967) to eliminate the ambiguity in speechreading by providing a variety of hand cues simultaneously with the spoken message. Just as letters and numbers can be used together to create a grid that specifies the exact location of a place on a map, the speechread pattern and the hand cues together can specify exactly which vowels and consonants are being produced by a talker. Hand cues are not associated with speech features like nasality, frication, or voicing. They are selected simply on visual criteria. Shapes that look alike on the lips are associated with different hand cues and hand cues that are alike are associated with lip shapes that look different. The hand cues are not signs. They have no intrinsic meaning and exist only to resolve the confusions that exist among the speech segments as they appear to a speechreader.

In Cued Speech, four hand positions differentiate the adjacent vowels that can be confused and eight hand configurations help to specify the consonants that look alike on the lips. The diphthongs are cued by moving the hand from one vowel position to another. The way that speech sounds are coarticulated (see Chapter 2) is reflected in the cueing of consonants as the hands move to or from the various vowel positions, a feature that allows a well practised person to cue and speak at a normal rate. The cues are simple to learn and an average person can become completely familiar with them (but not fluent in their use) in less than ten hours.

It has been demonstrated that Cued Speech can permit the reception of speech by totally or near-totally deaf school-aged children at extremely high (90 percent) levels of accuracy. So far, no comparable results with pre-lingually hearing-impaired children through the use of technological aids have yet been reported. A note of caution is in order here, however, for readers should not interpret such statements as unreserved endorsement of the system. There are several aspects of spoken language acquisition that Cued Speech may not support (see below) and it is suspected that Cued Speech and various technological aids may not interact beneficially. The type of information the two provide are not necessarily compatible.

The effects of Cued Speech on the communication development of children who have useful residual hearing are not yet known. There would appear to be no good reason for Cued Speech to be used with any child who has useful residual audition because (as shown in Table 5-1, p. 127) the cues obtained from well-used residual hearing can clarify the speechread signal and provide a great deal of information that Cued Speech cannot. Further, many professionals have reported that the system tends to encourage children to become so visual that they do not attend adequately to aspects of speech, such as prosody, that are best perceived through the use of residual hearing. Indeed, many professionals consider it an abuse of the system to employ Cued Speech with children who have useful residual hearing. These sorts of concerns are shared by those who are fitting cochlear implants and tactile aids to totally and near-totally deaf children. Such reservations can be supported or rejected only through further research. Further study is also required to define the age at which Cued Speech is best begun, and what level of intelligence children need for Cued Speech to be acquired successfully.

An undesirable feature of Cued Speech, or any system other than natural speech communication, is that it requires the talker to learn it specifically for interacting with hearing-impaired individuals. Unlike hearing aids or other sensory aids, which require only that the talker speaks clearly and, so far as possible, above the ambient noise level, Cued Speech has to be learned as a new skill by both caregivers and children, and practiced until very high levels of performance at normal speaking rates, and with normal speaking rhythms, are attained. If such levels of performance are not attained, dysfluencies will occur and impede communication, and possibly comprehension.

A desirable feature of any system designed to help hearing-impaired children acquire spoken language is that it should be helpful in both speech reception and speech production. Significant gains in the intelligibility of speech produced by children using Cued Speech were once predicted because all speech sounds can be so easily specified from the hand-lip associations. However, the expected superiority in the rate and standards of speech acquisition among children using Cued Speech has not been demonstrated. Indeed, many children using Cued Speech do not learn to speak intelligibly. This may be due to the way the system has been used or it may be due to problems within the system itself. For example, many children with whom it is used have been allowed, if not encouraged, to cue when they talk. Because the cues and lip shapes together so clearly define the vowels and the consonants, such children can be completely understood on the basis of the visual patterns they provide to their caregivers and peers even if they do no more than grunt as they communicate. With such communicative success they have little or no incentive to develop their speech skills further, because they are intelligible to those who know the system. Alternatively, it may simply have been used up to the present mostly by professionals and parents who have been so charmed by the system's capacity to develop English language that they have not attended to speech production.

The future for Cued Speech as an assistive procedure for totally and near-totally deaf children is not secure. It will depend on whether its unknown aspects will receive the study they deserve, whether its drawbacks can be resolved and whether its advantages will be more widely accepted. It faces intense competition from several quarters: from those who are developing technological aids to supplement speechreading, for their work provides children with pre-packaged sensory cue systems that do not have to be learned by caregivers, professionals or anyone else; from those who advocate sign language communication for such children even though sign is socially and linguistically more restricting; and from oral teachers who do not consider Cued Speech an oral system.

Many opponents to Cued Speech appear to hold the erroneous view that children brought up on it come to depend on it permanently. In fact, this is not so. The language such children can acquire through its early use and the social skills that can develop as a result of Cued Speech communication, can provide them with the means to supplement and interpret speechreading without the continued help of Cued Speech. (It will be interesting to see whether sensory aids will be discarded after initial use for similar reasons.) Further research on the system is required (a statement that holds true for all currently used systems), but it is prejudice rather than sound theoretical reasoning that discourages its more widespread use. Cued Speech clearly has much to offer, at least to those children and adults who are totally or near-totally deaf and cannot, or will not, for some reason, be fitted with a cochlear implant or wear a tactile device as an aid to speechreading.

visual aids

Many visual aids have been produced over the past half-century, but few have been designed to supplement everyday communication through speechreading. The few include eyeglasses that signal the presence of speech features such as voicing, frication, and nasality with tiny lights. These lights are situated around the edge of the lens so that they can be detected by peripheral vision. Such devices have not, on evaluation, proven to be generally beneficial. Most visual aids have been designed, not as communication aids, but as training devices for use with children, to provide them with feedback during speech lessons.

Devices for speech training that provide a visual indication of a single aspect of speech are not difficult to engineer. Most have featured the real-time (immediate) representation of voice patterns (duration, intensity and fundamental frequency), vowels, single consonants, or single words on a screen. Various visual indicators of voice pitch have enjoyed brief spells of popularity from time to time over the past forty years or so and each has been discarded relatively quickly as teachers and clinicians find that their immediate appeal does not translate into long-term gains in children's speech communication skills. In recent years, real-time speech spectrographic displays have been developed and applied in the teaching of speech to hearing impaired children. Evaluation showed them to be of some help to experts in supervising children's speech development, but did not offer a viable alternative to speech teaching undertaken by competent professionals.

The most serious problem with visual aids relates to the inherent complexity and integrity of the speech signal. The more complete the speech pattern displayed, the more difficult it is for children to use it to advantage; and the simpler the pattern displayed, the less adequately it represents speech. Speech is a very complex code and to break it down into components that can be displayed and interpreted can too easily result in teaching one skill to the detriment of others. For example, one can, by focusing on formant transitions on a spectrogram, clearly show how diphthongs should be produced but, by concentrating solely on this aspect, teach the child to ignore breathing and voice quality while doing so.

In speech training, as in all other aspects of learning, carry-over to real-life situations is most readily achieved when the components of the training situation are most like those that are to be met in everyday experience. Visual devices concentrate attention on aspects of speech that have little relevance in everyday communication and may, therefore, do little if anything to promote, and much to discourage, carry-over. Numerous children who, taught formally to say something correctly with the help of visual aids during a lesson, will leave the teacher or clinician pronouncing that same speech pattern in the way that it was pronounced before the lesson - for example, "teva" instead of "seven," or "ba-ba" instead of "bye-bye." To some extent this is because teachers do not develop adequate procedures for carry-over. But visual speech training aids are also unlikely to play an important role in the development of speech communication for another reason; namely, that hearing aids, tactile devices and cochlear implants can function better as communication aids than visual devices can serve as training aids. Moreover, a skilled teacher or clinician can provide speech models, feedback, and training that will transfer to real life more efficiently and far more simply than any visual device.

feeling speech

Whenever we talk, we create speech patterns that can not only be heard and seen, but also felt. Indeed, just as every speech pattern in English sounds different to the normal listener, it feels different to the practised speaker. Those of us who have normal hearing are not very aware of how our speech feels when we talk. We attend more to how it sounds. But, unconsciously, we are very tuned in to the way our speech organs touch each other (create tactile sensations) and move (create kinesthetic sensations) as we speak. This is clearly shown by those who are unfortunate enough to lose all of their hearing as adults. They do not stop talking. Nor does their speech become unintelligible. They continue to talk, and can do so because they are guided by the tactile and kinesthetic sensations they have long been accustomed to perceiving, perhaps without knowing it. In contrast, children who lose their hearing when they are too young to have had extensive experience of tactile and kinesthetic sensations may, in the absence of appropriate help, also lose their speech because they have insufficient history of proprioception (perception of self-generated sensations that provide awareness of the position of parts of the body) to guide them when audition has been lost.

articulatory coding

One of the most important aspects of work on speech development with hearing-impaired children is to establish articulatory coding - a repertoire of tactile and kinesthetic sensations that can, even in the complete absence of hearing, serve as a reliable guide for speech production. If appropriate training promotes awareness of the way correct speech patterns feel, both the children who become totally deaf following meningitis or some other disease and those who have been profoundly hearing-impaired from birth, can learn how to produce intelligible speech through self monitoring. At first, this may require the sensations created by speaking to be the focus of their conscious attention. Later, when speech becomes an automatic act, attention is more usually concentrated on what one is saying than on how one is saying it (see also Chapter 6).

external touch

Feeling one's own speech is not the only way in which the sense of touch can be used in speech reception and speech production. One can encourage children to feel what certain speech patterns are like when others produce them. Voicing can be felt on the chest, pitch can be felt as an elevation of the larynx, the tongue's position for various vowels can be felt with a finger in the mouth when the lips and teeth do not permit it to be seen, the burst of air can be detected when plosives, such as /p/ and /t/, are sounded out and the flow of air can be felt on a wet finger tip when fricatives like /s/ and /f/ are produced.

Natural touch can also provide the child with an analog of a sound's duration or intensity as a finger is drawn slowly or quickly, lightly or heavily down the arm or across the palm of a child's hand. Speech rhythms can be similarly indicated by tapping the pattern on the child's wrist or knee. More formalized way of using touch (for example the Tadoma method) have long been used to convey speech to deaf/blind children. Indeed, Annie Sullivan's use of touch to teach Helen Keller will be known to most readers. Specific uses of touch in relation to the teaching of particular speech sounds or speech patterns (utterances) will be suggested in Chapters 9 - 14.

The less hearing children have, the more necessary the use of touch will be to convey the subtleties of the spoken word to them. Helping hearing-impaired children to talk through the use of non-invasive touch demonstrates the close relationship that must exist and the intense caring that must underlie a speech development program for those who need supplementary or alternative channels to compensate for their inadequate audition of spoken language. All of our senses can function either passively or actively. We can use our ears to hear, but we learn when we listen. We use our eyes to see, but we learn when we look. Similarly, we can touch things or things can touch us, but we can learn about their characteristics only by feeling them. When we use direct touch actively (as in the process of feeling something) the sensation obtained does not wane over time to the same extent as that obtained through passive touch. Tactile devices are placed at a given location on some part of the body and the information they present may be largely passive. Active touch is, therefore, potentially more useful in speech acquisition than passive touch. Active touch is, however, potentially invasive and its use should always be treated with caution. It is only when children initiate or respond positively to speech presented through direct contact that one can be sure they are seeking to learn through the skin.

tactile devices

The information presented above shows that a great deal of information on speech can be transmitted through the skin. However, natural, direct touch is a close sense - one that can only operate over a limited distance. It has some disadvantages for speech transmission on this account. Normally, touch functions only when there is direct contact between one part of the body and another, or with another person. Electronic devices essentially change this, and allow touch to function, along with hearing and sight, as a third, distance sense. A microphone can be made to feed an amplifier which, in turn, can be made to feed a receiver of some sort that will vibrate the skin, or energize electrodes that will cause a small electric current to flow onto the skin. The quite distant acoustic events that surround us can thus be brought to the body and represented as a series of tactile stimuli. A variety of tactile devices have been created to transmit speech through touch over the past sixty years.

aspects of touch

The design of tactile devices has been complicated and impeded by several important aspects of the sense of touch. Perhaps the most important - and a blessing as far as everyday living is concerned - is that all parts of the body are not equally sensitive. Vibro-tactile devices are, therefore, likely to fulfil their function better when they are placed where there is adequate sensitivity; for example, on the hands, on the forearm, or near the face, rather than on the abdomen, the chest or the back.

Another complication of touch is that it does permits only gross differences in frequency to be perceived, and it becomes less and less effective for the detection of stimuli as they increase in frequency. Touch is at its most sensitive to very low-frequency sounds; and very little, if anything, is felt of stimuli beyond 1000 Hz. As many of the crucial components of speech lie around and beyond this frequency (see Chapters 2 and 3), some form of transposition of high-frequency sounds is required to render them tangible (detectable). But transposing (i.e., shifting) high-frequency sounds down so that they can be felt is not enough. To render different frequencies discriminable, speech frequency information has to be presented to different locations on the skin.

A third complication with the sense of touch is that it tends to accommodate quickly to initial stimulation. This means that stimuli that can be detected will, if continually presented, appear to fade away and become intangible. The difficulties in making devices that had sufficient power to produce strong enough and low enough vibrations to overcome these complications and were, at the same time, portable, held back the production of wearable vibro-tactile aids until recent years, when the miniaturization of components essential to this task was at last achieved. The components that have proven hardest to miniaturize have been the power source (batteries) and the transducers (the component that changes the electrical energy flowing from the amplifier into mechanical or other energy that can be sensed).

vibro-tactile devices

The earliest, and most simple, wearable vibro-tactile devices to be used with hearing-impaired children were hearing aids that drove a bone conduction vibrator worn on the wrist. Such devices presented the whole spectrum of speech to the skin even though it was known that the high-frequency sounds thus transmitted would be intangible. Later, the time-intensity envelope of speech (speech energy from which frequency cues are excluded) was transmitted through similar, single-channel instruments. These simple instruments did not, in themselves, make speech intelligible, but when the information they provided was added to speechreading under good acoustic conditions, significant gains in speech reception resulted.

More recently, instruments that function in much the same way, but have two or more vibrators have come into use. Two-channel vibro-tactile devices are usually worn in such a way that they present low-frequency information to the back of the wrist through one vibrator and transposed high-frequency information to the front of the wrist through the other. This sort of instrument provides even more supplementary information to speechreaders. A seven channel vibro-tactile device has also been produced that presents information on the second formants of back, mid and front vowels. This instrument is designed to be worn around the arm above the elbow. The design of vibro-tactile devices has, therefore, advanced in recent years, but there are still limitations imposed by their size and power requirements. Some work has also been done with vibro-tactile instruments that function with piezoelectric transducers (receivers that contain crystals that vibrate when an electric current is passed through them). So far, no such device has been developed for widespread use.

electro-tactile devices

In order to reduce size and power requirements, devices have now been introduced that present information on speech by delivering mild electric current to the skin through small electrodes. Although such instruments are called *electro-tactile devices* it is not clear that the delivery of current to the skin stimulates only - or even mainly - the cutaneous nerves that are involved in tactile sensation. Be that as it may, electro-tactile stimulation is much more efficient than vibro-tactile stimulation. It can deliver sufficient energy with greater precision to almost any area on which the electrodes may be placed - the fingertips, the wrist, the arm, the leg, or the body. The use of this form of stimulation as compared with that provided by the more traditional vibro-tactile instruments does not necessarily lead to better results in speech dis-crimination. They both provide much the same sort of information, but in different ways. Thus the two types of transducers, vibro-tactile and electro-tactile can be, indeed have been, used in a single device. The sensation that one receives through electro-tactile stimulation, the awareness of a small electric current, is best described as a tickle and is to touch much as a fricative is to hearing.

the state of the art

Single-channel tactile devices provide much less information than most multi-channel instruments. Single-channel devices essentially provide cues on the duration and intensity of vocalization. They transmit little or no spectral information, and reliable cues relating to duration and intensity can be effectively masked by the presence of noise. The thrust in recent years has, therefore, been towards the production of multi-channel devices.

Few of the numerous tactile devices that have been designed have found their way into general use. In part this is because power requirements and bulky components still prevent the design of wearable instruments that will deliver the large amount of information that some designers would like to have transmitted. It is also because designers are not yet sure which of the various aspects of the speech signal should be coded for optimal transmission of information, the most economical way to encode them, and the best way to present them to the skin. Some form of coding is essential if speech is to be transmitted via the skin because, as mentioned above, the skin is incapable of receiving and permitting the discrimination of the intensity, duration and, particularly, frequency components of speech in their raw form.

Numerous different strategies can be adopted to encode speech for tactile transmission. For example, different frequency bands can be presented in the form of tangible signals to different locations on the body, such as the arm, thigh, or abdomen. It has been suggested that the division of speech into many narrow bands is preferable to its division into a few wide bands. The accuracy of this notion is still open to question, however, and the optimal number of bands for tactile speech processing remains to be determined.

An alternative to such narrow-band frequency division is the extraction of the significant components of speech (see Chapters 2 and 3 and 4), such as F_0, F_1, F_2, the nasal murmur, fricative turbulence or plosive bursts (to mention a few of the most obvious) and their transmission through a number of different channels. Even if there are efficient ways to present all such coded information it is by no means clear that it can all be received by someone wearing the device. How well such information can be received will depend not only on the components selected for coding, the coding system employed, the number of channels used, their arrangement on the skin, and the form of the signal chosen, but on how efficiently it can be detected, discriminated, identified, and comprehended by the wearer. Wearable tactile devices currently in use are, then, their designers' best guesses on how to present what they consider to be the key aspects of speech in the most economical ways. In practice these devices are also the product of compromise between the realities of having to conserve power and to use components that are often less than satisfactory, particularly with regard to size, and the various needs of potential wearers.

devices in use

A brief description of some of the devices that have been designed to code speech components and present them to the skin may be helpful. At one extreme, there are devices that present a few selected cues through one channel. At the other, there is a device produced in the U.S.A. that divides the speech spectrum into 36 bands and has its 288 electrodes arranged in an 8x36 matrix to be worn on the abdomen. In between, there is a Canadian device that has sixteen channels through which subjects can discriminate between words without speechreading. It has been reduced in size to make it portable, but it is not small enough for a child to wear.

The most recent wearable multi-channel vibro-tactile device is the one mentioned above that was developed in the United States to divide the speech frequency range into seven channels and to present the information by means of that number of transducers strapped to the arm above the elbow. The most recent wearable multi-channel electro-tactile device to become available was created at the University of Melbourne, Australia. The device, known as the "Tickle Talker" has one reference electrode placed on the wrist and eight active electrodes. The active electrodes are placed over the nerve bundles located below the knuckle on each side of the four fingers on one hand. The device presents coded information in the following manner: F_2 by electrode position, the lower of these formants towards the index finger and the higher ones towards the pinky; F_0 by electrical pulse rate, at half the frequency of F_0; and amplitude envelope by pulse width. The microphone of the device is contained in the shell of a behind-the-ear hearing aid, and the instrument containing the electronic components driving the electrodes will fit comfortably into the top pocket of a boy's jacket. The electrodes are held in position with a mitten-like arrangement so that the upper part of the fingers are not covered and the hand can move reasonably freely. Figure 5-1 is a sketch of a parent helping her child to discriminate between familiar sentences presented without speechreading through the Tickle Talker.

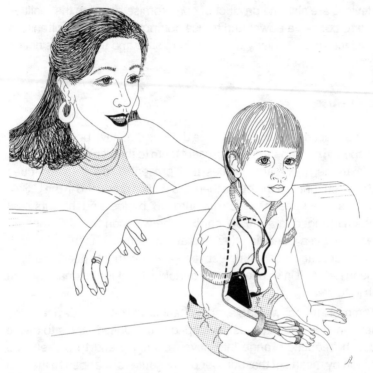

figure 5-1. A parent helping her child to discriminate between sentences routinely used in everyday life through the electro-tactile device known as the Tickle Talker (with permission of Prof. G. M. Clark and Dr. P. Blamey, University of Melbourne).

evaluation of effectiveness

Laboratory studies, usually with equipment that is neither portable nor wearable are a necessary preliminary step in the development of most devices for the several reasons given above, and it is important, before taking steps to miniaturize a device to know whether it will do what its designers expect it to do. There are no constraints on the size or complexity of instruments that can be used for training tactile speech reception in the laboratory or in a school, but there are constraints on what sort of training and how much testing can be done with subjects under laboratory or school conditions. In training their subjects, researchers present language materials ranging from syllables to running speech, using procedures that require discrimination within closed sets (choices from a limited number of items) to comprehension from open sets (linguistic situations that provide an unlimited number of items and no extrinsic cues). The most common open set procedure to be used is tracking. By means of this technique (described above, in the section on speechreading), one can measure the number of words per minute that a subject repeats back from a story.

Work to date has shown that tactile speech reception requires extensive training before the effectiveness of a given device can be established. For this reason, it is very difficult to make direct comparisons of various designs. Furthermore, it is difficult to assess the effectiveness of a device unless one initially uses normally hearing or adventitiously hearing-impaired adults to appraise it, because otherwise the results of training may be contaminated by additional variables, such as age, language skills, type of schooling, and communicative experience. However, the long-term goal is to produce wearable devices for hearing-impaired children, so once a device appears to provide a significant amount of help in various aspects of speech reception with adults, it must be miniaturized and then evaluated as a wearable device that can also be a speech production aid for children.

The differences in evaluation procedures that are possible within the laboratory and in real life are quite important, because the devices under the latter conditions serve as communication aids rather than training instruments and permit informal learning rather than formal teaching to contribute to the outcome. Evaluation of a device under real life conditions weakens many facets of experimental control, but strengthens the impact that a device may have through enhancing the pragmatic aspects of spoken language acquisition.

overall results

Results of testing a wide range of wearable tactile devices have consistently shown that they can permit the detection, discrimination and even the identification of some of the speech components that they were designed to transmit when used without any other form of input. However, comprehension of running speech has not yet been achieved from the use of tactile devices alone. Comprehension of running speech can, however be achieved when such devices are used as a support for speechreading. Most tactile devices developed to date provide a less effective supplement to speechreading than hearing aids, except for totally or near totally deaf individuals. For such children, however, tactile aids can usefully supplement the limited visual information present in speech and should be used to help them with speechreading, particularly under good acoustic conditions. It is perhaps even more important with tactile devices than with hearing aids to ensure that speech signals are presented to the children relatively free from noise.

Tactile devices can also supplement the information received by children from more than one other sense modality. Indeed, research published by the writer and a colleague several years ago showed that when a tactile cue on the presence of fricatives was added to the degraded speech signal received by profoundly hearing-impaired children through aided hearing and speechreading, they were able to make use of the extra information provided in this third sense modality.

Tactile devices are in their infancy and there is little doubt that new and more effective instruments will be developed and become available as research and development proceeds. Future work with such aids will involve miniaturizing their components, maximizing the information presented, finding effective ways of adjusting output levels to the individual needs of very young infants, and reducing or eliminating the adverse effects of noise, perhaps by the use of FM coupling procedures as with personal hearing aids. An important source of input to designers of tactile devices as they come into more widespread use will be reports on the children's speech development from the professional personnel and caregivers involved in habilitation programs. Those aspects of speech that are most readily developed (or not) will reflect the presence (or absence) of crucial components of the speech signal provided through speechreading and the tactile mode. The rate of development of these devices is not likely to be fast and caregivers would be well advised not to wait for greatly improved models if they have children who need some form of tactile assistance now.

cochlear implants

Some two hundred years ago, in 1790, Alessandro Volta put a metal rod in each ear, connected the rods to some batteries, and reported, once he had recovered, that the experiment had caused him to hear sound. But it was not until just over thirty years ago that two French doctors directly stimulated the auditory nerve of an anesthetized, totally deaf patient, and thus enabled him to hear the rhythm of speech. Since then, hundreds of devices known as cochlear implants have been built and surgically fitted so that totally or near-totally deaf individuals can hear something of speech and receive information on the acoustic events that surround them through electro-acoustic stimulation.

Totally or near-totally deaf individuals may lack most or all of the sensory components of the cochlea that convert sound vibrations to nerve impulses, but this does not necessarily mean that they have no nerve fibers that work. Some have inner ears that are filled with bony tissue or a cochlea that will not accept implants for some other reason, but most have nerve endings that can be stimulated electrically. Cochlear implants can therefore be used to convey sounds to most individuals with no useful residual hearing, not acoustically as do hearing aids, but electrically, through the insertion of one or more electrodes onto or into the inner ear (cochlea).

Cochlear implants are not a reasonable alternative to hearing aids for children having average hearing levels of about 90 to 95 dB or better in both ears. Such levels in and of themselves do not represent near-total deafness (here defined as being present in children who can detect high-level acoustic stimuli mainly through vibro-tactile sensations). There are many children with average levels of 90 to 95 dB who can, given appropriate auditory learning opportunities, process speech through audition alone under good acoustic conditions. The use of a multi-channel cochlear implant with a child who has no hearing beyond 1000 Hz in one ear and no audition whatever in the other should not be rejected, however: some spectral information that would not otherwise be available could be provided to the acoustically deaf ear that might thus supplement the residual hearing in the other. Children may be considered as having near total deafness when they can respond to a few steady state pure tones at high levels of intensity, but cannot learn to use that hearing for any communicative or social purpose following several months of intensive auditory stimulation.

components of cochlear implants

Cochlear implants consist of several parts, some worn externally, and some surgically embedded in the cochlea or otherwise placed in the skull. In all forms of implants, sounds are detected by a microphone and then delivered at appropriate power levels in some way through the device to one or more electrodes. The raw (essentially unchanged) speech signal can be delivered to one electrode inserted through, or placed adjacent to, the round window of the cochlea. The more nerves that are present, such as those that have survived a disease such as meningitis, the better the results with any sort of implant are likely to be. Typically, 10 to 50 percent of the auditory nerves survive following meningitis, even though all of the sensory receptors (hair cells) in the cochlea may have been damaged.

Most totally or near-totally deaf individuals inevitably have decoding problems that relate to the damage sustained in the cochlea so, while they can be made aware of sound through the use of a cochlear implant, speech patterns would not be normally intelligible to them. An alternative to delivering the raw speech signal to the damaged cochlea is to present information in a coded form through several electrodes rather than one. Such coding permits the transmission of particular aspects of the speech signal, such as the F_2 of different vowels, to various sites on the cochlea, because the organization of the inner ear favors the detection of high frequencies near the round window, and increasingly lower frequency sounds further away from it.

As shown in Figure 5-2, the external parts of cochlear implants are the microphone, the processor that changes the signals in various ways, and a special receiver, usually a coil worn behind the ear, to which the processor is usually wired. The internal parts are a coil (and possibly some micro-circuitry in the case of multi-channel implants) and the electrode(s). The microphone feeds the speech processor, which in turn sends electrical signals to the external coil that must be situated exactly over the portion of the device embedded in the bone (the mastoid) behind the ear. In some cochlear implants the implanted portions are controlled and powered by externally provided radio-frequency energy. In other types of implants, the internal parts are powered by induction. In such devices, the electric current that flows in the external coil creates a magnetic flux that causes similar current to flow in the other (internal) coil to the electrodes put in place by the surgeon.

By the two hundredth anniversary of Volta's experiment, recipients of cochlear implants, who know that these devices cannot provide them with normal-sounding speech, will be counted in thousands. While these data indicate that many people are benefitting from them, there is no guarantee that a cochlear implant will work even moderately well for any given individual. Nevertheless, the majority of cochlear implant recipients have been helped by them, some to such an extent that they can discriminate between various speech sounds and follow some speech without the support of speechreading. A few patients have received no benefit at all, a few have suffered temporary dizziness, and some have experienced facial nerve involvement that has caused twitching or facial pain. A few such devices have failed and have had to be replaced. There is always a risk of infection, as with any surgery, but so far, no deaths or serious adverse after-effects from cochlear implantation have been reported.

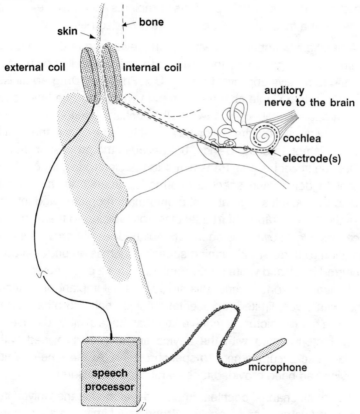

figure 5-2. A diagram showing the main external and internal components of a cochlear implant.

Different aspects of speech are transmitted through different types of cochlear implants, and the extent to which children - even those with similar backgrounds - can process sounds has been found to vary. Much greater variation in performance has been found in comparisons of pre-lingually and post-lingually hearing-impaired children. Differences among children in relation to age at onset of hearing impairment strongly influences the type of learning experiences that they need and the outcome of their habilitation treatment. Description of all of the devices currently in use is outside the scope of this book. The purpose here is simply to introduce the reader to devices that may be met in the treatment of hearing-impaired children, and the effects that cochlear implants may have on the development of spoken language. To provide a more adequate framework for the later discussion of these issues, background information on two quite different sorts of implants - one a single-channel, and the other a multi-channel device - are provided below.

The single-channel cochlear implant developed at the House Ear Institute in Los Angeles was the first one to become well known, widely used, and to receive approval from the U.S. Food and Drug Administration (FDA). It is a single channel system in which the one electrode is placed through the round window into the cochlea. Because it is a single channel device, it stimulates all of the available nerve cells in the cochlea at once. It is not a coding device, but because the processor radically changes the speech signal transmitted to the electrodes, it permits the recipient to derive little spectral information apart from fundamental frequency. It provides a great deal of information on time and intensity across the speech range of frequencies from voicing to the turbulence of fricatives. On its own, this cochlear implant does not provide enough information to understand running speech. Much as an under-exposed and blurred black and white photograph provides a poor representation of an intricate, colorful scene, this single channel implant provides the listener with a very limited representation of speech and other sounds. However, a blurred picture is much better than none at all, and those who are satisfactorily fitted with the device are thereby provided with a potentially useful supplement to speechreading. At the time of writing this device had been provided for several hundred children.

The multi-channel cochlear implant developed at the University of Melbourne, Australia, and Cochlear Proprietary Limited is a 22-channel device. It was the second cochlear implant to receive FDA approval. The external parts of the aid are a microphone, speech processor, and an external coil that, as in the House Ear Institute implant, is held in place by a magnet contained in the internal coil. The implanted parts are an internal receiver-stimulator and the electrodes. The implanted portions are controlled and powered by radio frequency transmission through the skin. The electrodes are platinum bands 0.3 mm wide, spaced at 0.7 mm intervals along a single strand that is inserted through the round window into the cochlea. At any time, only two electrodes are used. The electrical current flows from one electrode to the other so that there is little spread of current between the two electrodes. This feature limits the range of nerves that will be exposed to the electric current produced when any given electrode pair is stimulated. The amount of stimulation provided by each electrode pair differs from one recipient to another because their nerves differ in sensitivity, and the electrodes are not always in the same position relative to them. How much stimulation is provided by each electrode pair must therefore be measured and adjusted for each recipient. The device uses a speech coding scheme. Speech-processing circuitry in the device estimates formant frequencies and amplitudes, and codes this information in relation to the electrodes that are used to stimulate particular sites within the cochlea. F_0 is transmitted as the pulse rate of stimulation, F_2 is coded in relation to electrode position, and intensity as the amplitude of the signal. More recently, in addition to coding intensity, F_0 and F_2, F_1 has also been coded and transmitted in the same manner as F_2, through stimulating two electrodes in quick succession. This additional coding does not require changing anything that is already implanted. Coding procedures can be changed simply by making alterations to the speech processing component that is worn externally. In short, this cochlear implant was designed to permit reception of several aspects of speech: the fundamental frequency, the durational, and the intensity components of prosody, information on vowels, as well as provide some manner, place, and voicing distinctions among consonants. At best, it permits some recipients to identify a number of words without speechreading, and to achieve excellent rates of speech tracking. Only adults were fitted with this device before 1986, and two years later, less than a dozen children had it implanted.

the choice of device

Most of the comparative data on tactile devices and cochlear implants has been obtained from adults. Studies indicate that there is considerable variation in speech-reception performance levels among individuals implanted with or wearing the same type of device. They show that some individuals can do as well with single-channel as with multi-channel devices, but that those most satisfactorily fitted with multi-channel instruments out-perform the others. There are good reasons for expecting similar findings with children. The bases for selecting one type of device over another will change as new cochlear implants and tactile devices are marketed, and as improvements are made to the many single- and multi-channel devices of both sorts. Such advances are likely because of advances in technology and findings suggesting that if even more information on speech can be coded and presented in appropriate ways, higher levels of performance than have so far been obtained will probably result.

Tactile devices and cochlear implants both provide a new code for children who have total or near-total hearing impairments. Those who acquired their language through audition before they lost their hearing have usually been able to associate the code provided by most cochlear implants with the speech patterns they once perceived through normal hearing. For this reason, most adventitiously hearing-impaired persons can be expected to do better with cochlear implants than with tactile devices. One cannot, however, conclude from such an observation that cochlear implants are intrinsically superior to tactile devices for pre-lingually deaf individuals. They may be so, but whether better results can be achieved by pre-lingually hearing-impaired individuals fitted with cochlear implants or tactile devices that provide an equivalent amount of information remains to be seen. The relative advantages and limitations of such devices can only be judged in relation to the quality of the habilitation program provided, and the demonstrated abilities and needs of particular children. No one device or procedure can possibly satisfy the requirements of all individuals.

At present, findings in relation to learning difficulty suggest that the acquisition of speech reception skills through tactile devices of all sorts is a very slow process. This situation may be ameliorated by the production of improved devices, but it also suggests that, if tactile devices are to be employed with children, it would be advantageous to use them throughout the first years of life when the acoustic conditions are most favorable (see Chapter 3), and when there is less competition with learning spoken language skills from other forms of activity (see Chapter 7).

There is good reason to hold that children are less and less likely to be able to process speech through hearing if they have not had the opportunity to receive auditory stimulation before adolescence. The earlier they receive such stimulation, the better (see Chapter 7). There is no evidence relating to optimal or critical periods for receiving tactile stimulation, but there is reason to think that learning through any sense modality would be similarly affected by age. But fitting complex devices to children in early infancy poses problems at present. In providing multi-channel instruments, particularly cochlear implants and electro-tactile devices, the sensitivity of each electrode must be adjusted to provide optimal stimulation; and strategies to determine the best levels for each channel have yet to be devised and applied to infants. This should not be an insuperable problem, because there are electro-physiological tests that could be used for this purpose once their application has been sufficiently researched.

The great advantage of tactile devices over cochlear implants is that invasive surgical procedures are not required to fit them. A possible advantage of cochlear implants is that they exploit the auditory system which, in most animals, is the natural sense for processing sound and it may, on this account, prove to be superior to touch as a supplementary or alternative modality in speech reception. For adventitiously hearing-impaired children (i.e., those who lose hearing during childhood rather than at or before birth), cochlear implants may be the instruments of choice. For the pre-lingually hearing impaired, one must, unfortunately conclude that, at present, the choice between them is more a matter of faith than of reason.

criteria for decision-making

The criteria for deciding whether to use a tactile device for a particular child relate closely to those for deciding whether to use electro-cochlear hearing. Tactile devices do not require invasive surgery, as cochlear implants do. They are also much less expensive to purchase. On the other hand, they are less likely than cochlear implants (that are selected following due consideration of all known variables) to substantially improve an adventitiously hearing-impaired child's chances of learning to communicate effectively through spoken language. Pre-lingually hearing-impaired children may perform equally as well (or poorly) with a tactile device as with a cochlear implant. It is difficult for parents to decide whether a child should have a single-channel implant at one year of age in order to be exposed to the acoustic patterns of speech through electro-cochlear hearing during most of the early years, or whether to have the child use a tactile device for some years until a multi-channel cochlear implant can be provided that might be a better aid to speech reception at a later stage. There are difficult ethical considerations relating to such decisions. Rigorous decision-making procedures are therefore required. Some of the criteria that should be considered in opting for or against cochlear implants as compared with tactile devices are suggested below.

1. *Cochlear implants should be considered only for children who have no residual hearing.* Although cochlear implants can transmit useful information on speech, they should not be considered as alternatives to hearing aids on three counts: first, they presently provide less information except in unusual cases; second, the electrode or electrode bundle inserted into the cochlea destroys whatever residual hearing exists; and third, tactile devices can be used as a supplement to speechreading with children of any age.

It is conceivable that cochlear implants may eventually provide more information than hearing aids to some profoundly hearing-impaired children, but even the 22 channels of an advanced device is considerably less than the thousands of receptors that are normally present in the cochlea, many of which may remain useful to profoundly hearing-impaired children. This criterion would certainly be open to question if it could be convincingly argued that a child with usable hearing would certainly be able to achieve better speech recognition with a cochlear implant than with the continued use of an optimally selected hearing aid. An exception to this criterion might be a child with hearing in only one ear. A cochlear implant in the completely deaf ear might well supplement speech reception through a hearing aid in the other.

2. *Children should be considered as candidates for cochlear implants as soon as they can be positively identified as having no useful residual hearing.* Children who receive auditory stimulation in early rather than later childhood can follow more normal paths in the acquisition of social skills and spoken language. Those who do not receive early auditory stimulation may suffer loss of useful central nervous system (CNS) function through auditory deprivation. Such children may learn to do without hearing as they organize their perception through other sense modalities. Current behavioral and electro-physiological tests provide sufficiently reliable measures of an individual's hearing levels by about age two. However, the accurate fitting of very young infants with multi-channel instruments at this age and younger requires further research because objective ways to ensure appropriate adjustment of each available channel have not yet been determined. Tactile devices can be fitted from the earliest stages of infancy.

3. *Children must be known to have the physical requisites before cochlear implant surgery is recommended.* Cochlear implants require the presence of a cochlea that is not filled with bone, a cochlea that permits the auditory nerve to be stimulated. Children with these requisites who have no useful residual hearing must also be able to tolerate the surgery that is involved. Tactile devices are a viable option for profoundly hearing-impaired children who do not meet the physical requisites for cochlear implant surgery.

4. *Children should want to communicate through speech, even at the most elementary levels, if a cochlear implant is to be provided.* All children can be encouraged to communicate verbally from early infancy (see Chapters 1 and 7). Older children who have grown away from speech communication (for example through extensive emphasis on sign language) are unlikely to succeed in learning spoken language unless they are strongly motivated to do so. Using a cochlear implant along with sign or even together with Cued Speech is unlikely to yield optimal results unless their use is dropped for a major portion of the child's waking hours. This is because the complete visual communication Cued Speech permits will compete too strongly with the less familiar spoken form in situations that demand comprehension. It is advisable to arrange a pre-operative evaluation period of some months, during which the child's ability to respond to tactile stimulation are observed, and the child's actual and potential drive to communicate by speech are determined.

5. *Caregivers must be prepared to support the use of a cochlear implant by their children.* Learning to understand others' speech and to monitor their own speech production through any type of implant is a long and difficult task for children, particularly those who do not have language previously acquired at least to some extent through hearing. Their acquisition of the necessary speech

reception skills will require several years of communication in situations that are carefully structured to provide adequate learning opportunities, contextual supplements to promote comprehension, and the necessary socio-educational support (see Chapter 7). The same level of support is required for successful use of a tactile device.

intervention strategies in relation to devices

The three essential features of habilitation are the use of effective devices, the provision of opportunities for optimal learning, and the objective assessment of changes brought about by them. If all devices were to provide adequate information on all aspects of speech, as good quality hearing aids might do for children with moderate hearing impairment, then sufficient experience of speech communication in completely informal, unstructured situations would usually and quickly lead to excellent spoken language performance. However, the less information devices provide (and the less information of any type a sense modality can transmit), the more structured learning situations must be if hearing-impaired children are to attain spoken language proficiency. The type of intervention strategy that one adopts must therefore be geared to reflect the extent of information that the instruments are capable of transmitting. However, the children's perceptual systems, as well as the instruments are involved. Helping children to process the information transmitted is just as important as knowing what information an instrument can present. Only through reference to the results of valid evaluation can one rationally select and/or change either the instruments or the procedures used in the habilitation process.

system integrity

Once cochlear implants or tactile devices have been selected and adjusted, they should, like hearing aids for other hearing-impaired children, be regarded as part of each child's sensory system, one that begins at the microphone of the instrument and ends at the cortex. The integrity of this system is inevitably in doubt from the outset, for individuals tend to differ, for various reasons, in their ability to receive information transmitted. Those providing or supervising habilitation programs must, therefore, be constantly alert to what form of stimuli are being provided to the children in their care, what responses the children are making to them, and what sort of inferences may be drawn from their observations.

There are two types of data that one must seek in order to determine the efficiency of the instrument and the integrity of the system, one direct and the other indirect. The direct data is evidence of discrimination, identification, and comprehension of speech patterns. The indirect data is the presence of the various components of spoken language in the corpus of utterances produced by each child. Satisfactory tests are not difficult to construct for older children with whom spoken language communication has been established. But neither direct nor indirect evaluation procedures are easy to carry out with very young children, because formal tests of discrimination and identification for infants are not well standardized, and evidence of comprehension is based on inference. Evidence of perceptual skills derived from utterances produced by hearing-impaired children at any age is likely to be con-taminated by motor speech problems. Meaningful data of any type can be obtained only following extensive exposure to spoken language communication prior to testing. It is essential to guard against attributing results that are generated by the adults' and peers' interest in a new instrument to the characteristics of the instrument or of the habilitation procedures used.

language learning through supplementary or alternative channels

The spoken language used with children of any age should not, in general, be broken down into segments of less than a sentence (see Chapter 7) because meaning is most completely and commonly carried in sentences rather than sounds or words. Individual sounds and words can be derived from isolated sentences, but the reverse is not true. There is always a temptation to concentrate attention on sounds or on words when it is known that they will be used as stimuli in the assessment of the efficiency of a device. However, concentration on discrimination and identification of sounds and words in intervention programs can too readily serve as a substitute for efforts towards building comprehension skills. The engine that drives children to perceive and to learn any of their language skills is comprehension - success in deriving meaning from what is said. Exercises in discrimination and identification may also tend to focus attention on trivial aspects of perception to the detriment of more important ones, and any gains that result are difficult to carry over into everyday communication. Specific training in discrimination and identification should be provided only when particular elements of spoken language do not develop spontaneously when adequate opportunity has been given for such development.

The language patterns provided for all young children on initial fitting of a cochlear implant or a tactile device should initially relate, through commentary and interaction, to their interest in the objects and events that constitute their everyday experiences. From such verbal interaction children will derive the meaning of what is said and, at the same time, find the most effective perceptual strategies that allow them to derive the information the speaker intended to convey. Neither the meaning of spoken language nor the best ways for children to perceive it, can be taught by an adult as effectively as they can be learned by young children. Furthermore, children will not use speech as a means of communication unless it serves their interests (not those of adults) to do so.

Spoken language communication with somewhat older children on initial fitting of a cochlear implant or tactile device should not necessarily be a continuation of the strategies formerly employed. For example, supplementary visual information in communication should be much more consciously limited to that provided through speechreading. Conversation and other forms of verbal interaction should be made to focus very specifically on making the utmost use of the device. Games and stories in which the features provided by the device have to be attended to, the use of the device alone in contexts that permit speechreading to be dropped, and the child's awareness of contrast in speechreading performance with and without the device can all be used to augment everyday communication and, where applicable, schoolwork. Some such activities will permit the more speedy evaluation of the device as an integral part of an older, as compared with a younger, child's perceptual system.

assessment of intervention

Spoken language reception through the use of cochlear implants or tactile devices is likely to be much slower with pre-lingually than with post-lingually hearing-impaired children, and more difficult to assess in the early stages. Nevertheless, evaluation is an essential part of any efficient habilitation program. Comprehension can be assessed in relation to various behaviors in real life situations, various aspects of discourse including questions, the understanding of stories and conversation, as well as specially structured tests. Discrimination and identification can be tested informally in the course of interaction or formally through tests and structured games. The components of interest in evaluating progress and assessing the extent of system integrity are the same: the perception and production of all aspects of spoken language; namely, the suprasegmental aspects (intensity, duration, and voice frequency control); all segmental aspects (vowels, consonants, and consonant blends); vocabulary and word pronunciation; the syntactic, semantic and pragmatic aspects of sentence use; and different types of discourse (see Chapter 6).

suggestions for further reading

The standard books on various aspects of speechreading include those by Jeffers and Barley (1971), and Berger (1972). Since they were published, a considerable amount of research has been carried out and reported, principally in journal articles. *The Journal of the Acoustical Society of America*, *The Volta Review*, and *The Journal of Speech and Hearing Research*, among others, frequently contain accounts of speechreading research (see, for example, Breeuwer and Plomp (1985). Recent and comprehensive texts on speechreading have been edited by Dodd and Campbell (1987), and by DeFilippo and Sims (1988).

Cued Speech was introduced by Cornett (1967). The most comprehensive study on Cued Speech so far undertaken is that of Nicholls (1979).

The sense of touch in teaching hearing-impaired children to talk has been discussed by Ling (1976), and reviews of tactile devices and tactile perception have been provided by Carney and Beachler (1986),

DeFillipo (1984), Proctor (1984), and Sherrick (1984). Blamey and Clark (1985) report the development of a recently developed tactile device. There are some books and many articles on cochlear implants and those by Berliner and House (1981, 1982), Clark et al. (1987a), and Owens and Kessler (1988) provide excellent background materials. Some comparisons of cochlear implants and tactile devices have been made by Pickett and MacFarland (1985), but the first use of multi- channel cochlear implants with children has been more recently reported by Clark et al. (1987b). All aspects of speech reception that have been covered in this chapter are currently being studied by numerous researchers. While the basic information presented in this chapter can be accepted as written, advances in the design of cochlear implants and tactile devices are being made quite rapidly. It follows that details relating to specific devices will require constant updating. See References, pp. 433 ff.

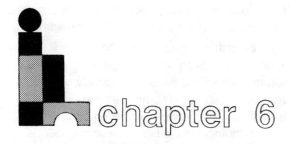

aspects of
spoken language.

introduction

Widely used languages have all of the features that are required for precision of expression. English is no exception. Because English has absorbed words from many other languages, it has a very rich vocabulary. It is also an extremely flexible language, so there are often several ways to express the same idea - perhaps with a lot of sentences, each truly simple, or with one or two sentences, each highly complex. All spoken languages have much in common, mainly because the people who speak them are more alike than different, and because the majority of human beings have similar communication needs. But all languages also have major features that are unique to them; a different range of sounds, different ways of making up words from those sounds, different ways of making up sentences from those words, and different ways of putting sentences together in communication. Our concern here is with spoken English.

Spoken language is a vast topic. To cover what is known about it would take several dozen volumes. To discuss theories of language and language acquisition would take many more. In this one brief chapter, therefore, only the barest of outlines of the major aspects of language can be provided. Discussion of each is intended to indicate the types of relationships that exist between language and speech, and the ways hearing-impaired children can perceive and acquire them. The material presented is not intended to be comprehensive; its purposes are to serve as a foundation for later chapters, and as a stimulus for further reading.

Four major aspects of English as a spoken language will be discussed - sounds, words, sentences, and discourse. Speech relates to all of them. Just as we need to have sound patterns (prosody, vowels, and consonants) that conform to those used by others around us, so do we need to have clearly articulated words, well-expressed sentences, and the ability to use several sentences together to develop notions about particular topics. Speakers must also be able to use acceptable ways of entering into, and terminating speech communication with others.

Of course, children learning a language usually acquire most aspects of spoken language in parallel. They learn *how* to understand and say things at much the same time as they are learning *what* to say, and even *when* to say it. To be successful at developing spoken language in hearing-impaired children, we must follow a similar parallel pattern. Speech is not just a skill to be learned, but a system of communication through which we learn.

One of the most important stages in a child's acquisition of language is learning to understand and to use sentences rather than just words. This stage may take quite a long time to master, but before even the simplest of sentences is used, verbal communication tends to be vague, related to objects that are present, or concerned with activities that are ongoing. Words outside the structure of a sentence are often hard to interpret. For example, the little child in Figure 6-1 has said two words - "box," "car." The adults, who have just come onto the scene, and know nothing about the box or the car, or how they came to be where they are, can place at least six different interpretations on the child's words. (For example, "A box fell from the car," "The box was taken from the car," "This box should go in the car," "There's another box in the car," "I want the box in the car," and "Your box is in the car.") Precise meaning cannot reside in utterances smaller than sentences without the support of context provided either by non-verbal cues or by additional verbal information. All aspects of spoken language discussed below are concerned with what goes into the making of sentences, and the integration of sentences in discourse.

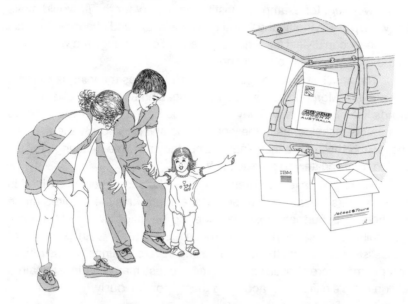

figure 6-1. **A child pointing and saying "Box, car." The scene provides the parents with too few cues for knowing which of several possible ideas she wishes to express. For the parents to use two-word sentences to the child would often be no more meaningful to her than her utterance was to them. The practice would also deny her opportunities to learn the decoding strategies that she needs for the development of language.**

In this chapter the reader will meet some of the terms used in linguistics. The special vocabulary that is used to talk about language is worth knowing, and will be explained or illustrated with examples as each section is introduced. Words that are explained in the text are also included in the glossary (Appendix D).

morphophonemics

Loosely translated, *morphophonemics* means "the form and meaning of sounds." The way that the many sounds of speech can be combined to form meaningful units is governed by a set of rules. For example, some sound combinations, such as *twi*, are permissible, and others, such as *wti*, are not.

The smallest meaningful sound in a language is called a *phoneme*. In the word *tip*, for example, substitution of a /p/ for the /t/ would make the word *pip*. Changing the vowel could yield *top*, and changing the final consonant could yield *tin*. Since each sound can change the word, each of the three sounds is a phoneme.

The smallest word or part of a word that has meaning is called a *morpheme*. Morphemes can be free (meaningful in themselves) as in words like *bird* and *play*. They can also be bound (added to a word to change its meaning) as in the words *birds* and *playing*. By themselves, the /s/ and the ing are meaningless, but they become meaningful when added appropriately to an existing word.

Hearing-impaired children may need the sort of help described in later chapters to learn how to perceive and produce the required range of phonemes. Further, most may need to be made aware of the rules governing the use of bound morphemes, such as /s/ in plurals and possessives, and both the /s/ and the ing in verb endings. These bound morphemes were chosen as examples because many hearing-impaired children have difficulty in acquiring them spontaneously.

morphophonemics and speech

In order to speak effectively children must be able to produce most - preferably all - of the speech patterns that occur in their language. This repertoire should include the prosody (tunes and rhythms), as well as all of the phonemes and morphemes, such as the /s/ that signals plurals and possessives, the word-final /t/ and /d/ that signal past tense, the ing that signals present continuous tense, and so on. To reduce the difficulty of the task for hearing-impaired children, and to encourage their acquisition of all of these patterns, the utmost care and attention should be given to the selection, use, and maintenance of the most appropriate sensory aids - hearing aids, tactile devices, or cochlear implants - as discussed in previous chapters.

In helping hearing-impaired children to acquire spoken language, speech sounds may first be taught without reference to meaning. This is termed teaching at a *phonetic*, rather than at a *phonologic* level. At the phonetic level one is simply developing the motor and feedback skills that are required for mastery. Only when speech sounds are used in words do they become phonemes and part of our phonology - part our meaningful speech. (Development of the sounds of English at both phonetic and phonologic levels is discussed in all future chapters.)

vocabulary

Words are the building blocks of language. Just as one cannot have a house without bricks, one cannot have a language without words. Only when bricks are organized into larger structures do buildings take shape, and only when words are organized into sentences do language forms emerge. Vocabulary consists of content words and function words. Content words represent objects, events, and actions. They include nouns and verbs. Function words are those that have no single meaning on their own, but give meaning to sentences, as shown below.

Both function words and content words have to be included in sentences and arranged in a particular order if language is to be meaningful. For example, even if one read the words *man ladies gave boys ice-cream* in different orders, their meaning would not become clear. Function words are essential for precision. Function words, such as *a, the, and, not, some, for, all, but,* and *to,* are needed if one is to know whether *the man and the ladies gave all the boys some of the ice cream,* or whether *the man with the ladies gave some of the boys all the ice-cream.* Children may begin by saying single words in context, and the first of them may be a function word like *up,* or a content word like *dada,* but in order to learn spoken language they must come to understand and say more than words. Certainly, they need to acquire words, but they must also learn - at much the same time - about the many ways in which words can be put together.

Young children - hearing-impaired or normally hearing - enjoy learning content words through naming games. Most parents like to track their child's gaze and to name the objects being looked at. Some parents deliberately indicate and name objects for their children. Young children who are great imitators will then often point to objects with the expectation that the parent will become an instant naming machine. Function words cannot be learned in this way. In order for children to learn function words, and thus acquire the tools for precise expression of meaning, they must be spoken to in sentences. In the sketch presented as Figure 6-2, the hearing- impaired child's father is using a book as the basis of a bed-time story. Some evenings, most of it may be read; other evenings, all of it may be read; but every evening, until the child's interest in it has waned, it is used to promote verbal interaction involving well- modulated speech patterns, most of them several words in length.

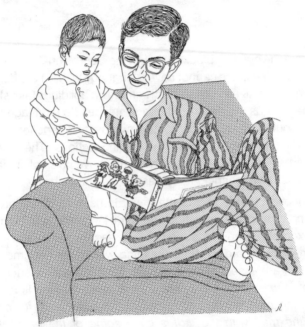

figure 6-2. A father reading and explaining a story to his hearing-impaired son, and thus using this bed-time situation to stimulate sequences of both verbal and non-verbal interaction - the foundations of discourse.

Most words, content or function, are best learned through their inclusion in sentences spoken to children about interesting events and objects in the context of repetitive, everyday experiences; for example, in questions and statements, such as "Can you find your coat?", "Do you want to take your coat off?", "Let's put your coat on!", "Oh! Your coat's dirty!", "Put your hand through the sleeve!", and so on. Similar commentary, in which both function and content words are used, should accompany all routine activities and include the many words associated with each of them. Word-by-word teaching is a much overworked strategy for developing vocabulary, and it does little to encourage the growth of language. In the above example, it can be see that a child talked to in sentences could learn words, such as *coat, sleeve, pocket, collar,* and *button*, just as easily, and from an early age, as parental commentary accompanies dressing and undressing. Even more important is that language - ways to express meaning - can be learned from commentary presented in normally constructed sentences. Naming is not, of course, without some merit, but words in isolation provide much less meaning than words in sentences, particularly if they are spoken with appropriate prosody. Single words and naming should, therefore, be regarded as the exception rather than the rule in language acquisition.

vocabulary and speech

Every speech sound occurs in the vocabulary used in the normal course of an extensive conversation. However, the sounds in speech do not occur equally often. Nor do they begin and end words with equal frequency. Some sounds, like ch are used much less often than /p/, and some sounds like /b/, occur much more frequently at the beginning than at the end of words. Among the most common sounds in words - at the beginning, in the middle, or at the end of them - are the lingua-alveolar sounds, sounds made with the blade of the tongue against the alveolar ridge like /s/, /l/, /n/, /d/, and /t/. These most frequently occurring sounds are not the simplest to make. It wastes time and causes frustration for both the children and their teachers if one tries to teach them before simpler sounds have been mastered. The order in which speech patterns are best mastered, so that each creates a stepping stone for others, is discussed in Chapter 8.

The importance of the function words has been emphasized above. To produce most of these words accurately, the lingua-alveolar sounds mentioned immediately above are required. The most obvious of reasons that hearing-impaired children sometimes omit these words in their utterances is that they cannot detect these sounds unless they have appropriate sensory aids that are functioning optimally all day and every day in an environment that focuses on speech as a means of communication. Because function words occur so frequently, attention to their perception and production can significantly help the development of both speech and language.

syntax.

Syntax is the system of rules that govern how sentences can be constructed. It is the aspect of language concerned with form as compared with function. Many people learn second languages through formal study of its grammar and syntax. But it is not easy to learn a first language that way. Children usually learn their first language through abundant experience of its reception and production, and in situations that are interesting and meaningful to them. They acquire their knowledge of syntax unconsciously as they communicate. As far as possible, hearing-impaired children should follow a similar path. Many such children acquire language that is syntactically perfect without having to be taught through reference to grammatical structures. Others may need to supplement informal language learning with formal teaching in order to achieve this end (see the next chapter).

It is trite but true to say that hearing impairment can be an enormous impediment to a child's development of language - and in particular to the acquisition of syntax. Utterances, such as "The baby he cry floor," and "Man he a the hit run away ball," may be produced by some hearing-impaired children even following many years of schooling. Many possible reasons for this widespread problem have been suggested by various professionals in the numerous books and articles written on the subject. The following represent some that are commonly put forward: "Hearing-impaired children are not given optimum experience of speech communication in many programs, partly because their hearing aids are often out of order." "Hearing impairment filters out the unstressed and hence less audible 'function' or 'relational' words of English, such as *so, how, to, and,* and *at,* that are syntactically important." "Function words are not only difficult to hear, they are also difficult to speechread." "Many children's syntactic difficulties are caused by mixing American Sign Language and Spoken English." "Too much emphasis is placed on the acquisition of single-word vocabulary so that opportunities to learn how words are put together are limited." "Most hearing-impaired children are taught single and simple sentence constructions rather than discourse skills, so they do not learn how to use the definite article 'the,' and pronouns, such as 'him' or 'they,' that occur mainly in multi-sentence units." " Most hearing-impaired children are taught language as a grammatical exercise, and do not, therefore, internalize the syntax, or generalize the rules to real life situations." Some, if not all, of these observations may be true, but such evidence and speculation have not yet led to a resolution of the problem. Fortunately a good many hearing-impaired children taught in programs that emphasize the use of spoken language can, and do, acquire not only highly intelligible - and sometimes normal - speech, but normal syntax as well.

Syntax remains one of the major areas of interest in the field of language. Widespread enthusiasm for syntactic analysis was spurred by the publication of N. Chomsky's (1957) book entitled *Syntactic Structures*. Chomsky considered sentences to be the basic units of language. He demonstrated that a finite number of syntactic rules could be used to generate an infinite number of sentences, and proposed that the sentences we produce are the surface representation of underlying "deep" structures. (For example, *The brick was thrown by the boy* and *The boy threw the brick* are different surface structures that result from "transformations" relating to the single deep structure, a structure that includes the concepts *boy, throw,* and *brick*.) He suggested that the various types of syntactic transformations that can be made include:

addition, e.g., adding a negative as in "The boy was not tall;"

conjoining, as in using "and" to join two different ideas;

deletion as in "didn't" and "don't" instead of "did not" and "do not", or "I want to go home and eat" instead of "I want to go home, and I want to eat;"

embedding as in "The girl who was sick went home" instead of "The girl was sick. The girl went home;"

rearrangement as in changing statements to questions or the reverse; and

substitution as in the use of pronouns to replace nouns.

syntax and speech

Being able to perceive the speech patterns that express the syntactic structures of language as clearly as possible is a basic essential (see Chapters 4 and 5). Being able to produce the speech patterns that permit the expression of these rules can be very helpful. For example, question forms require the production of h (as in how and who) and /w/ (as in which, where, when and why); negation requires n (as in no more, no, not me, never, nobody); deletion requires the word-final t (as in wasn't, didn't, and couldn't). The list could go on. Speech patterns help children to learn syntactic rules and transformations because they provide a means of rehearsing them. Similarly, learning to deal with morphemes and syntax in spoken language helps speech acquisition because the sounds children produce can thus be used in a meaningful way.

The most important relationship between syntax and speech is not how vowels and consonants relate to particular structures, but how prosody provides cues on syntactic structure. These cues do not just help differentiate questions and statements. Pauses mark sentences, and stress and intonation mark phrases and sentence boundaries. Prosody just as clearly defines exclamations. Particular rhythms suggest the presence of negatives, and other rhythms, prepositional phrases. Prosody in spoken language is not a random addition to an utterance. It is a well-organized system that helps carry meaning. Tradition has it that Julius Caesar issued the order "release, not execute" in response to a request for instructions on how to deal with a prisoner. The prisoner unfortunately lost his life because the messenger did not use appropriate prosody, and was understood to say "release not, execute."

developments from earlier work on syntax

During the thirty years since Chomsky's first works were published, a great deal of research and thought have been devoted to the development of his theories of grammar. The dominant theory at the present time is termed "government-binding theory." It appeared in its most comprehensive form in a book by Chomsky entitled *Lectures on Government and Binding* in 1981. It is, essentially, his extended theory of how the human mind represents language. The interaction of mind and language has been a consistent feature of Chomsky's thinking. He has long held that the deep structures of language reflect the structure of the mind. He also considers that children have an innate predisposition for "growing" language and thought, providing that the necessary conditions prevail, much as children grow limbs under normal, favorable conditions. The necessary conditions for spoken language growth have yet to be fully defined, but those suggested in this book are most certainly among them. The consistent use of appropriate hearing aids from an early age in an environment that features abundant speech communication are widely recognized as important conditions for facilitating such growth. Quantity and quality of perceived spoken language from an early age correlate closely with linguistic and mental growth. Indeed, it is now widely accepted that language and thought (cognition) are closely related and that children's language in particular reflects their understanding of the world around them. Research on the application of government-binding theory to hearing- impaired children is to be expected in the years ahead, because many aspects of it can readily be examined through applied research.

The awareness of syntax that Chomsky's earlier work encouraged has been a significant force in the education of hearing-impaired children who have received formal teaching. It is generally accepted that mastery of the language requires that its syntactic rules must, in some sense, be known by a child. However, since Chomsky's first contribution to language theory, others have argued that syntax is not separable from semantics - that meaning in language is, indeed, more basic than syntax. Before moving into a brief discussion of semantics, however, let us be reminded of the fact that, next to poor speech, weaknesses in syntax are among the most common and serious problems in the expressive language of hearing-impaired children.

Perhaps the best way to deal with - or, better still, prevent - syntactic weaknesses, is to ensure that language is acquired primarily through meaningful communication about topics that are relevant to the child, and serve some evident purpose. The structure of language (its syntax), its meaning (semantic properties), and its purpose (pragmatic function), can all be integrated through communication. This approach is consistent with the view that children talk about their experiences using words and word-ordering rules that mark meaningful relationships between people and things in a consistent manner. These relationships can as easily be defined in semantic terms (agent action) as in a syntactic description (subject - verb).

semantics

The semantic aspect of a child's language is concerned with the use of meaningful referents. (For example, when we refer to a boy or a box, we use the words "boy" and "box" to refer to the actual person or thing. The words in this sense are referents.) Semantic properties exist at both word and sentence levels. At a word level, the semantic aspect (the meaning) resides in the morphemes mentioned above. In essence, word meanings are of the sort defined in dictionaries. At the sentence level, each word in the sentence must relate to every other word in a meaningful way, or the semantic intent of the sentence may be utterly obscured. This is why the semantic purpose of the incomplete sentences children produce at an early stage in their language development can be extremely difficult to interpret (see Figure 6-1). Of course, to encourage children in their early attempts to communicate, such utterances should be interpreted by caregivers through reference to the context in which they are produced. However inadequate the utterances children make, contexts usually allow adults or peers to interpret what is meant by them. Analysis of utterances produced in a variety of situations suggest that they closely reflect a child's organization of knowledge about self, other persons, objects, events and the relations among them.

Sentences can be classified according to their semantic content by specifying what sort of relationships exist between persons, objects, and events. The meaning of the terms used in semantic analysis become evident when one looks at the classifications of a sufficient number of different sentences. This is demonstrated by the semantic relationships specified in the following examples:

The girl ran (mover-action).

The horse grew (experiencer-process).

The house collapsed (patient-action).

The boat sank (patient-process).

Joan broke the window (agent-action-patient).

The brick broke the window (instrument-action-patient).

Jack planned his retirement (agent-action-complement).

Dan liked the violin (experiencer-process-patient).

Jane thought of a plan (experiencer-process-complement).

The man owns the cow (beneficiary-process-patient).

The garden needs rain (patient-process-instrument).

Joe Higgs is the professor (entity-stative-entity).

The garden is green (entity-stative-entity).

George is in the garden (entity-stative-locative).

George is late (entity-stative-temporal).

Garden produce is good for you (entity-stative-reason).

This produce is for Emily (entity-stative-beneficiary).

The examples above represent a range of the semantic relationships that is to be found in the sentences that make up our language. Mastery of spoken language requires that all of the semantic relationships illustrated in the above sentences be understood and used. The earliest and simplest of a child's utterances can be classified according to its semantic properties. Children start talking by using a few semantic classes, and then including more and more of them as they map language onto their experiences. The linguistic changes that occur as the child develops more complex forms of utterance is a product of the interaction between syntax (form) and semantics (meaning).

semantics and speech

Semantic notions are about meaning, and the use of suprasegmental cues - the tunes and rhythms that are intrinsic to an utterance - is one of the most important ways in which meaning can be - and usually is - enhanced in spoken language. Take, for example, the statement "The boy travelled by train to see the air show last week." Intonation and stress patterning can enhance different parts of the information it contains, namely about *who, how, why* and *when*. The vowels and the consonants are much less closely linked with meaning. Other than /z/ for the stative (as in "is"), there appear to be no particular speech sounds associated with any of the semantic classes.

pragmatics.

In a narrow linguistic sense, pragmatic concepts refer to the truth and logic of sentences, and how appropriate they are to the situation of a speaker. Here, the pragmatic aspects of language are treated in the broader, socio-linguistic sense to include the reasons for speaking, and the purposes that may underlie the production of an utterance. We use spoken language to encourage people to respond to us, and to influence their attitudes and actions.

There are many "pragmatic" ways in which such social purposes can be achieved. We question, we command, we express our needs, we answer, we call, we plead, we collaborate, we discuss, we inform, we protest, we repeat, we greet, we argue, and we demand attention; in short, we interact verbally in an enormous number of ways. Speech serves primarily social purposes, and there are social rules that govern most of the purposes for which language is used. If we are unaware of the logic of an utterance in relation to the particular situation of the speaker, we are likely to misunderstand it.

When we work to develop the use of speech by a hearing-impaired child, we must ensure that the pragmatic functions of the utterances produced by ourselves and the child reflect reality, and have social integrity. An example of communication failure that can result when pragmatic aspects are commonly ignored was once provided for me by a hearing-impaired child who, looking high in a cupboard for some chalk, turned and asked the teacher "Where should I look"? The teacher replied "Lower." The child's response was not to direct his gaze down, but to repeat the question in deeper-pitched voice. Such (perhaps less evident) misperceptions as to the purpose of spoken language commonly occur if pragmatic reality in everyday communication is not an integral part of the speech acquisition process.

pragmatics and speech

The context in which we teach speech, if speech is to be more than an exercise, must reflect the contexts in which spoken language will be used in everyday life. One of the reasons that speech skills taught in formal lessons are often not generalized (are not carried over into everyday use), is that many speech lessons do not incorporate the spoken language components that relate to the real life situations in which the child needs to communicate.

Formal lessons that involve development of phonetic level speech skills should be planned to begin and end with abundant communicative interaction between adult and child. Such interaction should take place in settings designed to provide experience of the various pragmatic functions of spoken language, and should include communicative use of the phonetic level skills featured in the lesson. A speech lesson in which a child only sits at a table and repeats sounds for analysis and reinforce-ment, either by a teacher or by a teaching machine, provides few if any opportunities for spoken language experiences that have social and pragmatic reality. Of course, the best contexts for developing the prag-matic functions of spoken language are those that occur in real life settings. Such settings usually feature a variety of places, activities, objects, and people.

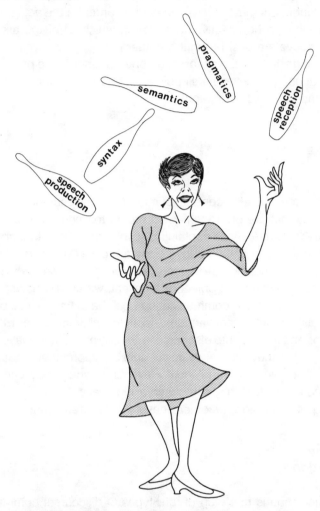

figure 6-3.   The juggler, in keeping several pins in motion, is represented as undertaking a task similar to that required of caregivers who are helping a hearing-impaired child to develop spoken language. Success requires that all the pins - all aspects of meaningful speech communication - receive attention.

No one aspect of spoken language should be promoted to the detriment of another. Just as speech reception and speech production are an integral part of spoken language, so are the syntactic, semantic, and pragmatic components of language inextricably linked. As the juggler depicted in Figure 6-3 suggests, all of the different pins (aspects of spoken language) must receive attention in order for the act (speech communication) to be effective. The way in which all of the aspects discussed above are best brought together is through discourse - the use of language that employs more than one sentence in the process of communication. The several well-defined forms of discourse are discussed in the following paragraphs.

discourse

Most communication consists of more than one sentence. Just as several words that are put together according to underlying rules are called sentences, utterances containing several sentences that are put together according to certain conventions are called discourse. When we engage in conversation, tell a story, ask for information, provide an explanation, or describe an object or an event, we usually use several sentences to achieve our communication goal. Each type of discourse follows a distinct set of conventions. To help children to learn these conventions and to enter into discourse in socially acceptable ways, one must ensure that they receive sufficient sensory information about the communicative events around them - events in which they can participate, and events that they can observe. Optimally selected and well-functioning hearing aids, or other sensory aids, are essential in this respect.

conversation

Conversation is made up of four types of discourse: comments, requests, acknowledgments, and answers. Conversation can involve every type of discourse, including narration, questions, explanations, and descriptions, but for the sake of clarity, and because it is important for parents and for professionals in the various types of programs to ensure that children develop skills in each aspect of discourse, we shall treat them separately below.

When we are engaged in conversation, we take turns with our listeners according to rules that permit it to be an effective and pleasurable activity. The first step is to establish contact by exchange of greetings. A topic is then introduced by a speaker, who ends the first segment of the exchange by signalling to a particular listener to carry on. The signal can be verbal or non-verbal. For example, the speaker may ask a question of a particular listener, and this effectively prohibits another listener from responding; or, alternatively, the speaker may glance at a listener and, by addressing the last sentence to that person, identify who is to make a response.

Should there be a sufficient gap at this point, another person may respond instead. The next turn goes back to the original speaker unless somebody else quickly intervenes. Such intervention is a delicate matter, and if it involves speaking over another participant, or jumping in too often, it is regarded as rudeness. Conversations move to a close, as do episodes within conversations, by a listener making a non-committal response, for example, "uh huh," or "I see!" This signal offers the speaker the chance to close the conversation by a similar response, and either to part by using a "goodbye" statement, or to move to a different topic. These conventions are widespread, and if they are ignored, the quality of conversation suffers, or communication simply fails to occur.

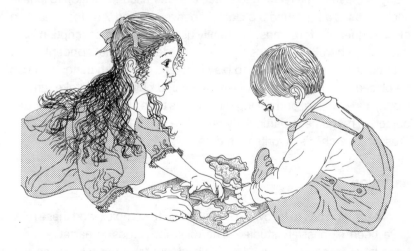

figure 6-4. **A young hearing-impaired child and his slightly older sister engaged in activities leading to the development of conversational skills.**

Conversational skills grow out of encouragement of children's vocalization and turn taking in the production of voice patterns long before first words are acquired. Once verbal interactions take place, conversation can be encouraged by responses to any utterance - acknowledgments with words or smiles, questions for clarification, or dropping one's own pursuits in order to join in those of the child. Conversation relating to a child's interests and pursuits is not normally limited to adult-child interaction; it is also to be observed and encouraged between children. It is particularly important to encourage conversation between hearing-impaired children and their normally hearing friends or siblings. This form of interaction, illustrated in Figure 6-4, is not only socially desirable; it can lead to significant advances in spoken language development.

description

Description tends to be more space oriented than time oriented. To describe a house, a room, or an object calls for definition of the position of one thing in relation to the position of others. This type of discourse also requires specific vocabulary, particularly prepositions, such as "near," "above," and "around," as well as "higher than" and "lower than." Many of these terms relating to space are later used in relation to time in such phrases as "around 5 o'clock," "between 6 and 7 o'clock," and so on. The question form most frequently used to clarify a description is, of course, "where?" An excellent way to develop the concepts and vocabulary for description is to play hide and seek with things that can be placed around the house. Caregivers and children can take turns in hiding and seeking, and asking for clues as to the location of the hidden objects. The game is particularly attractive when the hidden object is a present, or a child's favorite type of toy.

narration

Narration has to follow rules that are quite complex, and these rules have been extensively studied. The different stages in narration have been labelled as shown by the italicized words in the discussion that follows. To tell a story, one must begin by providing a *setting*, such as "Once upon a time there was...," or "When I was walking... ." Having begun, one must *initiate* the topic of interest, specify the *event* that makes the topic interesting, express the *internal* thoughts or feelings of those concerned, indicate the *response* to those thoughts or feelings, continue discussion of such *internal* thoughts or feelings, outline a *plan* of action for the character(s) in the story, give an *account* of the action taken and its *consequences* and, finally, state the *reactions* of the participants to the outcome, such as "and she felt very happy to see her mother again."

Narration can, of course, be a part of a conversation, as when a speaker recounts a personal experience. Children learn narration skills by having stories, or accounts of experiences not only told to them, but asked of them. Their initial attempts to tell stories, or to report experiences will not include all of the steps outlined above. Increasingly full narration will occur as children are asked questions (And then what did he do? How did he feel about that?), or provided with prompts (So then they were frightened, I suppose!) that help them to fill in the details.

Children's narration skills should be encouraged as soon as they are able to put a sentence together. They can begin with the chaining of sentences first with, and later without, the prompting of caregivers. Prompting and questioning by caregivers help children to begin to sequence their narratives according to the order in which events naturally take place. This stage is a very important part of children's acquisition of time-related concepts. Later, at about the same time that true "why" questions are being asked, causal relations can be expected in narration. The more cause and effect become part of narration, the more interesting it becomes. There are three important ways in which caregivers and professionals can encourage children's development of narration skills: the first is to provide them with commentaries about events as they unfold in real life; the second is to ensure that they are given the variety of experiences (accompanied by commentaries) that they need so that they come to understand the world around them; and the third is to read stories in abundance so that the inherent structures of narration can be derived by the children from the numerous examples provided for them (see Figure 6-2).

questions

A question may be considered as discourse even if it is formed from a single sentence. This is because a question requires an answer of at least another sentence. Questions are best treated as a means of seeking new information. The person using questions simply to elicit a response from a child, and not to acquire new information, may be providing that child with a misconception about the purpose of questioning. For example, questions, such as "What color is that?", are not appropriate if it is clear to the child that the questioner knows the answer. Getting a child to name a color or an object can be just as effectively done by using ellipsis (deliberate omission of a word or words), as in "That's a green one, that's a red one, and that's _____." This technique tends to elicit responses that are longer, and just as accurate, without confusing the child as to the purpose for which questions are used.

Children develop the ability to use questions according to the difficulty of the concepts that underlie them. Thus "who" and "what" questions are fairly concrete compared with the more abstract "when," "how," and "why" questions. They tend, therefore, to develop sooner. A wide variety of questions can be developed by playing guessing games with a child. For example, the adult can hide objects or pictures, and encourage the child to ask questions in order to identify the object or the content of the picture. Children and adults can take turns at hiding and asking, so that the question forms become familiar to the children, and both understood and used by them effectively. Everyday experiences also offer many opportunities for the development of all sorts of question forms.

The most appropriate way for children to learn how to question is for caregivers to use questions in their conversations with their children. Questions should be asked that fit the situation regardless of whether or not children can understand them for, over time, the context in which they are asked will lend them meaning (e.g., "Are you hungry?" "What would you like to eat?" "Do you want some more?" "Who is that at the door?" "Would you like ... or ....?" "When will you play with Joe?" "How did you hurt yourself?" "Why do you want that one?"). Also, if there is doubt that the child understands particular questions, one can simply provide the answers. (e.g., "Where's your coat?" "Oh! Here it is in the cupboard!"). Initially, one must be more concerned with children's experience of questions than with their complete understanding of them, for experience has to come before meaning can be deduced. Experience in questioning can also be provided by having the child relay questions to another member of the family (e.g., "Go and ask Daddy where he put the hammer. Say 'Daddy, where did you put the hammer?' O.K. Off you go.") The type and complexity of questions can be extended as the child's competence increases.

explanation

Explanations involve the ability to recall a sequence of happenings. This form of discourse can be developed only when the child has a sufficient concept of time in relation to events, and a quite specific time-related vocabulary. To explain how to do something, for example how to make lemonade, or how to put a model together, calls for sequences, such as "First...", "then...", "and after that...", "but before...", and so on. Certain forms of explanation also require the concepts and vocabulary in relation to cause and effect. The question forms most likely to be used to clarify such explanations are "how?" and "when?"

Directions on how to get from one place to another are closely related to both explanation and description. They demand concepts of both space and time; for example, "after ten minutes, you take a right turn towards the church." Ability to give and to follow directions involves advanced skills.

cohesion in discourse

There are many devices used to hold sentences in discourse together, whether the discourse is on an aspect mentioned above, or whether it is a discussion, a monologue, a lecture, or a debate. Sentences in discourse are held together by anaphora (making a sentence relate to a previous utterance: for example, by using pronouns, such as *she*, *they*, *his*, and *its*; and conjunctions or disjunctions, such as *and*, *so*, and *but*). Unless sentences in discourse are given such cohesion, they become disjointed, and the discourse is rendered inefficient, or fails. Children learn devices that lend cohesion to language by being exposed to them, and by being expected to use them. Just as hearing- impaired children may fail to acquire sentence grammar if they are exposed to just single words, or phrases of only a few words, so will they fail to absorb the rules of different forms of discourse if the focus in communication is mainly or exclusively at a single sentence level.

speech patterns in discourse

The suprasegmental patterns of speech are of great importance, and they help to determine how successfully some aspects of discourse are used. Very different stress and intonation patterns are usually employed in explanations, descriptions, stories, questions, and conversations. All speech patterns (suprasegmentals, vowels, consonants, and blends) are required in discourse, but some consonants are more frequently encountered in certain aspects than in others. For example, the /w/ and the /h/ are very common in questioning. To point this out is not to suggest that spontaneous discourse should be used for formal speech development lessons. The purpose of discourse is to interact meaningfully. If speech teaching and speech correction are imposed in such interactions, a child's development of discourse skills will not be optimally encouraged. Children's approximations to adult speech patterns should be accepted unless repair to utterances is essential for understanding the content of the communication. The primary objective of speech communication is to produce and to understand spoken messages effectively. Acceptable pronunciation of speech patterns is but a means to this end.

learning spoken language

normal language acquisition

Normally hearing children usually acquire all of their speech, and most of their language, informally. As argued in the next chapter, it is learned rather than taught. Children respond to sounds differentially from birth, and rapidly associate speech with meaning. Hungry young babies will, for example, look for food when a cup from which they have been fed is stirred with the usual spoon; quiet down when mother, not a stranger, speaks from another room; and choose to ignore sounds that have no personal meaning for them. They search for meaning in the sounds around them from the earliest moments of life, and this search is enhanced through their interaction with caring adults in their environment.

Not only do very young babies recognize differences between and among sounds, they also produce differences as they cry from discomfort, vocalize in anticipation of a routine event, and gurgle with pleasure. Later on, they babble a wide range of sounds that they will come to use in their spoken language. Both speech perception and speech production have their foundations in these behaviors. It is also in the context of the routines of their early life that hearing-impaired babies begin to differentiate objects and events, as well as sounds, and gain their initial concepts of the world around them. One of the many familiar routine situations that offers abundant opportunities for parental commentary and the encouragement of a child's vocalization is depicted in Figure 6-5 in which the mother is (a) bathing and (b) drying her hearing-impaired baby. Note that the baby's hearing aid is worn through both operations, and that only perceptual-oral communication can be used in the course of such activities.

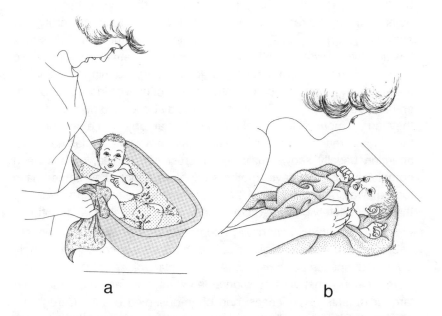

a   b

figure 6-5.   Communication taking place as a mother: (a) bathes and (b) dries her hearing-impaired baby.

Concepts can only develop when children begin to perceive that the world around them is relatively stable, and that it offers a range of experiences relating to objects and events that have consistent features. Such awareness of environment must be present before any child can begin to understand the nature of objects and events, what they mean, and what sound and/or speech patterns go together with them. At first, of course, all babies' interests are limited to their internal needs, but this changes quickly, and within a few months normal babies and their mothers spend a great deal of time sharing their attention to, and communicating about, externally located objects and activities that clearly captivate the babies' attention. Professionals should determine whether mothers of hearing-impaired children do spontaneously share attention to things with their children and, if they do not, help them to relate with them in this way.

All communication is accomplished through sharing. Sharing between babies and their mothers is achieved through mothers' attending to what their babies are gazing at, reaching for (later pointing towards), and vocalizing about. Mothers talk mainly about things that interest their babies. They talk while sharing their gaze, as they hand them nearby objects, and as they attend to their needs. Mothers straightforwardly, and apparently correctly, infer from the beginning that their children's acts towards things external call for them to communicate about them while they are looking at them. What the child is seeing, touching, or tasting is enhanced by a *simultaneous* commentary. Not until children are considerably older, and spoken language is already becoming meaningful, do they turn to mothers for verbal comment on an object or an event. Until this stage is reached, babies' turning away from whatever has held their attention usually shows that their interest has waned, or has been completely lost. Whatever mothers might say once their babies have turned away may, therefore, be less relevant to their language learning than incompletely perceived commentary that parallels their attention.

Spoken language normally becomes a familiar accompaniment to babies' attention. As caregivers talk to them, they become increasingly aware that speech patterns, not just particular voices or tones of voice, have meaning; that, to a considerable extent, familiar words map onto familiar objects, experiences, and often-observed events. Caregivers' commentaries about objects and events given as they and their children share attention to them is the major force in helping children to begin breaking the language code that does, indeed, become their mother tongue. (Language is, indeed, a code - words can be used merely to refer to, or describe, external objects, events, or features; they are not, themselves, the things to which they refer).

Speech that is addressed to a child after the event is less meaningful than speech that goes on as the child's attention is focused on it. Providing that the hearing-impaired children are able to perceive caregivers' voices, differentiate most vowels, and recognize some consonants through hearing or other sensory aids, caregivers' commentaries without speechreading can often become just as meaningful to them as they are to normally hearing babies. Even profoundly hearing-impaired children who need speechreading to make sense of what is said, need voice contact in the early stages of communication *while they are attending to objects and events*. Such contact is likely to provide a better base for their spoken language development than waiting until their attention can be fully focused on what their caregivers want to say.

Once children have developed awareness of the meaning embedded in mothers' vocal commentaries, understand that objects do not disappear when their gaze is averted, and begin to vocalize in response to stimuli, they begin to alternate visual attention between things that command their interest and their mothers' faces. At this stage they also begin to point to things of interest as they vocalize. Only from then on can mothers' parallel (ongoing) commentaries on objects and events become less frequent, and serial (separate and later) commentaries begin. Together with use of first words, mother-child communication that follows shared attention to an object or event, signals the onset of dialogue and the beginning of turn-taking.

All language learning must initially be focused on concrete experience. For babies, it is usually exclusively related to what is present and ongoing in their immediate environment. The environment provides a context for the sound patterns, vocabulary, and sentence structures of their mother tongue, and it is this context that allows the children to find meaning in what is said and discover for themselves how language codes work.

Once sufficient language has been acquired in immediate contexts, children discover that it can be used in slightly modified forms to refer to less immediate contexts, namely familiar experiences that have just completed or are about to take place. Eventually, through stages where it relates to situations that are more and more distant in both space and time, language develops to the point where it can be used without the support provided by situational contexts. At this stage, children can display their imagination by beginning to use more abstract language.

Children do not readily develop abstract thinking, and abstract language to accompany it, unless they have had extensive opportunities to manipulate language in more concrete contexts at an earlier stage. For example, unless they can verbalize about being in a bath, in a car, or in any given location, they cannot be expected to use the same sort of language to specify the closely related but more abstract notions of being in a muddle, in a hurry, or in a rage. Nor can they express having more concern about one thing than another if they have not had a verbal concept relating to such experiences as wanting more candy or more ice-cream. Further discussion of the concrete foundations required for the development of abstract notions will be provided in the section on formal language teaching in the next chapter.

early language and hearing impairment

Language development tends to be delayed among hearing-impaired children because they tend to receive spoken language patterns that are distorted in some way. For some children, whole syllables or words may be missing from an utterance addressed directly to them. Even more of an utterance addressed to others may not be perceived at all. Such impoverished speech reception can be a great disadvantage, because many normally hearing children learn much about language and the way it is used in conversation by overhearing the people who talk in their presence. Be that as it may, opportunities for learning spoken language at a very early age can be provided for most hearing-impaired children through the use of techniques described in this book (see Chapter 7).

Language can more easily be learned informally by younger than by older children. When children learn language in relation to the context of their ongoing real-life experiences during infancy, words become an integral part of their concepts. In contrast, when children acquire their verbal skills in later childhood, the language related to the objects and activities with which they have been familiar from early childhood rarely becomes an intrinsic part of their conceptual development. This disadvantage is reflected in the difficulty that many hearing-impaired children who are late starters experience in dealing with abstract notions and abstract language.

Language learning, regardless of a child's age, must be supported by good audiological services, and by collaboration between professionals and parents. Language learning among young children can best be promoted through caregivers who are with them for most of their waking hours. To promote language learning among older children may, however, require the best efforts of both parents and professionals. As more formal language teaching is introduced, a greater amount of direct attention from professionals is inevitably required. Strategies to encourage the learning of spoken language are best applied in an environment where most of a hearing-impaired child's peers communicate by speech.

Hearing-impaired children attending some special schools are expected, from an early age, to learn more of their language through reading and writing than through speech communication. Some such children - those who are unable to obtain sufficient sensory information about speech - may need print and writing coupled with formal speech teaching in order to lay the foundations for later speech communication. But they are a minority. Language development among hearing-impaired children usually benefits to a greater extent from verbal interaction than from desk-top teaching, however carefully structured that interaction has to be. If formal strategies are unnecessarily adopted in a school, they can inhibit rather than enhance spoken language development. It is through speech communication rather than through the written form that language learning is best fostered in the early years of schooling. Basic reading and writing skills should, to the greatest extent possible, be related to spoken language skills that are already acquired. Reading instruction does not provide an optimal framework for language growth among children whose language skills are delayed or deviant at the outset.

Reading is a poor means of acquiring initial language skills. To learn a significant amount of language through reading, children must already have basic visual word recognition skills, a good vocabulary, an awareness of syntactic rules, understanding of the semantic properties of words and sentences, and extensive experience of the world around them. Only if such knowledge and skills are present can children search a text for meaning and extend their understanding of the conventions of language for themselves. Many academic subjects, as well as social situations, can provide opportunities for interactive communication with the teacher, and it is such interaction rather than attention to paper and print that should be made the major feature in education programs for children with impoverished language.

Reading is also a poor means of acquiring speech and spoken language. To relate speech sounds (phonemes) to written letters (graphemes) is to teach the false notion that speech is a series of distinct sounds, when in fact it is a stream of blended sounds. To use early reading as a means of teaching speech is to overload the child with two unmastered tasks: reading and speaking. Such overload destroys the rhythm and cadences of speech that are so essential to its intelligibility. Reading aloud before speech is mastered also has adverse effects on the acquisition of reading skills because reading practice should be primarily aimed at helping the child to obtain meaning from the written form. Adequate attention cannot be given to the meaning of a written passage if children have to concentrate mainly on how they are pronouncing it. This is a poor teaching practice known as "barking at print."

In reading and in the reception of spoken language, it is important that most - perhaps as much as 95 percent - of the material presented is understood by a child. Caregivers may well question this statement, and ask, " If this is so, then how can children ever learn to make sense of either spoken or written language?" The answer lies in the proportion of comprehension that is contributed by context.

In acquiring spoken language, all children are spoken to by adults who use words that initially mean nothing to them. However, *the intent of a communicative act can be clearly understood in the absence of word knowledge if sufficient contextual cues are present.* The context surrounding (i.e., external to) the communication in such a case contributes all that is necessary for the child's deduction of its meaning. Even the tone of a parent's voice can convey sufficient information for a child to understand the intent of a message. As spoken language develops, less and less external context is required to provide the necessary clues to meaning because more and more of the actual words in an utterance are understood. A similar situation exists with reading.

Only when children have enough knowledge of the words used in a text, and can draw sufficiently on their knowledge of the world around them, can they be expected to understand a text. The introduction of too many unfamiliar words can destroy comprehension, even in the presence of such external context as explanatory pictures. Text based on topics of interest involving familiar concepts can assist children in their early steps towards reading. However, at all stages they must be able to interpret the meaning of the few new words that are introduced in a text in the light of previously known vocabulary, language knowledge, and life experience if reading skills are to grow. Talking effectively to hearing-impaired children, and ensuring the development of their reading skills both depend, therefore, on presenting them with enough that is new to challenge them, and on ensuring that they have sufficient context of one sort or another to permit them to derive its meaning.

Once reading, language, and cognitive skills have progressed beyond a certain stage, children's linguistic achievements can be enormously increased by silent reading. Indeed, an explosion of language and thinking skills is frequently encountered once children can do grade-three- and grade-four-level work. The ability not just to read, but to learn through reading should be expected by teachers of normally hearing and hearing-impaired children at and beyond these grade levels. An explosion of language and thought can only come about when children have first obtained an adequate foundation for the abstract notions they will meet in various texts. This foundation can only be ensured through providing the child with extensive experience of communicative and, to a lesser extent written, language in its more concrete forms. The concrete bases of abstract language and thought will be discussed further in the sections on formal language teaching in the following chapter.

suggestions for further reading

Several introductory texts on the psychology of language and normal language acquisition are available. Those that have had, or are having, significant influence in the education of hearing-impaired children (though not written specifically with this group in mind) include books by Blank, Rose and Berlin (1978), Bloom and Lahey (1978) Clark and Clark (1977), Fletcher and Garman (1986), Owens (1988), Pinker (1984), and Snow and Ferguson (1977). The communication of infants during their pre-speech years has been discussed by Bullowa (1979).

Parental involvement in language development for children with various types of language disorders has been addressed in several books, outstanding among which are Bromwich (1981), Fey (1986), and Rees (1984).

Ling and Ling (1971) provide a helpful vocabulary and language thesaurus that lists five thousand words commonly used by young children by situational contexts met in everyday life.

The works on syntax by Chomsky (1957; 1981) mentioned in this chapter are both highly technical and theoretical. Easier reading about modern work on syntax is provided by Hyams (1986) who proposes ways in which Chomsky's theories can be examined through research with children. The acquisition of syntax among hearing-impaired children is discussed by Kretschmer and Kretschmer (1978), Quigley (1978), and Quigley and Paul (1984). The importance of suprasegmentals to various aspects of spoken language is discussed by Crystal (1981), and scales for the assessment of simple and complex sentences produced by hearing impaired children have been prepared by Moog and Geers (1975; 1979; 1980; 1983).

Semantic theories and semantic analyses applicable to hearing-impaired children are also discussed in Kretschmer and Kretschmer (1978). Pragmatic issues in relation to assessment and intervention (but not with hearing-impaired children) are extensively treated in Gallagher and Prutting (1983).

Cohesion in discourse has been discussed by Halliday and Hasan (1976), propositions in discourse and their meaningful representation in memory have been discussed by Kintsch (1974), and the social implications of discourse have been more recently considered by Stubbs (1983). An interdisciplinary journal for the study of discourse entitled *TEXT* has been published by Mouton since 1981.

The development of various aspects of language through conversation with hearing-impaired children of various ages is discussed extensively by Van Uden (1980).

The development of spoken language by hearing-impaired children in the pre-school period has been discussed in a very readable text by Grant (1987). Spoken language acquisition through interaction with young children is particularly well addressed by various authors in a book edited by Ling (1984a), which includes chapters by Beebe, Pearson and Koch, by Clezy, by Cole and Paterson, and by Pollack. Cole and Gregory (1986) describe stategies for both development and assessment of emerging language.

Various language curricula used in school programs for hearing-impaired children are reviewed in Bunch (1987), and teaching practices that may enhance or impede the development of spoken language of hearing-impaired children during their early years in school have been insightfully addressed by Wood, Wood, Griffiths and Howarth (1986). See References, pp. 433 ff.

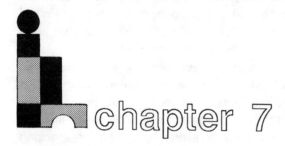

chapter 7

informal learning
and formal teaching

introduction

Helping hearing-impaired children to acquire spoken language is a task that can be carried out with emphasis on informal learning, formal teaching, or a mixture of the two. Whichever way one choses to work, the goal is the same: *to develop children's spoken language so that they can communicate effectively and intelligibly with those around them.* The range of knowledge and skills that children have to acquire in order to achieve spoken language are also the same: *they must learn to understand and use well-formulated sentences in all aspects of discourse.*

informal learning and formal teaching

For the purposes of this chapter, *learning* will be regarded as something done by the child, and *teaching* will be considered as whatever a parent, clinician, teacher, or other adult does to assist the child in the learning process. Both learning and teaching can be informal, in that one can learn or teach as a by-product of an apparently unrelated activity; or formal, in that one can deliberately set out to learn or teach something in a direct and methodical manner. This chapter, for reasons given below, will be concerned with informal learning and formal teaching. *Informal learning* will be treated as something that children do without deliberately giving it attention. In contrast, *formal teaching* will be defined as specific, goal-oriented, educational and therapeutic practices consciously adopted and applied by professionals.

Of course, formal learning and informal teaching can also be observed. For example, children of a certain age can consciously set out to understand and solve a problem or acquire particular knowledge (for example dates in history) through formal learning. This sort of learning is, however, more appropriate for acquiring facts than for acquiring speech communication skills. Informal teaching also occurs, and includes the practices parents commonly engage in to promote their children's learning in everyday situations. Such informal teaching is, without doubt, one of the most important components of child rearing. This chapter, however, suggests ways in which both parents and professionals can enhance a child's learning of specific speech and language skills. So, while the importance of formal learning and informal teaching are recognized, neither will be considered in any detail in the following paragraphs.

To enhance a child's learning of spoken language through either informal learning or formal teaching, the adults concerned must provide carefully structured situations that promote the acquisition of speech-communication skills. This means that they must plan activities - and, above all, social interactions - to achieve selected and specific goals. The targeted behaviors in such activities must provide a base for the child's further development, and consolidate previously learned skills. The adults must monitor the child's progress, and base their future activities on what the child has achieved as a result of their efforts.

To structure learning opportunities, or to teach to a plan, does not imply the imposition of a dull and restrictive regimen. To promote informal learning, caregivers can lend emphasis to various aspects of interaction in some way. For example, informal learning can be promoted by:

- ensuring optimal acoustic or alternative sensory input;
- engaging the child as frequently as possible in verbal activities;

- introducing new vocabulary or concepts in the course of everyday living;
- providing the child with a range of vivid, different experiences that contrast with everyday living, and extend vocabulary; and by
- using every opportunity to respond in an appropriate way to the child's verbalizations during activities.

Informal learning usually begins in the home as a result of one-on-one parent-child interaction, whereas formal teaching is usually carried out in an educational setting (clinic or school) by one or more professionals interacting with one or more children. Whether the child is being helped to acquire spoken language predominantly through informal learning or formal teaching, skillful guidance should be available to parents or other caregivers if optimal progress is to result.

Some children's needs are best met through informal programs, and others are best catered to in more formal ones. Neither type of program alone can possibly meet the needs of all children at all stages of their development. Young children, and those who have mild or moderate hearing impairments, generally benefit most from informal strategies; and, through informal learning, most such children can reach linguistic milestones at an appropriate time. Those who are older and have the most severe hearing impairments usually need more formal programs. They may take considerably longer than normally hearing children to acquire their language. The majority of children who have more than moderate hearing impairment require a mix of both types of input. It is not unusual for children to need brief spells of formal teaching in order to acquire particular skills that they would otherwise fail to learn or take longer than necessary to master.

choosing between formal and informal strategies.

There are no generally accepted guidelines for the selection of formal over informal strategies or *vice versa*. Some hearing-impaired children may, therefore, find themselves in programs that needlessly permit them to develop faulty patterns of spoken language that, over time, become habitual because the professionals working with them either do not know how to use formal procedures, or are averse to using them. At the other end of the continuum, formal speech teaching may be premature if attempted with young hearing-impaired children when they have not yet developed even the most elementary concepts about spoken language, or a drive to communicate through its use. As a rule of thumb, formal procedures for teaching any aspect of spoken language should be adopted only if a child does not acquire it within a reasonable time frame when given optimal opportunities to do so in the course of everyday living and learning. The need for formal teaching is thus likely to differ from child to child. It might also be needed at different stages of a particular child's development. The following discussion is not, there-fore, aimed at promoting one type of strategy to the detriment of another, but rather at promoting the more widespread use of the most suitable procedures - those that can best meet each child's needs.

In this chapter, both the similarities and differences between infor-mal and formal procedures for developing speech and spoken language will be explored, and some assumptions relating to current clinical and educational practices for the development of verbal behaviors will be discussed. It will be stressed that all informal learning or formal teaching must be supported by the consistent use of appropriate sensory aids - hearing aids, tactile devices or cochlear implants - in an environment in which speech is a major mode of communication. It will be proposed that young children (certainly those from zero to four years, and probably those from zero to six years), should initially learn through the use of informal strategies; that the formal teaching of both speech and language skills should broadly reflect normal sequences of acquisition (the hierar-chy of skills that is to be observed among normally hearing children); and that all skills, whether developed through informal or formal strategies, should be integrated into real-life communicative interactions as they are acquired. It will also be suggested that formal teaching, when appropriate, will allow us to reduce the period otherwise required to attain successive benchmarks of spoken language development, and to elevate the levels of its mastery above those generally achieved by hearing-impaired children.

factors influencing progress

The major factors influencing the achievement of perceptual-oral and educational skills - progress through speech communication - can be considered under three headings, as shown in Figure 7-1. Some are intrinsic to each child and cannot be either changed or greatly improved through direct intervention. These include hearing levels, visual acuity, age at onset of hearing impairment, and so on. Other factors involve abilities that we want the child to acquire - abilities that are the focus of the informal learning opportunities that we provide for the child, or of the formal teaching that we undertake. They include auditory, visual, and tactile skills, different aspects of spoken language skills, academic knowledge, thinking skills, and personal/social skills.

INTRINSIC FACTORS	ACQUIRED ABILITIES	EXTRINSIC AND INTERACTIVE FACTORS
hearing levels	auditory skills	hearing aids cochlear implants
visual acuity	visual skills	glasses
	auditory-visual skills	
tactile acuity	tactile speech reception	tactile devices
		socio-educational experience
	language comprehension	environmental communication modes
age at onset of hearing impairment	language expression	parental collaboration
	speech skills	
neurological status	academic attainments	teacher/clinician competence
intellectual potential	thinking skills	adjustment of child
	personal/social skills	child's contact with peers
		child's cognitive functioning

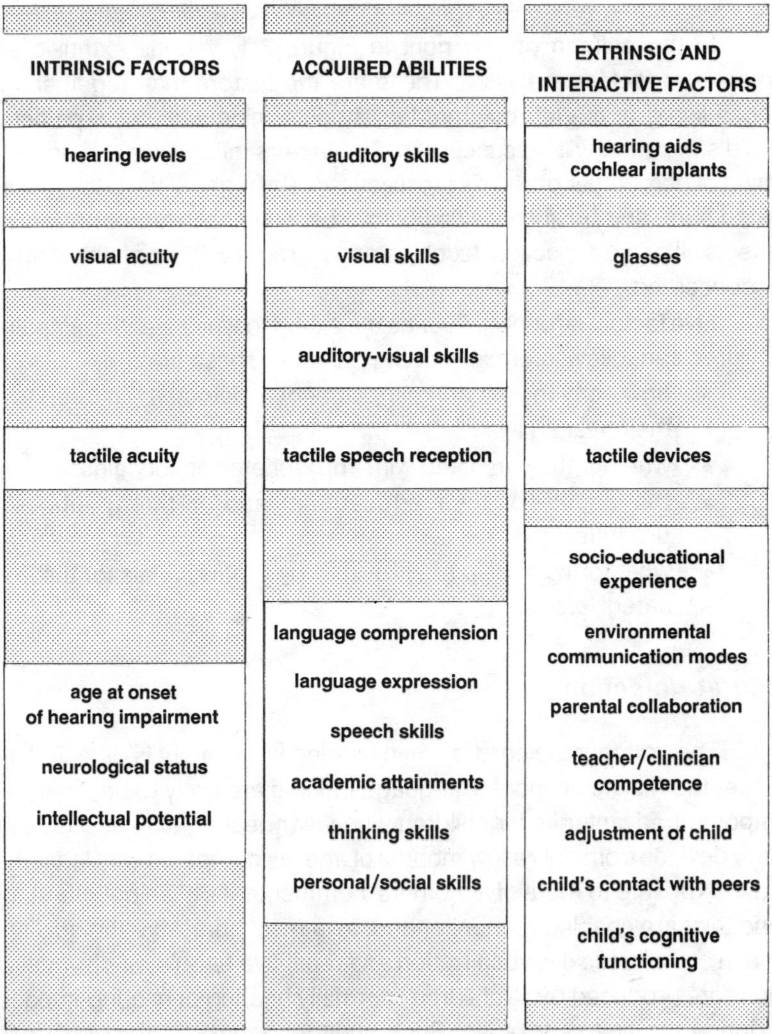

figure 7-1. **Factors influencing the development of perceptual-oral skills.**

In order for each one of these aspects of development to receive appropriate attention, one must evaluate and plan educational and therapeutic programs according to the demonstrated needs of each individual child. It is tempting to overlook the overall needs of a child as a whole being when dealing with the prevention or remediation of a deficit that threatens his or her development. However, the whole child is not only more important than his or her sensory impairment, but the effectiveness of a program for a special child will depend on the extent of consideration given to all aspects of that child's development.

In the column on the right in Figure 7-1, various extrinsic and interactive factors are listed. These are the factors that, together with those listed in the left column, largely determine whether a particular child's program will be successful. The factors influencing the development of perceptual-oral skills are discussed throughout the book, but are listed here, and briefly reviewed below, because each factor profoundly affects all of the aspects of teaching and learning with which this chapter is concerned.

Five factors strongly influence the extent to which hearing-impaired children can follow informal learning patterns. These are :

- how early their hearing impairment is detected;
- their hearing levels;
- whether they are fitted with appropriate sensory aids;
- the quality of their educational and/or therapeutic programs;
- what forms of help are provided by professionals for the caregivers.

age at detection.

The younger the child is when hearing impairment is detected, the better the results of spoken language training are likely to be. There are important advantages for children who wear hearing aids or other sensory devices from only a few months of age, as compared with later: they have exposure to more of a mothers' commentaries at an optimal stage; and they are enabled to monitor and, as a result, preserve the quality of much of their reflexive vocalization and repetitive babble. Such vocalizations are produced by all children - normally hearing or hearing-impaired - during the first year of life. Such auditory access to their own early utterances promotes their production of an extended range of vocalization, provides them with the essential foundations for feedback on the quality of their voices, and ensures that spoken language is an integral part of their overall development.

Most children who start using hearing aids or other sensory aids during or after the second year of life can also be expected to benefit from informal language learning in the context of everyday activities, particularly those that take place in their homes. Indeed, it is rare to find children of less than three years of age who can profit more from formal than from informal teaching in any environment. Even beyond age three, most children continue to require extensive exposure to the acoustic riches associated with the routines of life at home. Experiences based on daily living within a family usually contain a wealth of opportunity for children of all ages to extend their understanding of the language that surrounds them. This is not to say that it is advisable to postpone habilitation. There are, as shown below, good reasons to avoid such a delay.

Children who are not aided until after their first birthdays have missed an enormous quantity of auditory experience of their own and others' voices. They have also begun to learn how to live without spoken language. Additionally, children have fewer opportunities to listen to speech under ideal acoustic conditions after their first year. Children over one year of age usually move over considerable distances without help from or contact with their mothers. They therefore tend to have less speech addressed to them at close quarters.

To compensate for these differences, situations must be created that will allow older children to experience the quantity and quality of sound patterns to which younger children are normally exposed. Creating such situations does not call for formal work. Quite the reverse. It demands only that activities in and around the home become structured in ways that provide such children with more intensive and extensive natural learning opportunities.

The older children are before they are given the opportunity to begin acquiring spoken language, the less likely it is that informal learning will be sufficient to permit its spontaneous development. Children appear either to learn language spontaneously with relative ease as a result of having the right amount and the right sort of early experience, or to struggle with language acquisition through many years of formal teaching. Just as a child's body, given appropriate physical conditions, will grow because it is genetically programmed to do so, so it seems a child's mind will grasp language during the early years, providing the necessary conditions are present. True, no one has yet been able to specify what all of the essential conditions for spontaneous language acquisition are, but the child's age at first exposure to speech communication is certainly one of the most important.

hearing levels

If diagnosis is made sufficiently early, children with aided hearing levels that permit the reception of most speech sounds, can follow a virtually normal path of spoken language development. They may need no specific training to do this. The benefits of early, informal learning experiences need not, however, be limited to those with moderate or severe hearing impairment. During their early years, profoundly hearing-impaired children are equally good candidates for the provision of informal learning opportunities if, as suggested above, opportunities are structured to enhance their perception of spoken language.

Many children who have unaided hearing levels in excess of 90 dB can hear a great deal of speech when they are appropriately aided (see Chapter 4). The relatively small number of children who are near-totally or totally deaf may also become spontaneously aware of speech and other sounds in their environment when fitted with devices such as cochlear implants or tactile devices (see Chapter 5). The key to providing appropriate sensory experience for profoundly hearing-impaired children with useful residual audition is to structure their acoustic environments so that they are consistently within earshot of the acoustic events created by sound producing objects and talkers around them. When situated relatively close to the source of a sound or to a talker, or provided with a hearing aid coupled to an FM unit, speech patterns will be detectable to most of them. Speech may not be as distinct to them as to less severely hearing-impaired children, but much of it can, nevertheless, be rendered perceptible to them in one way or another, as the strategies described in this book clearly show.

sensory aids

Hearing aids can provide sufficient sensory input for the development of spoken language by most hearing-impaired children. Some such children may benefit from FM units as a supplement or as an alternative to their personal hearing aids in certain circumstances. Aided hearing levels that permit the various components of speech to be perceived were discussed in Chapter 4 and will receive no further comment here. For a minority of hearing-impaired children, cochlear implants or tactile devices will be required. Whatever type of instrument is used, additional information on spoken language will normally be supplied by speechreading (see Chapter 5). Children using any of the available types of sensory aids effectively may be expected, within the first year or so of obtaining them, to develop spoken language skills that reflect the amount of information their devices provide. For most, available devices should permit the development of voice patterns that vary at least in intensity and time, several vowels, and some clear words. Some of the words may not be as well formed as those produced by children who have less or no hearing impairment to contend with, but they should be close approximations to adult forms of speech, and appear within a stream of sentence-like utterances.

When left to assimilate what they can from an unstructured environment, profoundly hearing-impaired children wearing either hearing aids, cochlear implants, or tactile devices are not exposed to enough acoustic information for them ever to make sense of it. Children whose aided hearing levels do not permit them to detect sounds across the complete speech frequency range (e.g. those with no hearing beyond 1000 Hz) have to speechread as well as listen in order to differentiate among spoken language patterns (see Chapters 5, 10 and 11). Structuring situations so that the children can be within earshot of the caregiver, and can also see what or who is producing the sounds of interest is an essential step in providing them with the foundations for acquiring all aspects of spoken language. Ensuring that appropriate sensory aids are being well used, suggesting activities that relate to each individual child's levels of development, and helping parents to structure home situations appropriately while still preserving informal learning opportunities are among the most important contributions professionals can make in the habilitation of young and profoundly hearing-impaired children.

program quality

Program quality depends on abundant and systematic stimulation of each child. These are the essential foundations of any program aimed at the promotion and maintenance of cognitive growth and spoken language development. Four factors contribute to such stimulation: the knowledge and skills of the habilitation specialist (teacher or clinician), the full and vigorous participation of the parents and/or other caregivers, ongoing diagnostic teaching, and ready access to audiological services.

The knowledge and skills of the professional engaged in the task of developing spoken language skills in young hearing-impaired children must derive from an extensive theoretical base, and sufficient practical experience of working with children and with caregivers. Both professionals and parents must come to know how best to promote the optimal development of each child, and to expect their work to achieve the desired results. Without the confidence that perceptual-oral work will succeed, success cannot be expected. Such confidence can only be developed through ongoing diagnostic teaching, the outcome of which is used to guide each successive stage of spoken language development. Ready access to audiology services is a key element in high-quality parent-infant or school-based programs. This access is essential (see Chapters 4 and 5) because:

- ongoing selection of a hearing aid may have to be pursued;
- children's hearing levels are subject to change, and adjustments may have to be made to the hearing aids or other sensory device;
- rapid physical development affects how well earmolds fit, so earmolds may have to be changed;
- the performance of hearing aids may change due to their relative fragility. It is, therefore, important to have frequent and objective checks carried out to ensure their proper function; and
- a more appropriate hearing aid or an alternative or additional sensory device may have to be fitted.

Audiological services help professionals and parents meet the problem of hearing impairment head on - by direct prevention or reduction of the handicapping condition, and not by circumvention. Helping hearing-impaired children to use their residual audition and/or other senses to perceive and produce speech is the skilled audiologist's first concern. High-quality audiology programs, as well as extensive collaboration between audiologists and aural habilitation specialists (teachers or clinicians), are basic to the development and maintenance

of effective perceptual-oral skills. Such concern and collaboration ensures that each child is regularly evaluated. Without regular evaluation,
one cannot determine whether a child is responding as well as can be
expected to the wide range of acoustic stimuli present both in treatment
sessions and in everyday life.

forms of help provided in early habilitation

To facilitate young children's overall development, including their
communicative skills, three main avenues of support for parents must be
provided: counselling, education, and guidance.

Through counselling, parents of younger children can more readily
come to understand and accept the problems of hearing impairment.
Such acceptance is essential if they are to forge strong emotional bonds
with their children - bonds that provide the trust and self- assurance that
permit youngsters to explore and assimilate knowledge from the world
around them.

Education about hearing impairment cannot be successfully undertaken until parents voluntarily embark on a search for information. At
that point, they will look to the teacher or clinician serving as the aural
habilitation specialist to present the facts and implications relating to their
child's hearing handicap.

Most parents need a considerable amount of guidance in order to
ensure that specific day-to-day management of their child results in
progress. Guidance should include explanations and demonstrations of
strategies that can be used to promote particular skills, provide support
in the pursuit of a course of action, and offer opportunities to share any
problems encountered. Through guidance, parents can receive and
generate ideas on appropriate toys and activities that can help, and be
encouraged to involve themselves in new and appropriate activities at
each new stage of their child's development. Guidance can also help
parents and/or other caregivers become sensitive observers and accurate reporters.

For various reasons, some parents may not be able to help their
children to benefit sufficiently from the many advantages that early
home-based learning can afford. Single and working mothers have
particular difficulties in this regard. In such cases, professionals may have
to provide direct teaching services for the children in addition to counselling, education, and guidance for the parents. Depending on the needs

of the children, such teaching may be provided in either regular or special classes. Children who are placed in integrated settings with normally hearing children are expected to be able to learn both formally in set lessons, and informally at all other times. Children in special classes may also be able to learn informally, but such placements are usually made in the first place because at least some formal teaching is regarded as necessary. Children in either type of setting usually need extensive support services involving aural habilitation specialists. Placement of a child in a school setting, even on a full time basis, should not be interpreted to mean that the participation of parents is no longer needed. Parents usually need some form of support at each successive stage in a child's habilitative program so they can provide optimal opportunities for that child's development.

learning speech skills informally

Learning speech and acquiring language tend to be much more closely associated with each other in the early years of life than during a child's years at school. This is, of course, because talking and listening are the usual ways of communicating with young children, and it is through the process of communication that they usually learn all aspects of spoken language. Most normally hearing children communicate fluently through the use of speech by the time they enter school. After that, people do not expect their speech to undergo any radical changes, although continued language growth is usually expected to occur as an outcome of education. If the goal of informal learning is to be pursued with hearing-impaired children, then to the greatest possible extent they should be helped to follow the same broad patterns of development that can be observed among normally hearing children.

To promote a natural course of development, those involved with young hearing-impaired children must consciously create appropriate environments for their children. They must use strategies that will provide sufficient focus on speech perception and speech production skills to compensate for their children's levels of hearing impairment. These skills, regardless of the degree of focus required to promote their acquisition, will continue to be closely associated with the development of language.

Focus on speech production can sometimes lead to practices that are a barrier to the long-term goal of fluent communication through the use of spoken language. One such practice is to use a child's spontaneous attempts at conversation for speech correction. The purpose of using speech to communicate is to transfer information. This purpose should be respected. When a child wants to say something he or she should be allowed to say it without fear that the attempt to tell you something will be turned into a speech lesson; without fear that the adult's response will indicate dissatisfaction. Only if there is a breakdown in communication - if a child simply cannot be understood - should adults intervene, and then only to help the child express *what* it is he or she wants to say.

Criticisms of *how* children talk can be most discouraging to them, and can even reduce their drive to use spoken language in further spontaneous communication. Listeners can use several different repair strategies to help children who fail to get their message across in their attempts to communicate. Listeners can, for example, tell them that they were not understood, ask them to repeat, ask questions to clarify certain points, and recapitulate what was said to ensure that their understanding of it was accurate. These are the sorts of interventions that children clearly understand are concerned with the message - with the listener being concerned about *what*, and not *how* it has been said. There may be occasions when conversation can be staged with older children's consent as a means of formal speech teaching, but correction in the course of spontaneous communication should not be lightly undertaken.

Normally hearing children acquire most of their speech patterns in a broadly similar order over their early years. Basic control over voice production precedes vowel acquisition, which in turn precedes the mastery of most consonants. Most sounds are to be found in children's speech by age two, but some sounds, such as /s/, and several consonant blends may not be mastered by some late-developing children until they are six or seven years of age.

The order and approximate timing of spontaneously acquired speech patterns among normally hearing children should be followed with hearing-impaired children if natural language is to be achieved through informal learning. For example, it is inappropriate to focus strongly on the production of an /s/ sound by a three-year-old hearing-impaired child when it is a matter of no great concern that many older normally hearing children are blithely communicating effectively without

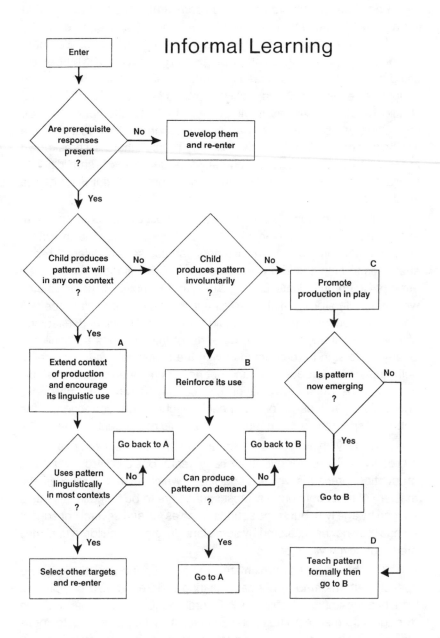

Informal Learning

figure 7-2. An algorithm depicting the steps and decisions inherent in the process of promoting informal learning.

it. When the natural hierarchy of skills underlying spoken language is ignored, young hearing-impaired children tend to become conscious of the adults' efforts to accelerate speech development and of their failure to meet the adults' wishes in relation to speech. This can lead to their reluctance to communicate. Adults must never put their efforts into developing speech skills at the expense of promoting communicative language. Sensitivity to this danger on the part of professionals, and appropriate guidance for caregivers, can prevent the development of such a situation. This should be borne in mind when reading the following paragraphs that describe a model to enhance the informal learning of particular speech patterns.

a model for informal speech acquisition

The diagram presented as Figure 7-2 indicates how one can provide structured but informal learning opportunities for hearing-impaired children to promote the acquisition of their speech skills. It can be used effectively only with children who use appropriately fitted hearing aids, or alternative forms of sensory stimulation through the use of tactile devices or cochlear implants. This model is appropriate for use during infancy and throughout the elementary school years. It indicates the pattern of focused intervention that can be adopted to promote acquisition of a given speech pattern at any stage of speech development. Let us work through the model using a couple of examples.

For our first example let us consider Joan, a three-year-old, profoundly hearing-impaired child, who started her informal learning program at eighteen months of age. She is enrolled in a parent-infant program that features informal learning activities. Our goal is for her to produce high- and low-pitched sounds as a preliminary step towards controlling the fundamental frequency of her voice. We begin by determining the level of development she has reached. Entering the diagram at the first column, we ask whether the prerequisite responses are present. Joan can vocalize spontaneously and on demand, but she cannot voluntarily produce differences in voice pitch, a skill that we now wish her to develop.

We recall that differences in voice frequency cannot be seen but can be perceived through audition by all but a very few hearing-impaired children. Joan is well aided, and has a reasonable amount of hearing under 1000 Hz. She can, therefore, be expected to hear at least gross differences in voice pitch. She does not, however, produce them in any communicative context. Following the diagram, we can answer "yes" to the first question in the second column. When excited, she involuntarily produces pitch changes in her vocalizations. We set out to imitate her pitch changes when they occur in order to draw her attention to them. This strategy succeeds, and soon she happily imitates a vowel sound with falling pitch as we pretend that the airplane she is holding is coming down to land. Going back to column 1, as directed in the diagram, we extend the use of this pattern into linguistic contexts, such as questions and exclamations, by ensuring that pitch differences are meaningfully used in everyday communication. A structured procedure, yes. A formal one, no.

For our second example, let us assume that another child, Sheila, with similar, profound hearing impairment, who makes no response to sound beyond 1000 Hz, is approximating sentences but has no ee vowel. This is the sound that we have targeted for development. She has (see column 1) the prerequisite behaviors, in that she can vocalize, and uses a variety of other vowels spontaneously. We expect the ee because she uses words that normally contain it. When they occur, however, she substitutes a neutral vowel with lips spread.

We recall that the second formant of the vowel ee is over 2000 Hz, and therefore beyond the frequency range of her audition, but the first formant is well within the frequency range of her well-aided hearing, at around 300 Hz. Thus we know that Sheila can detect the vowel, but does not yet discriminate or identify it through audition. Proceeding to column 2, we observe her closely to determine whether she ever produces an ee involuntarily. She does not. Proceeding to column 3, we play a lot of games with her. We then find that she produces ee when she giggles. Using similar strategies to those outlined above, we move to point B on the diagram, then back to point A and quickly provide opportunities for her to use this vowel in her spoken language.

It is rare, indeed, that one needs to teach young children formally (see point D on the diagram), and one should not consider doing so unless and until they attempt to communicate through approximation to mature patterns of spoken language. The speech patterns used as examples above could certainly be taught formally by using tactile cues (see Chapter 5), but formal strategies require voluntary behaviors and conscious learning, and are thus best used with older children. The long-term goal in spoken language is to be conscious only of *what* one is saying, not of *how* one is saying it. It is, therefore, an advantage if one can avoid late and conscious learning of speech patterns.

The informal process, like the formal one to be described below, can be regarded as consisting of seven components or steps that are basic. The first four relate to the planning that must be preparatory to learning and teaching. The remaining three are part of the learning and teaching process. They are:

1. ensuring the presence of *prerequisites*;
2. deciding on the *set* to be used;
3. selecting the child's most appropriate *sense modality*;
4. choosing the *strategies* to be used;
5. achieving *production* of the targeted speech sound;
6. providing *reinforcement* of the behavior; and
7. extending *production in other contexts*, including spoken language.

Informal learning has several advantages over formal teaching of speech skills. Children tend to be more relaxed when active than when seated in the traditional manner for formal teaching. Such features of informal situations tend to lead to much better breath flow and a more relaxed posture that, in themselves, encourage good voice quality and more abundant vocalization. This is not to say that formal teaching cannot be used to promote good breathing habits and excellent voice quality. It can. However, the teacher or clinician has to pay more attention to these features in a formal situation. Finally, in relation to Figure 7-2, similar algorithms can also be used to promote language patterns as well as speech skills.

formal language teaching

Formal teaching of any aspect of spoken language can be successfully undertaken only when children have already acquired some understanding and use of spoken language through sufficient exposure to informal learning opportunities. Spoken language, even at a most elementary level, must first of all be meaningful to them. Oral intent - a drive to talk - must also be established. If the development of spoken language has not been, or cannot be, undertaken in the home on a one-to-one basis with a caring adult, the professional must work directly with the child rather than with the parents. In such cases, the first requirement is to establish two-way communication through encouraging the child's vocalization and approximations to more mature forms of speech through informal interactive play.

For child-centered teaching to be optimally successful, one must create routine situations in the school that offer essentially the same crucially important elements as those that are more usually offered in a normal home. These include providing abundant one-to-one interaction, extending non-verbal communication to provide a base for later verbal interaction, and using every opportunity to clothe the child's interests with spoken language by following the direction of and interpreting their gaze, body posture, pointing, and vocalization. The professionals should, at least in the early stages, talk at the same time as the child's visual attention is directed to objects and events, as well as create and exploit routines that help the child derive meaning from the context of what is said. They must also, of course, ensure that the child they are working with is surrounded with excellent models of spoken language communication.

In some formal language teaching programs, children are expected to acquire their language skills primarily through reference to a grammatical framework. They are expected to learn the parts of speech, such as nouns, verbs, and adjectives, as well as where each should go in a sentence; all this at much the same time as they are learning basic vocabulary. This is stark contrast to the way that most children learn their first language. The majority of children come to a knowledge of grammar (if they learn it at all) through reference to a language *that they already know.* There is no evidence that hearing-impaired children who are required to learn a grammatical system and then fit language into it, end up having any advantage over those who acquire the underlying rules without conscious attention to them. Formal systems that are based on a syntactic framework simply cannot provide a child with all of the rules of language that must be learned in order to communicate effectively. The language required for effective speech communication and reading has too many facets to be adequately covered by simplistic systems. It may not be essential for a child to be consciously aware of grammatical rules, but teachers must know a lot about them if they are to be effective. Some formal language programs not only base their teaching on a grammatical model, but carry them out through written rather than spoken language.

Such procedures have to be questioned for the various reasons detailed in the following paragraphs.

formal programs

Numerous types of formal language development programs have been proposed, some designed specifically for children with hearing impairment, and others designed for children with language deficits due to some other cause. Workers with a background in behavior modification usually suggest very specific content and detailed training strategies in all areas of language development, but programs that focus more specifically on either semantic, syntactic, or pragmatic aspects are also available. Such formal language teaching programs should not be adopted for all children. They should be used only with children who are not acquiring their language skills spontaneously or rapidly enough through interaction, and even then they should be used to supplement, not replace, learning through communicative interaction.

The possible adverse effects of "plugging" children into pre-planned programs has led many professionals to provide intensive spoken language stimulation in which programs based on individual needs are planned and measured by "test and teach" procedures. Programs of this sort can help to avoid the unnecessary concentration by groups of children on what may be, for several of them, relatively unimportant features of language acquisition. "Test and teach" programs are not easy to manage. They require selection and administration of evaluation procedures that are geared to the age and approximate language level of each child, as well as careful planning of remedial or developmental strategies. Both can be enormously time consuming. Such programs, however, provide the best basis for promoting overall linguistic competence through interaction within a framework of meaningful communication, particularly if the evaluation procedures are based on samples of spontaneous spoken language.

"Test and teach" programs are based on the theory that there are broadly distinct, sequential stages in language acquisition that can be clearly defined - stages that a child should master in an orderly manner on the road to linguistic competence. Although not all aspects of spoken language appear at the same time or in the same order among normally hearing children, such broad sequences of events can be reliably observed in normally emerging spoken language. The writer, in the company of many other professionals, accepts that these sequences are the most appropriate guide in designing "test and teach" type programs for hearing-impaired children.

reading and language

The practice of focussing heavily on the use of written materials early on in formal language teaching programs is not supported in current educational philosophy. It is reasonable to teach reading and writing skills using language that is familiar to the child, and the use of computer-based programs for this purpose is expanding; but to confront children with two tasks - learning language, and learning to read - is to risk overload and invite frustration. Moreover, it is impossible to create reading books that follow normal, interactive patterns of language development and, at the same time, meet the requirements of meaningfulness, interest, and relevance of content.

Reading-based language work is also an unnecessarily slow process for most children. True, some of the outstanding oral deaf adults of today were taught through such a process before modern sensory aids were available. A child who can learn in less formal ways will be hampered by the snail's pace at which most reading-based work has to proceed. A significant amount of spoken language discourse relating to the pupils' interests and needs can be covered, and a considerable amount of teaching can take place, in the time it takes readers with a weak language background to understand all of the words and the phrase structures they meet in the first half-page of most books available to them. For similar reasons, hearing-impaired and language-delayed children can learn very little from, and can waste a great deal of valuable time being occupied with, most workbooks.

Workbooks often help teachers keep some children busy while they work constructively with others, but being busy is not necessarily being gainfully occupied. Written language should be based on the spoken form, and not *vice versa*. This is not to say that reading cannot open children's minds to new vocabulary, ideas, concepts, and experiences, as well as ways of expressing them. It can, but not until the children have mastered their basic language with its intricate rules and systems, and acquired considerable skill in reading at more fundamental levels. Several important long term goals in the curriculum, including fluent reading, are best reached by de-emphasizing them in the early years in order to build strong foundations for their later mastery.

language and learning

Special education is required for hearing-impaired children with no significant additional handicaps only because they have problems in spoken language communication resulting from their hearing impairment. If children are to overcome these problems through learning to understand and to use spoken language, then they must be provided from the outset with optimal opportunities to succeed. To this end, logic demands that their communication problems receive the utmost priority, and are met head on; that the teachers do not attempt to circumvent them, or engage in activities that leave no time for spoken language development through speech communication.

One reason that academic weaknesses among hearing-impaired children tend to persist throughout and beyond their school life is that their communication deficits have never been overcome, and therefore continue to undermine efforts to promote learning. Priority given to communication in the early years of school would not, of course, remove all of the problems posed by deafness. It would, however, prevent many of them from becoming as severe. The poverty of educational achievements reported among deaf school-leavers in numerous demographic studies is unnecessarily severe. Progress in academic subjects among hearing-impaired children under eight or even nine years of age is much less important than the development of their spoken language. Once children can communicate, they can catch up academically. Indeed, there is substantial evidence to indicate that the postponement of academic emphasis for a few of the elementary years has no serious long-term disadvantage even among normally hearing children.

Formal programs, then, should be designed to begin not with children who lack effective language skills and have no school experience, but rather with those who have an already established speech communication base and can readily cooperate with the teacher. Both of these requirements can be met only when the children's verbal and cognitive development are sufficiently advanced, so that whatever spoken language has to be formally taught can be "mapped onto" their concepts of the world around them. From that time, both formal and informal strategies can be used systematically to elicit, generalize, and automatize all aspects of spoken language at each successive stage of development. These strategies are described in general terms below, and in more specific terms in subsequent chapters.

communicative content

Several principles underlie all effective language programs. In brief, these are that children learn best when spoken language is:

1. related to their interests;

2. integrated with their prior linguistic knowledge in ways that are meaningful to them;

3. used communicatively; and

4. developed to high levels of automaticity.

As stated above, children communicate effectively through spoken language when they attend to *what* it is that they are saying, rather than to *how* they are saying it. Their spoken language must, therefore, be used until it becomes automatic. The proverb has it that practice makes perfect. This is not true. Practice makes permanent - or at least habitual. To prevent habitual errors in production, accuracy must be achieved for each spoken language target from the outset.

Adults must carefully monitor a child's production of recently acquired patterns to ensure that their accuracy is preserved as they are first used in communicative contexts. Only then can patterns be effectively practiced to perfection. Speed, economy of effort, and flexibility of production all follow on abundant and accurate use (see Chapter 8 for more detailed discussion of automaticity). Accurate production and automaticity can be achieved in good programs of all types. Once mastery of spoken language skills is truly achieved, whether by conscious or unconscious effort, conscious attention to any aspect of spoken language usage will be an option that can, but need not, be exercised.

The semantic intent of communication that embodies formally taught language should be made clear to a child. Such clarity can be achieved through the use of contextual cues, whether language is taught formally or informally. The strategies, materials, and situations contrived to teach spoken language in school should reflect real-life situations so that carry-over from the classroom to everyday communication is promoted.

The grammatical integrity of the spoken language patterns used by the children, their teachers, and by other caregivers is of particular importance and should be carefully monitored. Well-formed sentences are required for precision of expression. Only exceptionally does an utterance of less than a sentence have the information content and the precision required for meaningful communication (see Chapter 6). In some remedial programs for children with cognitive and linguistic deficits resulting, for example, from Down Syndrome, syntactically reduced models, such as "Push car" and "Throw ball," are deliberately used. Because children produce such two-word utterances in the early stages of spoken language development is, however, a poor reason for adults to provide them as models, particularly if they are working with hearing-impaired children who have no cognitive deficits. Unless children are exposed from the outset to somewhat more complex sentence patterns than they can produce, they will have no opportunity to derive and reconstruct the linguistic conventions that must be mastered for their eventual comprehension and use. Of course, just as unnatural forms of reduction must be avoided so must natural forms of reduction be encouraged. For example, it is more appropriate for children to respond to the question "Who has the ball?" with "I do!" or "I don't!" than "I have the ball." Similarly, questions such as "What color is the horse?" and "How old are you?" are usually answered with one word. Natural language must be used if the child is to acquire it.

experience-based learning

Language must have its origins in the real world of personal experience before it can be understood in more advanced forms. Only when a thorough understanding of many words has been derived from the concrete experiences of the "here and now" can they then be used with understanding in more abstract ways. Let us take common adjectives as our first example. The concepts associated with the words *soft*, *cold*, and *dirty* must have become thoroughly familiar through concrete experience before the more abstract notions of being *soft-hearted*, receiving a *cold reception* or playing *dirty politics* can be appreciated. For another example, consider children's experience with the everyday events, such as finding that mothers are pleased when milk is drunk rather than thrown on the floor, and that glass breaks when dropped on kitchen tiles. These experiences lead them to understand the concepts "if you drink your milk, Mummy will be pleased," and "if you drop your cup, it might break." In turn, these concepts, derived from concrete and verbal experiences in the routine situations of everyday life, underlie the more advanced and abstract notions of possibility and probability, such as "if this strategy can be used successfully to teach a hearing-impaired child, then it should also work on normally hearing children who have similar problems with their speech." This principle - that concrete ex-

perience provides an essential foundation for abstract verbal development - pervades all aspects of language.

Hearing impaired children who do not readily understand and
manipulate abstract ideas linguistically have not usually had sufficient
(abundant) prior experience of manipulating language in more concrete
contexts. Children need a wealth of practice at concrete levels in order
to learn how to use analogous language in abstract verbal thinking, and
to express abstract ideas. Of course, while such practice is necessary, it
may not be sufficient: children must also develop the sorts of imaginative
thinking skills that underlie abstract notions.

Several other examples of language skills that are frequently found
to be weak among hearing-impaired children, and that are best
developed through concrete action and interaction, include the use of
verb tenses, pronouns, and function words. These are briefly discussed
below, and will receive further attention in the later chapters that focus
on speech-teaching strategies. The persistence of weaknesses, such as
those described below, often reflects badly on the professionals involved.
It is a strong indication that a child's progress is not being adequately
monitored, and that the necessary adjustments are not being made to
the teaching program.

The exact meaning of utterances in English frequently depends on
the appropriate use of verb tenses. Verb tenses only begin to become
meaningful to children when they have developed concepts relating to
time. These concepts develop as a result of their day-by-day experience
of events and the relative order in which they occur. Most hearing-
impaired children old enough to require formal language teaching have
acquired at least vague concepts of time, but have yet to learn to express
them verbally through the manipulation of tense. The more exact understanding of time, and the precise use of tense, can only come about
through the children themselves being engaged in action. It cannot be
derived from books and pictures. For instance, the true sense of the
sentence "The boy is playing" cannot be accurately derived from a
picture because a picture depicting a boy engaged in a play activity could
equally well illustrate the sentence "The boy was playing." The numerous
verb tenses in English are an essential system within the language. Only
communicative situations in which a child's past, present, and projected
activities are discussed and reported can lead to the understanding and
appropriate use of these tenses. The routine experiences of everyday life
offer the best framework for developing notions and vocabulary relating

both to time and to the various forms of past, present, and future tense - because they are both repetitive and predictable. The range of things done yesterday, that are being done today, and will be done tomorrow or next week, provide the best context possible for the comprehension of tense. Communication relating to children's activities is a much better route to their learning about time than reference to a calendar!

Pronoun weaknesses also commonly persist throughout many years of special schooling. Only through communicative interaction - for which there is insufficient provision in many formal teaching programs - can children learn that in various situations they can be *I* or *me* to oneself, *you* when others address them, *he*, *she*, *him* or *her* when someone refers to them, one of a group called *us*, *they* or *them* under different circumstances, and so on. Similarly, the possessive pronouns *mine*, *his*, *hers*, *ours*, *yours* and *theirs* can only be learned through interactive experience. They cannot be learned through reading. The possessive adjectives *my*, *his*, *her*, *its*, *our*, *your*, and *their* are also sources of common error, and must be acquired through action and interaction to become meaningful.

A child's active involvement in a learning situation cannot always be observed. Thinking is a highly active process, and a time-consuming one, too. So, in working on any aspect of spoken language development with children, we must give them good reason to be involved, as well as sufficient time to absorb, synthesize, recall, and use the information we present. Indeed, we must give them even more time than it takes them to plan the answer to a question (three or four seconds?) if we are to encourage them to initiate the sorts of verbal interaction we seek to promote.

Among the most frequent errors found in the language of hearing-impaired children are those relating to the use of function words - those words that indicate the relationships that exist between other (content) words within sentences. They include the pronouns discussed above, the articles *a* and *the*, the determiners, such as *this*, *that*, and *those*, the common auxiliary verbs, such as *is*, *are*, *was*, *has*, *have*, and *will*, together with the prepositions *off*, *in*, *with*, and so on. These are not only the most frequently used words in English, but those that most effectively defy explanation. The only way one can arrive at an understanding of their meaning, and where they are acceptably placed in a sentence, is through experience with their use in concrete situations.

In part through their potential for providing analogy, function words help to create an essential foundation for abstract thinking. How can one be in a quandary unless one knows what it is to be in a bath, in a store, or in some other location? Function words also lend a precision to the language that cannot be achieved except through their use because they not only specify such things as quantity, identity, and location, but possibility and probability. They also differentiate between particular and general statements. For example, the differences between *it's glass*, *it's a glass*, and *it's the glass* cannot be understood unless the meaning of the articles in utterances such as "I saw *a* bird in *the* garden" are known.

required emphases in formal language teaching

The arguments presented above suggest that there is need for stronger emphases to be given to the following aspects of language in the early years of formal teaching:

1. Communication instead of writing.

2. Spoken language geared to each child's interests and needs.

3. Complete sentences and discourse as well as words.

4. Tenses, not just verbs.

5. As much attention to function words as to content vocabulary.

6. Promoting learning through active and interactive strategies.

Such emphases should provide hearing-impaired children with the least time consuming ways to learn the elements of English that can be exploded into accurate and higher level language, prevent them from arriving at, and adhering to, incorrect systems of comprehension and use, and ensure adequate preparation for further language learning and education through later reading. Coherent, insightful, formal language teaching should permit the conscious learner to perceive the successful mastery of sequential steps as a series of personal achievements. When achievements are thus regarded, a child is reinforced by the act of acquisition itself, becomes fascinated with the subject matter, and begins to use it intuitively and inventively. As much personal drive develops towards effective speech skills, too, when they are taught formally, effectively, and coherently. It is to this aspect of spoken language that attention is now directed.

formal speech teaching

The formal teaching of speech, like the formal teaching of language, should be based on careful evaluation. Formal teaching of any body of knowledge or type of skill requires the clear presentation of a systematically arranged, progressive sequence of activities; that is, teaching in a step-by-step manner.

The most basic step in all teaching is, of course, to be sure that the child is able to detect, discriminate, identify, and comprehend the stimuli employed. A check on auditory (or other sensory) function must, therefore, be carried out, and any necessary adjustments to hearing or other sensory aids made, before teaching is begun (see Chapters 4 and 5).

Two types of speech evaluations are required to provide the information necessary for the effective formal teaching of speech: a phonetic-level evaluation to determine which speech patterns a child can produce, and whether the motor skills required to produce others are present; and a phonologic evaluation to determine which speech patterns the child produces in the context of different aspects of spoken language communication. These forms of evaluation are described in Chapter 8. Once a series of speech teaching targets has been determined on the basis of such evaluations, a set of systematic procedures is required to elicit and generalize each target pattern and ensure its carry-over into communicative speech. A model suggesting how such procedures can, following speech evaluation procedures, be selected and applied is provided in Figure 7-3 and discussed below.

a model for formal speech teaching

The diagram presented as Figure 7-3 summarizes the sequences of thought and action involved in developing speech skills in hearing-impaired children through a formal teaching process. Such teaching can be used effectively once the child is spontaneously attempting to communicate through spoken language. Formal teaching that follows the format presented below is particularly appropriate in the elementary school years, when any deficits in spoken language skills should be identified and remediated before omissions and distortions are inadvertently practiced and become habitual.

Formal Teaching

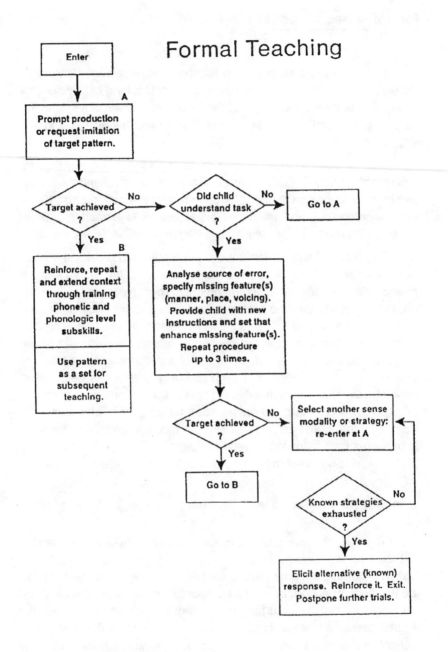

figure 7-3. An algorithm depicting the steps and decisions in formal teaching

The diagram shown as Figure 7-3 indicates the steps in intervention that can be followed for the formal development of any speech pattern. It is, in essence, a developmental and carefully sequenced "test and teach" program such as that described in the next chapter. It is, therefore, important to specify rather closely the order in which speech patterns are optimally presented for acquisition, and what previously learned patterns will provide the best base from which to proceed. Indeed, such previously learned patterns may be regarded as prerequisites for progressive teaching. Let us work through the diagram using a couple of examples. The first is with a boy called Jim who will help to illustrate the lines of thought and action that are taken to elicit a sound pattern, use it communicatively, and then have it serve as a prerequisite for further teaching.

Jim is a bright, profoundly hearing-impaired, six year old child who responds to low frequency sounds between 70 and 90 dB, but has no measurable hearing beyond 1000 Hz. He entered a special school for the deaf at five years of age after spending two years (since his diagnosis) in an informal learning program run by an inexperienced professional who did not ensure that he had been fitted with the most appropriate hearing aids, had not ensured that he made the most use of his residual hearing, and had not ensured that his parents received appropriate counselling, education or guidance. The school's audiologist had Jim's hearing aids changed so that sounds under 1000 Hz became optimally audible to him. Jim is now encouraged to use speech communication both at home (through better informed parents) as well as at school.

To teach Jim in accordance with the model shown, we must regularly assess his speech (see Chapter 8). On the basis of the phonetic level evaluation (PLE) we have found that he is using vocalization well, can control voice intensity and duration without problem, and can produce some vowels as well as some first step consonants. His phonologic level evaluation shows that he attempts simple sentences, but does not have the speech skills to produce intelligible words. The six targets identified include modification of voice pitch, production of three front vowels, and the first step fricatives. Our goal will therefore be to obtain discrete high- and low-frequency voice patterns as a preliminary step towards control of voice frequency. The prerequisite behaviors that underlie the production of vocalization on demand are available, but informal strategies have failed to produce voice pitch that is either higher or lower than the monotone that is typical of Jim's speech.

Before we can begin this teaching activity with Jim, we have to decide on the *set* we shall provide, what *sense modality* (hearing, vision, or touch) we shall employ, what *activity* to plan, and what *apparatus and materials* we shall need. These have to be decided for each target pattern, for while audition or some other sense modality may be most appropriate for sounds in one frequency range, it may be least appropriate for those in another. We recall (as we did in promoting Joan's informal learning of the same target) that differences in voice frequency cannot be seen, but can be perceived through audition by all but a very few hearing-impaired children. Jim is well aided, and has a reasonable amount of hearing under 1000 Hz. He can, therefore, be expected to hear at least gross differences in voice pitch. We decide to provide a set simply by asking Jim to vocalize, to work first through audition, to have him imitate the teacher's models, and to use teacher-provided cues instead of apparatus or materials.

The teacher first produces a model for Jim to imitate (see Figure 7-3, first box, column 1). She uses the vowel oo because it is already in Jim's repertoire and, because both of its formants lie under 1000 Hz, is optimally audible to him. The model is about three seconds in duration. About half way through its production, she abruptly raises the pitch of her voice and the height of her hand, which she holds to the side of her face. Jim is then asked to produce a long vocalization in imitation of the teacher. As usual, his voice does not vary in pitch, but he imitates the vowel. The target is not achieved (see first diamond in column 1). She then checks to see if Jim understands the task (see first diamond in column 2), and does this by telling Jim that his voice pitch didn't change and, to illustrate her point, she imitates Jim's flat-pitched vocalization and shows him, by moving her hand horizontally, that it did not vary as in the model she provided. She then asks Jim to try again (going back to the first box, column 1) and, again, he does not achieve the target behavior (first diamond in column 1). This time she is sure that he understands the task (first diamond in column 2), so she makes a quick analysis of the problem (first box in column 2). She suspects that Jim can hear the difference between a high voice and a low voice, and decides that her next step will be to check and, if necessary, train Jim's auditory perception for the task.

To check Jim's perception of the task the teacher produces a high voice and holds her hand high, then a low voice and holds her hand low. She repeats this procedure often enough to ensure that Jim is attending to both her hand and her voice, and has understood that her hand height and voice pitch are associated. Children must, through one sense modality or another, be able to discriminate the target sound from others before they can understand what pattern they are expected to produce. Accordingly, she then asks Jim to tell her, using his hand as well as speech, whether her voice is high or low. He does this first of all watching her closely and succeeds on each trial; but as she may be providing an extraneous visual cue on these trials, such as raising or lowering her eyebrows as she vocalizes, she then asks him to do the task with his eyes shut. On the first few trials he is unsure, so the teacher then takes his hand and raises or lowers it to correspond with the pitch of her voice on successive trials. She then asks him to identify the pitch of her voice, and signal it to her, as before, without her assistance. He then succeeds on most trials, she decides that the five minutes or so she has spent at this task is already long enough for one session, and they leave the training on a successful note for that day.

The next day, Jim and his teacher return to the task from a different vantage point. She begins by checking his perception of pitch change, and finds that he has remembered how to identify her high and low voice with eyes closed. She then asks Jim to produce high- and low-pitched voice as she signals the desired pitch with her hand (see first box, column 2). Small changes in the right directions occur (see second diamond in column 2), but Jim uses neck stretching to achieve a high voice, and shoulder hunching to achieve a low voice. The teacher recognizes that Jim has achieved the target, however, and reinforces him simply by saying "That's high (or that's low). Good!" However, she proceeds to repeat procedures to elicit the desired patterns by providing the child with new instructions until the production of a wider pitch interval is obtained without accompanying exaggerated movements - trials that will take only a few minutes several times a day over the next week.

Following error-free production, the teacher (returning to point B on the diagram) then reinforces the production, and extends it to other vowels (as shown in the last box in column 1). Intonation in meaningful speech requires continuous rather than discrete voice pitch changes. The discrete patterns obtained as above are prerequisite behaviors for obtaining them and, as soon as Jim can produce continuously changing patterns of voice frequency, they will be developed in the context of familiar, meaningful phrases and sentences that Jim already uses. At this point, the parents are alerted to Jim's newly acquired skill so that he can be encouraged to use intonation patterns both at home and in school.

Had this auditory strategy failed, it would have been possible to teach Jim through a tactile strategy (see first box in column 3). For example, we could have asked him to drink some water and, as he swallowed, feel his larynx rise and fall. Following that, we could have had him raise and lower his larynx without swallowing. When he could do that, we could have asked him to vocalize at the same time. This would have resulted in the production of a high voice when his larynx was high and a low voice when his larynx was low.

Should professionals exhaust their supply of known strategies in eliciting a particular speech pattern, they should temporarily drop the task rather than risk their own and the children's frustration with it, and have the child do something else that can be positively reinforced so that the session closes on a note of success. The teacher or clinician can then come back to the problem target again when they have planned a different strategy that has a good chance of working. Just as a feeling of success is important in the promotion of further learning, so is an experience of failure an obstacle to it. Avoidance of failure and achievement of success are essential elements of long-term motivation. Efforts to elicit particular sound patterns will, on most occasions, meet with success within minutes if the strategies suggested in this book are adopted.

In our second example, let us set out to teach another child, Jack, who has an educational history and profound hearing impairment similar to Jim's. Like Jim, he cannot respond to sound beyond 1000 Hz, but his parents have used an abundance of spoken language to communicate with him and, as a result, he is able to approximate simple sentences. A phonetic level evaluation shows that he cannot produce a th sound. He tries it in words, such as *with* and *thank you*, but produces *wi* and *tayoo* instead. We know, at the outset, that important components of this sound are not audible to Jack. The fricative turbulence has only high frequency acoustic energy that falls outside the frequency range of his residual hearing. He cannot imitate it because he can neither hear it nor see the turbulent breath stream that distinguishes the th from the /t/ that he substitutes for it. We need to provide a *set*, a pattern that has features in common with the target sound, choose the most appropriate *sense modality* and decide on what *apparatus or materials*, if any, we shall need for our chosen strategy. An adequate set for the breath flow is blowing, the sense modality of choice is touch, because he can neither hear nor see enough of the sound to imitate it (although he sees enough of it to process it through visual-tactile coding once he has learned about the turbulent breath flow). We decide to use no materials. Because there must be no undue tension for a fricative such as th to be produced well, and moving *to* a final fricative induces less tension than moving *from* a fricative to any other sound, we shall first seek to elicit the th in syllable-final and word-final positions.

The clinician first asks Jack to imitate ath as in *bath* (see Figure 7-3, first box, column 1). The target is not achieved. She is not sure that Jack understood the task, because she did not specifically indicate that the sound has to contain turbulent breath flow (first diamond, column 2). Next, therefore, she prepares Jack to meet success (see box 1, column 2) by asking him to wet his first finger (this makes it more sensitive), and to tell her if he can feel her breath stream when she blows on it. She presents several trials, sometimes blowing on the finger, other times not, until Jack responds with *yes* or *no* with certainty. She then asks Jack to wet his finger again, and she repeats the process, this time with the ath sound having or not having its appropriate breath flow. Again, she persists until Jack responds with certainty. Now she is ready to ask Jack for another imitation (see box 1, column 1). This time, she produces ath while allowing Jack to feel the breath flow on his finger. She then places Jack's finger in front of his mouth and invites him to imitate. He succeeds (second triangle in column 2). She then reinforces his success, and moves to extend the contexts in which he can produce the th (see box at B).

The first step in extending the context of the th or any other continuant sound is to require its production in repeated and alternated syllables, and in syllables with pitch differences (see Chapters 2 and 4). To repeat it with various vowels in syllable-final position is to lay the foundations of its production in word-initial and intervocalic positions. This is because the gap between the consonant and vowel is reduced as repetition rate is increased, so instead of producing ath ath the child produces *athathath* and this sequence contains both tha (word initial) and atha (intervocalic) examples of the phoneme. Alternating the sound with another and at different voice pitch will ensure that sound patterns can be blended together in the speech stream. Alternation of syllables and words that contain th with those that contain nasals, such as m, is an excellent way to prevent or remediate nasalization faults that are due to poorly developed velopharyngeal valving. (Further discussion of such teaching is provided in chapters 9-13.)

In none of the above examples would a skilled teacher or clinician work on the production of a target for more than a minute or two at a time. What is not achieved in one session is simply postponed to the next. Long periods of drill are not required for the mastery of any sound pattern. It is helpful to work very briefly on up to half a dozen phonetic level targets in any session, limiting each session to a few minutes' duration, and providing several such sessions each day. Such an arrangement permits spaced practice, which is superior to massed practice, and ensures that the children can experience success at the beginning and end of each session.

The interval between the first production of a speech pattern and its communicative use largely reflects the extent to which professionals in a program promote, and expect children to develop, spoken language communication. In most effective programs, a newly acquired pattern should be incorporated into particular words within a day or two of its first production, and its spontaneous use in a few contexts should be expected within days. Its use in all samples of spoken language may require considerably longer. Much will depend on the sensory salience of the sound pattern in question and on the morphemic load it carries in the language. For example, /s/ has to play many roles in English and not all of them may be known to children at the time they are learning to produce the sound.

required emphases in formal speech teaching

For formal teaching to be optimally effective, certain general requirements must be met. These include:

- the child's use of appropriate hearing aids (or alternative devices if necessary) every waking hour of each day;
- the creation of situations that permit optimal reception of spoken language;
- teaching by highly competent professionals based on phonetic, phonologic, and linguistic evaluations of each child;
- parental collaboration;
- the child's contact and communication with speaking peers; and
- the provision of abundant opportunities to learn and practise speech communication skills in all aspects of life.

Examination of the above list of requirements indicates how important parental involvement can be in several aspects of the formal speech teaching process. Apart from making sure that hearing aids or other sensory aids are functioning well all day and every day, parents can have the child rehearse speech targets at home (as specified by the teacher or clinician), ensure that he or she uses clearly spoken language patterns in the context of activities that are interesting and meaningful, arrange for optimal contact between their hearing-impaired child and his or her normally hearing and speaking friends in the neighborhood, and involve all members of the family - other children, aunts, uncles, grandparents - and neighbors in providing the child with a speech communication environment.

The materials presented in the previous sections also suggest that specific emphasis should be given to certain aspects of formal speech teaching and that a number of principles reflecting such emphasis can be formulated as follows:

1. Base initial formal teaching on informally learned patterns.

2. Select teaching targets on the basis of evaluation.

3. Ensure optimal use of residual hearing and/or other sense modalities at all times.

4. Choose the most appropriate sense modality for teaching.

5. Move from known to unknown speech targets, thus providing a set.

6. Work briefly on several targets in any one session.

7. Ensure that each child experiences success entering and leaving all formal teaching sessions.

8. Work on speech skills frequently for very brief periods.

9. Immediately generalize elicited patterns to broader contexts.

10. Use new patterns in function words as well as content vocabulary.

11. Promote use of all new patterns in spoken language communication.

12. Gear spoken language to each child's interests and needs.

13. Use training procedures that reflect real-life situations, because these will most readily carry-over from formal teaching.

14. Encourage self-responsibility for the quality of spoken language.

15. Identify and remove any obstacles to spoken language acquisition.

16. Integrate speech communication into all classroom learning.

17. Make formal speech lessons fun as well as functional.

18. Use drama and recordings to enhance speech communication skills.

19. Teach speech patterns formally only when the child has developed "oral intent" - the drive to communicate by spoken language.
20. Welcome communication events as such and do not use them as opportunities for formal speech teaching.

recommended further reading

Early and informal spoken language learning by hearing-impaired children is extensively treated by Grant (1987), Kretschmer and Kretschmer (1978), in a book edited by Ling (1984a), in a text written by Ling and Ling (1978), and by Wood, Wood, Griffiths and Howarth (1986).

Formal language teaching programs for normally hearing children that have been applied with hearing-impaired children include those by Bricker and Bricker (1970), Stremel and Waryas (1974), and Tate (1972). Those specifically designed for use with hearing-impaired children have been reviewed in Bunch (1987). Problems in carry-over have been addressed by Gerber (1973).

Tools for the measurement of language acquisition are presented by Crystal, Fletcher, and Garman (1976), Kretschmer and Kretschmer (1978), Moog and Geers (1975, 1979, 1980 and 1983), and Stickler (1987), among others. The nature and outcomes of early treatment of hearing-impaired children are reviewed in a text edited by Mencher and Gerber (1981), and common problems in the language of older hearing-impaired children are addressed by Quigley (1978), Quigley and Paul (1984) and in Schildroth and Karchmer (1986). The relationships between learning language, writing, and reading among hearing-impaired children have been addressed in Kretschmer (1985).

Strategies for informal speech acquisition have been described by Grant (1987) and by Stovall (1982). More formal speech teaching strategies are suggested by Calvert and Silverman (1983) and by Ling (1976), who provides an extensive treatment of the theoretical and practical aspects of the formal speech teaching procedures discussed in this chapter. The history of speech teaching for hearing-impaired children is covered in an interesting and easy-to-read book by Markides (1983). See References pp.433 ff.

chapter 8

crucial bases of
the Ling system

Numerous discussions with practitioners in the field have indicated the need for an in depth analysis of the major concepts underlying the effective use of the Ling (1976) system - hence the inclusion of this chapter. Response to the publication of the system has been overwhelmingly positive. Although differences in its application have become apparent, a consensus as to what is crucial in the system has gradually emerged.

Teachers and clinicians who are more inclined to use formal teaching methods have been apt to concentrate somewhat more fully on the development of phonetic-level skills (eliciting sounds and ensuring a sound base of motor control) than on phonologic-level development (meaningful use of speech patterns in communication). Experience has shown, however, that in most educational settings, both phonologic and phonetic level development have to be promoted if spoken language is to be acquired.

At the other end of the scale, some professionals have worked entirely on phonologic level skills and, often to the detriment of the intelligibility of a child's speech, have resisted phonetic level teaching.

Speech faults, some as obvious as they were simple to prevent or to cure, have thus been allowed to persist until they became habitual.

Several professionals treated the system as if it were exclusively oriented to older children who needed remedial work. Others have shown that it is highly applicable to young children who are able to benefit from a focused but informal learning program. In both types of programs, professionals have learned that parents' collaboration can substantially enhance a child's progress. The purpose of this chapter is not to dwell on the formal versus the informal applications of the system. These are considered in Chapter 7. In this chapter attention will be directed to the seven aspects of the system. In the course of ongoing review, these have come to be recognized as its most important basic elements. Each will be discussed in separate sections below:

1. the seven-stage model of speech development (progression and recursiveness in acquisition at both phonetic and phonologic levels);
2. criterion-referenced evaluation (targeting the first six phonetic or phonologic items failed for immediate attention);
3. the selection of the most appropriate sense modality as the channel for input and feedback of any pattern;
4. the provision of a set (moving from the known to the unknown);
5. working towards automaticity by ensuring accuracy, speed, economy of effort, and flexibility in the use of the targeted pattern;
6. ensuring generalization of a targeted sound from one context to another; and, last but most important,
7. ensuring that the speech learned with professional help is carried over into everyday communication through spoken language.

systematic seven-stage development

Speech skills progress from simple vocalizations to complex, intelligible spoken language through a series of relatively distinct stages. These stages are shown in the "bottom up" model presented as Figure 8-1. At each stage there are two levels of speech production to be considered: the phonetic level and the phonologic level. At the phonetic level, the neuromuscular coordinations required for the production of different speech patterns are developed. At the phonologic level, speech

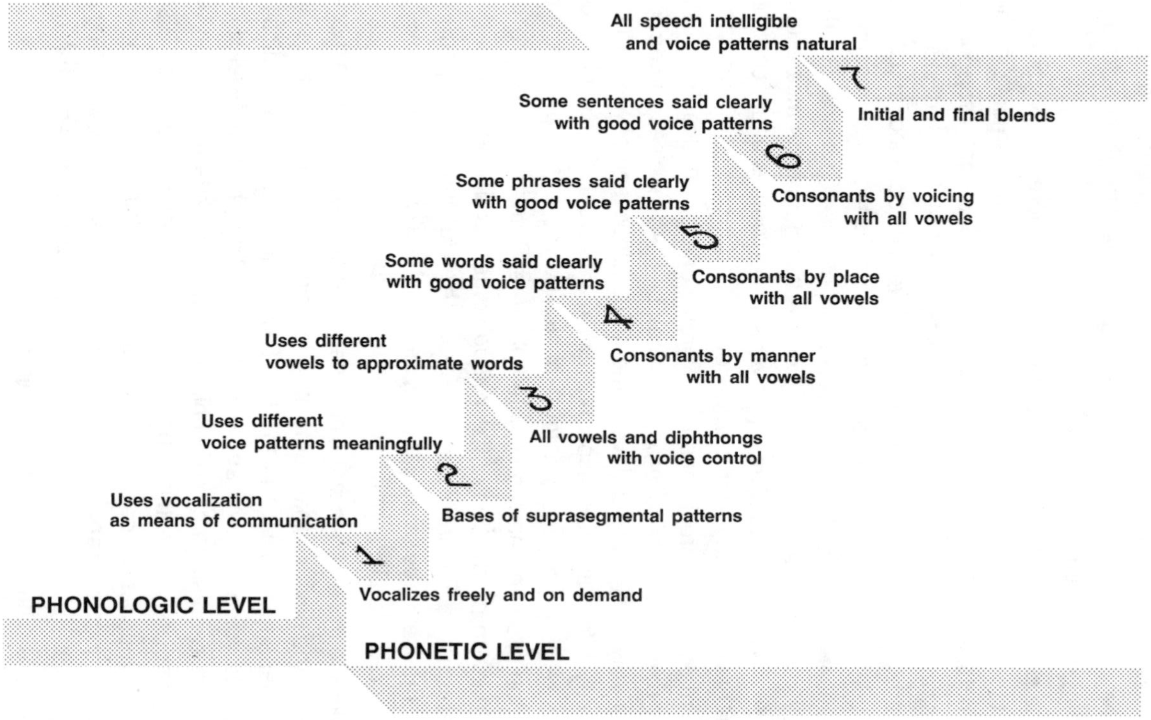

All speech intelligible
and voice patterns natural

Initial and final blends

Some sentences said clearly
with good voice patterns

Consonants by voicing
with all vowels

Some phrases said clearly
with good voice patterns

Consonants by place
with all vowels

Some words said clearly
with good voice patterns

Consonants by manner
with all vowels

Uses different
vowels to approximate words

All vowels and diphthongs
with voice control

Uses different
voice patterns meaningfully

Bases of suprasegmental patterns

Uses vocalization
as means of communication

Vocalizes freely and on demand

PHONETIC LEVEL

PHONOLOGIC LEVEL

figure 8-1. **The major stages of speech acquisition. The process of speech acquisition follows seven relatively distinct stages, each having both phonetic (motor speech) and phonologic (spoken language) components.**

225

patterns are used meaningfully in spoken language. In Figure 8-1, the phonetic level stages are depicted as being downstairs (foundation-related skills) while the phonologic level stages are depicted as being above the stairs (end-product skills - the speech patterns that are for use in meaningful spoken language).

The skills targeted for development become increasingly complex as the stages in the model are completed. The most fundamental of the stages in this model (see the numbered steps) is *vocalization supported by an adequate breath stream.* Acquisition of the targeted skills is demonstrated when the child vocalizes freely and on demand; and these phonetic level goals permit the child to use vocalization as a means of communication. *Second,* is the development of voice control skills - the *bases of suprasegmental patterns* - patterns that permit the meaningful use of prosody. *Third,* as diversity of vocalization comes under control, a range of *vowels and diphthongs* is developed, and these permit the child to make first approximations to words. *Fourth,* consonants initially having a different *manner of production* can be used to release, interrupt or arrest vowels, a stage of development that allows some words to be said clearly. *Fifth,* various consonants having a different *place of production* are reliably produced, a level of achievement that permits the production of some clearly articulated phrases. *Sixth,* the fine control of timing leads to production of the *voiced-voiceless* distinction that differentiates between pairs of consonants, such as /b/ and /p/, and permits some sentences to be said clearly. *Seventh,* and finally, consonant blends are mastered and all speech becomes intelligible.

Skills learned at one stage are integrated and extended with those learned at the next, so that cumulative learning is ensured. As a result, speech patterns acquired in the last few stages feature prosodically appropriate voice patterns and clear vowels. The phonetic level skills acquired at each stage provide children with new patterns that can be used immediately to extend their ability to communicate. They also create the foundation for the acquisition of new skills at a subsequent step, and incorporate and refine skills that have been previously learned. In short, each speech pattern grows out of previously acquired behaviors and provides a base for further learning.

Each of the seven stages shown in Figure 8-1 contains a variety of speech patterns that can be targeted for development. For example, suprasegmental patterns require control of the intensity, duration, and frequency of vocalization; there are over a dozen vowels and diphthongs to be mastered in English; and there are many more consonants than vowels that a child must acquire in order to achieve intelligibility. All major speech patterns, as well as formal and informal strategies for developing them motorically and in spoken language, will be discussed in the remaining chapters.

phonetic and phonologic levels of development

At the phonetic level, attention is directed towards gaining mastery over the basic mechanics of talking - speech reception, speech production, and feedback skills. At the phonologic level, concern is with using speech patterns meaningfully, in ways that convey thoughts and feelings. The two levels are developed concurrently. Teachers and clinicians should never succumb to the temptation to concentrate exclusively on the development of phonetic level skills during times assigned to "speech" lessons. Thus, when teachers, clinicians, or parents are concerned with reaching some advanced phonetic level targets, such as consonant blends, they should also be concerned with extending the phonological use of recently acquired consonants, as well as with refining the linguistic use of voice patterns (suprasegmentals), and the integration of previously learned consonants in all aspects of discourse.

At all stages of speech development, most normally hearing children spontaneously use their voices in two ways: to play with sound, and to convey meaning. Playing with sound is akin to phonetic level practice for hearing impaired children, for it helps them to attain control over vocalization, and to extend the range of sounds they can make. At the same time that normally hearing children play with sounds, they also gain phonologic experience by learning to use speech to communicate their needs and feelings.

Meaningful speech is not something that develops out of the blue. A lot of skills have to be acquired before intelligible words can appear. In much the same way that a variety of vocalizations and canonical (repetitive) babbling precedes speech in normally hearing babies, so do such pre-speech patterns help lay the foundations for hearing-impaired children to talk. Just as control over the production of a wide range of vowels and diphthongs precedes mastery of most consonants and blends in the speech of normally hearing children, so do they create a similar groundwork for the development of consonants in hearing-impaired children. The stages outlined above are broadly true for all children who are learning to speak.

All babies use loud demanding cries to tell the caregivers that they want something, and contented gurglings to indicate when they feel happy. It must be clear to children that their vocal efforts, from babyhood on, can be understood, if they are to acquire and maintain a drive to develop spoken language. This is particularly important for hearing-impaired children. Whatever their speech skills, they must constantly be encouraged to use them meaningfully, and be provided with appropriate responses to their efforts.

The range of speech patterns children have at their command may be very limited, but this should not prevent them from expressing their needs and conveying their feelings. Caregivers, as a rule, quickly learn to interpret a child's needs from primitive vocalizations and the context of ongoing activity. Such interpretation serves more than one purpose. It keeps the frustration of both caregiver and child at a minimum level, and it encourages the child to make further attempts at communication. Early speech patterns may be as simple as a cry or a gurgle, as vague as a string of vowel sounds with the prosody of speech, as unclear as an unintelligible approximation to an adult sentence form - but the interpretation of their meaning by caregivers within the context of ongoing activities is one of the most important keys to the child's further growth in speech, and his or her mastery of skills at subsequent stages. Professionals may need to help parents of young children to respond appropriately to their children's early attempts at self-expression, particularly when the diagnosis of hearing impairment has been made recently.

the stages as guidelines

The stages outlined above should be seen as guidelines rather than distinct steps that imprison effort. It is, for example, often necessary to attend to the refinement of some suprasegmental aspects - perhaps voice pitch - at the same time as one is encouraging acceptable production of a certain vowel or setting out to elicit a consonant. One should never concentrate on one speech pattern to the exclusion of others. To ensure the necessary variety that will maintain a child's interest in acquiring spoken language skills, and frequently lead to him or her being (and feeling) successful, it is best to focus on several different patterns in the course of any given day. These patterns could be phonetic and phonologic targets within one stage or across a couple of stages. While rigid adherence to a stage-by-stage approach is not advocated, neither is a random attack on a variety of stages. In the past, failure to realize that certain sound patterns logically precede others, has led to a considerable waste of time, effort, enthusiasm, and effectiveness.

criterion-referenced evaluation

Ongoing evaluation must underlie all developmental or remedial speech work. Following the initial diagnosis and the various assessments that must precede treatment (pediatric, otologic, neurologic, audiologic, etc.), repeated evaluations have to be carried out to assess whether the treatment plan is succeeding. The most important information for teachers, clinicians and parents is provided by answers to such practical questions as:

- What level of skill has the child acquired so far?
- Are skills, once learned, being retained?
- Are both phonetic and phonologic skills progressing?
- Is the rate of skill acquisition satisfactory?
- Are skills being carried over from training to real life?
- Are caregivers sufficiently knowledgeable and involved?
- Is satisfactory progress being made?
- What particular problems (if any) are impeding progress?
- What skills should next be developed?

The answer to each question calls on someone to make a judgement based on a criterion acceptable to those working with the child. Such evaluation is therefore termed "criterion-referenced evaluation." Another sort of evaluation, one used principally in research rather than clinical or educational treatment, is called "norm-referenced evaluation." Such evaluation compares one child's performance with that of a large sample of others. In teaching and therapy, as long as our goals are clear, our primary interest is not in knowing what other children of a similar age, sex, or family background can do, but rather in defining and meeting the immediate speech acquisition needs of each child in our care.

Three types of evaluations relating to speech production skills should be undertaken at the outset: an oral-peripheral examination, a phonetic-level evaluation, and a phonologic-level evaluation. Effective administration of these evaluation procedures demands appropriate use of each child's abilities to use residual hearing or alternative sense modalities in the perception of speech. Thus tests of speech reception (such as the Five-Sound Test described in Chapter 4) should be used immediately ahead of any speech assessment procedure. Usually, the oral-peripheral examination needs to be undertaken just once - before treatment is begun - but should there be an unexpected lack of progress following a period of treatment, it would be wise to repeat it. Because these evaluation procedures have been discussed in detail in earlier writing (Ling, 1976), only brief descriptions of the procedures and the reasons for them will be provided in this text.

oral-peripheral evaluation

An oral-peripheral examination is designed to evaluate the structures that are involved in speech production (lips, jaws, teeth, tongue, and palate). To determine whether there are any abnormalities of form or function that might prevent a child from learning to talk is very difficult to determine unless the examination includes observations that show how these organs are used in producing a range of speech sounds. This is because perfectly normal speech can be produced by a person with a somewhat abnormal speech mechanism or abnormal speech movements.

It used to be thought that to be deaf was to also be dumb (that is, unable to speak). The (mistaken) idea that deafness affected the speech organs as well as the ears came about because, years ago, most hearing-impaired people were simply not taught to talk. Even today, there are quite a lot of hearing impaired children who do not learn how to speak intelligibly, but this is not because their speech organs are abnormal. Most such children are simply not being given optimal opportunities to acquire spoken language.

phonetic-level evaluation

A phonetic-level evaluation is used to determine the extent to which a child can control breath, and produce vocalization, voice patterns (non-segmentals) vowels, consonants or consonant blends on demand, and in imitation of the examiner. Vowels and consonants are elicited as single, repeated, and alternated syllables, and in conjunction with different voice patterns (high or low, loud or quiet, voiced or whispered, long or short). If a child is unable to produce the different speech patterns at a phonetic level, he or she is unlikely to be able to use them in everyday speech communication. This evaluation is therefore intended to show how far controlled production of speech patterns has been mastered, and whether adequate neuromuscular coordinations for the various speech patterns have been established. It is particularly important to determine whether each speech sound can be alternated with others, because running speech requires rapid transitions from any given phoneme to a range of different ones.

Phonetic level evaluations can be repeated time and time again. Indeed, they have to be if one is to provide a systematic remedial speech program. When a teacher or clinician is familiar with this test, and uses it to determine what phonetic level speech patterns should be targeted for immediate attention, only items from the child's known stage of development need be selected. This permits a half-dozen or so target patterns to be identified in a matter of a few minutes. Because the evaluation is based on sequential acquisition through the seven stages outlined above, the first items failed on this test are the first to be taught. Teaching at a phonetic level, though necessary for many hearing-impaired children, is not sufficient to ensure that patterns thus acquired are being used in meaningful speech (see Chapter 7).

phonologic-level evaluation

Phonologic-level evaluation is carried out through the analysis of a tape-recorded sample of a child's everyday communication. It is designed to identify the speech patterns used consistently and correctly, those used inconsistently, and those not used at all. With children at a pre-linguistic stage, the purpose is to determine whether sound patterns that will be required later in spoken language are consistently emerging. With children who have already developed some speech communication skills, the evaluation is carried out by recording a session with the child in which five different aspects of discourse are explored: conversation, description, narration, question, and explanation (see Chapter 6). The writer chose to use these categories because the type and complexity of language, the types of sentences, and the child's articulation all tend to vary according to which category of discourse is sampled. A transcription of the recorded samples is made, and this is phonetically and linguistically analyzed. These analyses show how far speech patterns are used in both phonetic and phonologic contexts, which patterns taught at a phonetic level have not been satisfactorily transferred to phonology, and how one might best plan to develop the child's spoken language skills. Unlike the phonetic level evaluation, this procedure may take two or three hours to complete.

While full scale phonologic level evaluations are required from time to time, many professionals argue - and with good reason - that they simply do not have time to carry out such time-consuming procedures. Although a full scale testing is recommended on an annual basis, there are less demanding alternatives that can be used in day-to-day management. One that the writer has found to be feasible involves the following steps:

1. Tape-record at least ten utterances relating to each aspect of discourse listed above and described in Chapter 6;

2. Play it back up to seven times (depending on the child's stage of speech acquisition). On each run listen for, and mark down which of the speech patterns in each of the seven stages described at the beginning of this chapter is used acceptably, beginning with vocalization and ending (if possible) with blends;

3. Plan phonologic work based on the outcome of this procedure, assigning priority according to the order of the stages tested. The first items failed should be the first patterns to receive attention. (See the section on generalization at the end of this chapter.)

In the early stages of speech acquisition, the average number of words in each utterance, the ratio of morphemes to words, and the ratio of function words to content words should steadily increase. These ratios should be determined and carefully noted when carrying out an alternative (less than a full scale) phonologic evaluation, and taken into account in planning phonologic work, because language skills are the essential foundation of meaningful speech.

evaluation procedures

The evaluation procedures outlined here are illustrated in a series of videotapes entitled "Ling Programs" that can be obtained from the Instructional Communication Center, McGill University, 815 Sherbrooke Street West, Montreal, P.Q., H3A 2K6 Canada. The topic is also treated in considerably more depth in the Ling (1976) text *Speech and the Hearing Impaired Child*. Printed forms for both phonetic and phonologic evaluation are available from the Alexander Graham Bell Association for the Deaf, 3417 Volta Place N.W., Washington, DC 20007.

selection of the sense modality for speech reception

Hearing-impaired children must function through one or more of the sense modalities available to them - hearing, vision, and/or touch - if they are to understand what is said to them, and if they are to be able to monitor what they themselves are saying in the most effective manner. The modalities used in everyday life should also be used in teaching if carry-over is to be ensured. To select the most appropriate sense or senses through which to develop a speech pattern targeted for development, one has to make use of the information provided in Chapters 2, 3, and 4. To develop the pattern through the selected modality, one has to make use of the information provided in Chapters 5 and 6. A given modality may be emphasized more with one child than another, and more for one speech pattern than another. For example, a child who can best learn the nasal consonants primarily through audition may be unable to learn the fricatives except through the combined use of vision and touch.

In teaching the various speech patterns, the auditory, visual, or tactile channels can be used to provide either direct or indirect information on production. Aided hearing and cochlear implants, by permitting the detection and higher level processing of the sounds themselves, make direct use of the auditory channel. Speechreading provides direct visual information on certain aspects of many speech patterns. Tactile information on a targeted pattern can be provided directly from a tactile device, but is always present in the child's oro-sensory patterns (tactile and kinesthetic patterns of sensation produced in the mouth as one speaks). Less direct use of the tactile modality is often made when the child is instructed to feel, for example, the breath stream on the finger, vibration in the chest when using voice, or where the tongue is placed for the production of an ee vowel.

Prompts and hand cues can be effective in providing a visual analog of the intensity, durational, and/or frequency characteristics of a targeted pattern, or indicating its place of production. Explanation of how or where to place the tongue, shape the lips, or move the jaw is the least direct way of helping children to acquire speech sounds. A child's acquisition of speech and spoken language skills is most efficiently fostered only if teachers and clinicians select and use the most appropriate sensory channels with the utmost care.

The professional, using the sort of information provided in the previous chapters, begins by recalling first what the device(s) worn by the child (hearing aids, cochlear implant, or tactile aid) can provide; second, what the acoustic characteristics of the speech pattern are; and third, whether the child, using the device(s) with which he or she has been provided, can *detect* the speech pattern, *discriminate* it from others, *identify* it and/or *comprehend* utterances in which the pattern is a key element. No attempt should be made to teach the pattern formally if the teacher or clinician is not utterly familiar with all aspects of such information. Furthermore, no spoken language pattern should be specifically taught if a child can acquire it spontaneously without incurring undue delay in its development.

steps in the selection of the modality

In preparation for the formal or informal teaching of a speech pattern, a professional has to ensure that whatever sensory aids the child is wearing are functioning correctly. This can be accomplished by using The Five-Sound Test or a similar procedure. Prior to promoting the informal learning or planning the formal teaching of any spoken language pattern, professionals should automatically consider the series of questions suggested below to which they can, on the basis of their existing knowledge of the sensory aids, the target speech pattern, and the child's response levels, respond *yes* or *no* as follows:

1. Can the child detect all essential components of this pattern through hearing aids or through the cochlear implant?

Yes   No.

Use audition (A).   Go to 2 (audition and vision).

2. Can the child detect all essential components through audition and vision together?

Yes.   No.

Use A + V.   Use A + V + Touch.

If the child has a tactile device instead of hearing aids or a cochlear implant, the professional would ask:

3. Can the child detect all the essential components with the tactile device and speechreading"?

Yes.   No.

Use V + Tactile device.   Use A + V + natural touch.

Where no tactile device is provided, and natural (i.e., unaided) touch is required to convey particular components, a further decision must be made as to which tactile strategies should be employed. Appropriate strategies for each speech pattern are suggested in subsequent chapters.

steps in using the selected modality

The first step in using the selected sense modality is to consider the characteristics of the device or devices used by the child, the properties of the speech pattern, and the child's responses to previous tests. If the device(s) is functioning as it should be, and all of the components of the target pattern can be detected by a child through one or more of the available sense modalities, then teachers or clinicians can, using the selected sense modality, straightforwardly ask a child to produce the pattern in imitation of a model they provide in a context that facilitates its production (see Chapters 9 through 13). If this procedure does not meet with success, the next strategy is to enable the child to move from the *detection* of the target pattern to its *discrimination* from another (reference) pattern - preferably one that has already been acquired from among those in the same stage of development - and then repeat the process.

Development of discrimination skills and production of the target patterns through the selected modality can be encouraged informally in games, or by means of formal teaching. Formal strategies for teaching a child to discriminate between two speech patterns need involve no more than the following four simple steps. As an example, consider teaching Peter to discriminate between /b/ and /m/ through his new hearing aid. *First*, associate the selected target pattern (/m/) with one hand (or a colored block), and the reference pattern (/b/) with the other hand (or a block of a different color). This can be done with Peter watching any additional cues or prompts that may have to be provided in order for the task to be understood. *Second*, produce the target and reference patterns in random order, and ask Peter, who is listening carefully, to indicate the hand (or the block) associated with each pattern. Provide feedback on correctness on each trial. *Third*, continue this procedure until he responds reliably (at least 5 occasions in six trials). *Fourth*, repeat the task without any additional cues or prompts until he again responds reliably. The purpose of this maneuver is not only to make certain that he can perceive the main characteristics of the target pattern, but to provide him with the speech reception skill required for feedback in the learning process. (The process can be reversed in order for Peter to learn to produce the two sounds distinctly.)

Discrimination between any speech sounds can be taught by a procedure such as described above if an appropriate sense modality is selected for the task. Of course, if a child's hearing is not adequate for the task, one follows the same sort of procedures with hearing + vision, or hearing + vision + tactile device. If none of these permits discrimination between the target and a reference pattern, then a natural touch strategy can be selected. As soon as a child develops the ability to discriminate a given speech pattern from all others, the production of that pattern can be expected to follow at the appropriate stage of development.

selecting and using different modalities: some examples

To provide some examples of selecting and using the various modalities in the development of a particular speech pattern, let us briefly describe how teachers and clinicians can adopt the procedures outlined above in teaching children who have been fitted with different devices. For purposes of comparison, the target sound in each case will be the stop /p/ in word-final position. We know its acoustic properties; namely, the presence of rapid vowel-to- consonant F_1 and F_2 transitions that precede abrupt cessation of voicing. We need to know, in each case, what the child's responses to sound are, and what device is worn. We can then infer what each sense modality will provide, and hence what strategies will be most effective in eliciting and developing the use of the sound.

The first child to be taught is Abby, a four-year-old girl who has a profound bilateral impairment with no hearing beyond 1500 Hz. She wears a hearing aid that allows her to detect something of all voiced sounds and vowels. She approximates a great deal of speech, has good voice patterns, clear vowels, and several consonants. However, she substitutes /m/ for a stopped /p/ so that the word *up* is pronounced *um*. She attends a regular nursery school class and a clinician sees her together with the mother in her home three times a week. The clinician knows that Abby cannot hear all components of the target pattern. She also knows that, with this profound hearing impairment Abby will be able to hear the sudden cessation of the sound, perhaps some F_1 transitions depending on the vowel, but few F_2 transitions. The range of acoustic cues she can receive will not permit her to differentiate the unreleased stops, /b/, /d/, or /g/, but she should be able to discriminate between the /m/ and the /p/ through audition alone, because they differ on two major dimensions - voicing and nasality. The clinician therefore guessed (probably correctly) that the causes of Abby's problem were over-reliance on vision (the two sounds look alike), and insufficient attention to their auditory components.

In this case, the clinician decided to play a "tidy up" game with Abby that required each of them to put objects away on shelves in locations specified in phrases that included (as italicized) the pattern in a prominent position (Put it over there, *Put it up there*, Put the rabbit down there, *Put the horse on the top shelf*). The clinician and the child first had to listen (without speechreading) in order to focus on the temporal form of the acoustic pattern. As the toy rabbit was moved towards Abby, she was enjoined to say *hop, hop, hop*. Then, when more things were found to put away, the roles were changed so Abby was the first to direct the operation. If Abby used an /m/ instead of a /p/ no move was made to follow the direction, but the clinician would provide a correct model if Abby needed one to complete the task. The word-final /p/ was learned and then used in other language contexts within a few days.

The second child to be taught is Bill an eight-year-old boy with the same sort of hearing aid as Abby, but with a somewhat more profound hearing impairment. Bill did not start school until he was five, and received little encouragement to speak until recently when the family moved from the country into a distant town to have him participate in an oral program. He has developed good voice patterns, vowels, several consonants, and many approximations to sentence forms. He is keen to improve his speech, and enjoys formal lessons with his teacher. Bill uses a /p/ in word final position, but his problem with it, and with other word-final stops, is that he always releases them, so that a sentence like, "The tap went drip drip all night" comes out as, "The tap^{ha} went^{ha} drip^{ha} drip^{ha} all night^{ha}." The teacher thinks that Bill's problem stems from the teaching he had previously received, in which speech sounds were taught by reference to written forms, a strategy that often misleads children into intrusive release of plosives when /b/ is learned as b^{uh} and /p/ is learned as p^{ha}. She decides that Bill's difficulty, though more conceptual than perceptual in origin, cannot be cleared up through audition alone, because he cannot easily detect the presence or absence of plosive bursts with his residual hearing.

The teacher, in this case, decided to use audition + vision to correct Bill's faulty /p/ pattern, and then to provide discrimination training through audition alone to help him differentiate the unreleased /p/ from other sounds. She followed four simple steps to correct the pattern. *First*, in order to use his plosive release of the /p/ as a basis for developing the target pattern, she asked Bill to watch her raise her hand as she started to say the word *up*, and drop her hand quickly as she produced the plosive burst. She did this several times, each time pausing longer at the height of her hand movement before dropping her hand and releasing the burst. *Second*, she asked Bill to say *up*, and to watch her hand movements as he did so. When the teacher saw that Bill was, without difficulty, following the visual directions she was providing, she stopped her hand in its raised position and kept it there. Bill realized her intention, and did not release the /p/. *Third*, having reinforced Bill's success with a nod and a smile, the teacher then provided Bill with several models of the word *up* as she raised her hand and arrested both its movement and the /p/ simultaneously. *Fourth*, she asked Bill to do the same. A further nod and a smile with the comment "That's good" were provided when he succeeded. As Bill was now able to produce this unreleased stop, the teacher went on to rehearse it and contrast it with the released stop so that he had the opportunity to feel how the two patterns differed when he produced each of them. She then asked Bill to listen (without speechreading) to the rhythm of some written phrases that contained word-final /p/ sounds (such as *up the wall, my hip pocket,* and *hop to it!*) as she read them with and without releasing the /p/ so that he could hear the effect of intrusive plosion on speech rhythm, even if he could not hear the intrusive plosion itself. She followed this up with having Bill read and produce similar phrases correctly and incorrectly, so that he himself learned to monitor this aspect of speech through the tactile and kinesthetic sensations he generated as he spoke. Finally, she helped Bill use stops correctly in communicative speech by adopting several different procedures for ensuring carry-over (see the section on generalization below).

The third child to be taught is Carole, a five-year-old girl who was born with normal hearing, but became totally deaf following meningitis at two years of age. Immediately on recovery she was enrolled in a total communication program. No attempt had been made to preserve and extend her spoken language by systematically building on her existing awareness of articulatory sensation of speech patterns. Her parents wanted her to communicate by speech rather than sign, however, so they arranged for her to receive a single channel cochlear implant at age three. By this time she had lost most of the speech she had acquired prior to her hearing loss. During the two years since she received the implant, she has been enrolled in a parent-infant program run by a teacher of the hearing-impaired who is skilled in perceptual-oral development. As a result, Carole has begun to revive her speech skills, and is now again able to speak in sentences. She has, however, developed many of the faults that can occur with speechreading.

Carole's problem with the unreleased /p/ is that she releases the plosion through her nose, rather as if it were an unvoiced /m/. Her teacher was aware that Carole could not directly detect this through the single channel cochlear implant or through speechreading. He had undertaken an oral-peripheral examination, and therefore knew that this problem, one often met in children having cleft palates, was not due to an organic deficit. He decided to treat the problem through touch and, by analogy with an unreleased word-final /b/, knowing that the most important difference between an unreleased /b/ and an unreleased /p/ is the length of the preceding vowel, and that any nasal escape following a /b/ would be perceived through her cochlear implant and speechreading as /m/.

The teacher followed a seven-step procedure. *First*, he asked Carole to listen and watch as he said *cub*. To carry out this step, he also raised her hand to his mouth so that she could feel that there was no release of plosion for the /b/. *Second*, he repeated the procedure but, this time, released the plosive burst onto Carole's other hand, so that she could feel it distinctly. *Third*, he repeated both the previous maneuvers, and then asked Carole if there was a difference. She recognized that there was. *Fourth*, he asked her to make the comparison herself, feeling the effect on her hands as she had done when he provided the models. She succeeded in doing this. *Fifth*, he asked her to repeat the released vs. unreleased contrast several times. *Sixth*, he showed her pictures of a cub and a cup, and asked her to feel that neither word-final sound was released and, *Seventh*, asked her (by saying "Show me the cub" or "Show me the cup") to identify each with speechreading and (implant) hearing together. Next session, he asked her to identify them without speechreading, which she could do on the basis of durational cues. The task was then reversed and she successfully asked him either to "Point to the cub" or "Point to the cup." It was a mere *hop, skip,* and a *jump* before Carole was using the unreleased /p/ appropriately in everyday communication.

Totally deaf children using either a multi-channel tactile device or cochlear implant might well have avoided developing these three types of faults (but might have developed others instead). Most such instruments are capable of providing sufficient direct information on nasality (the problem with Abby), and plosive release (the problem with Bill). Indeed, a single-channel instrument that works well should also provide enough direct auditory information on the sudden cessation of sound pressure that normally signals an unreleased stop. That such an instrument did not provide it for Carole within two years of use was good enough reason to clear up the problem of inaudible nasal release with the help of other modalities before the fault became habitual. The selection of sense modalities pervades all aspects of spoken language acquisition. In the above examples, the focus has been more on the selection of an appropriate sense modality for speech reception, but such selection also has an important influence on speech production. In the section that follows, the effects of using carefully selected sense modalities in providing set will be shown.

provision of set

The provision of sets is one of the most powerful tactics that can be used in teaching spoken language. It is based on the principle that most learning requires moving from the known to the unknown. When features of two previously acquired behaviors (Part of A and Part of B) are present in a new, target behavior (C), then a clinician or teacher can have the child rehearse A and B in order to promote the child's awareness of the nature of the target (C). This procedure is known as providing a set. When an A + B set is provided, a child's chances of successfully producing the target behavior C are greatly enhanced. The concept of set is closely related to generalization, a topic that will be addressed later in this chapter.

some examples of sets

For our first example of set, let us see how a /z/ was first elicited from Teresa. She knows how to voice for several seconds at a time (pattern A) and has been taught to produce the /s/ (pattern B) in chains of syllables or words such as *us us us us us*. Teresa is asked to rehearse patterns A and B, and is then asked to say *us us us us us* with voicing throughout. Doing this she straight away succeeds in producing *uz uz uz uz uz* (pattern C). The focus on A and B immediately before attempting C enormously increased Teresa's chances of achieving C because human beings can generalize from particular, and especially immediately prior, experiences.

Before proceeding to further examples of the use of set in teaching, let us illustrate the power of set by turning to an example that can be used for amusement. Tell people that you are thinking about a child's card game, and then say, "I want you to fill in the missing pieces when I pause. First (A) I want you to tell me what these two letters say when you sound them out together. The letters are a and p, and they say __. Good. They say *ap*. Second, (B) another name for a short sleep is a ___. Good again, a *nap*. Now, (C) you are playing cards with a child, and when two different cards come up at the same time, you say_____." The effect of set is extraordinarily compelling, so under most conditions it will take several seconds of silence before it is realized that the answer is not *snap*. In the following paragraphs, and in the next chapters, we shall see how the provision of set can influence the acquisition of many different speech skills.

The use of anticipatory set need not, of course, be limited to the teaching of speech. It can be used for teaching any aspect of spoken language and, indeed, many other physical or intellectual skills. Here, a few aspects of spoken language will be used as examples. From these, generalizations can be made to other areas of knowledge or skill.

The clinician or teacher has to choose a set carefully in order to achieve the desired result, because many hearing-impaired children can only know whether or not they have achieved the desired behavior from feedback on correctness initially provided by the professional. Later, when the sound has been practiced, they will be able to tell the sound apart from all others by the features that characterize it for them as individuals - the cues that are available through whatever sense modality they are using, including the oro-sensory and motor patterns that they experience with saying it, and their awareness of its use as a morpheme in particular words or language structures. If only one (A or B) speech pattern is available to provide set, then a second one can be taught, or appropriate cues can be given by the clinician or teacher through another modality. Visual hand signals or tactile cues can be useful in this regard, and some of these will be described later. When sets are successfully used, children look forward to speech or language lessons because when A and B patterns have been appropriately chosen, C patterns result in a matter of minutes, if not seconds. Most children revel in the speedy accumulation of skills and, as more and more speech skills are acquired, the faster the process can go. If set is not carefully planned, unexpected outcomes will occur that can confuse, frustrate, and mislead the child.

sets and spoken language

Sets can frequently be used to turn a simple correction of grammar into the learning of a language principle. For instance, if, in a conversation, a hearing-impaired child used the construction "He didn't want me go," one could choose a convenient time to point out that the correct form is "He didn't want me to go." (It tends to discourage the very effort you want to see the child make if you use conversation as a vehicle for speech or language correction.) The portion "He didn't want me" (A) is acceptable, but the use of the infinitive to complete such sentences (B) had to be taught. Left at a simple correction, there would probably be no long lasting effect. However, used as a set, other sentences of the same (C) form as "He didn't want me to go" can be developed, and their use in real-life situations encouraged; for example, "He didn't want me to fall" (to run, to walk, to swim, to ride, to play).

Creative clinicians and teachers can also use sets for the promotion of concepts and the prevention of common errors. For example, many hearing impaired children do not spontaneously learn when to use a to signify "one from more than one,", and when to use the to signify "the only one." Confusions of these determiners are not uncommon even in the written work of some hearing-impaired children of high school age. To promote the concepts underlying a and the, and to prevent confusions in the use of these words in later childhood, clinicians often provide opportunity for young children to learn this important linguistic concept as they play with, and help put away, several similar objects, say toy animals, different colored sticks or different sized books (and, at a later stage, different sized, shaped, and colored buttons) on display, with one of a particular sort, and many of other sorts.

To illustrate establishing a set from which the concepts relating to *a* and *the* can be derived, let us use the following toy animals: one sheep, three horses, one cow, and four pigs. With the teacher (and later the child) asking (A), "Pass me *the* cow (or sheep), please," and (B), while there are still more than one, "Pass me *a* horse (or a pig), please," the principle is first illustrated. The next time, of course, the numbers of animals must be changed to (C) several horses or pigs, and only one cow or sheep, in order to ensure that *a* and *the* are seen to relate to the number of objects rather than the objects themselves. Once the notion is mastered, the set provided by the experience is immediately applied to another lot of objects, and the process repeated and extended. To ensure that the correct use is carried over into everyday life, the set is used in extending the concept to clothing, sorting cutlery, choosing furniture, and identifying other types of household objects that are in common use.

set and speech development

In speech development, every pattern that is learned by the child can be used to provide a set for the development of further speech patterns. For example, in the previous section on selection of the sense modality the unreleased /p/ was featured. This may seem a trivial sound to be so concerned with, but it is not. Once established, it helps to provide a set for the production of unreleased /t/ and /k/ sounds. The production of both are important in preserving the natural rhythm of utterances, but the unreleased /t/ is also as important as its released counterpart in signalling past tense, and it is the most important component in differentiating ch and sh.

The ch sound is initiated by the unreleased /t/, so that the main acoustic difference between these sounds is that the ch is characterized by a sudden, and the sh by a gradual, release of energy in the octave band centered on 2000 Hz. Depending on the hearing levels of the child and the type of device worn this difference may or may not be audible. When it is not, providing the unreleased /p/ as part of a set (A), a sound that permits the speechreader to see and feel that there is no release of breath after vocal tract (lip) closure, and showing the child that the desired sound is produced by arresting the breath stream with the tongue and not the lips (B), indicates exactly how the unreleased /t/ (target C) is to be produced. In turn, the unreleased /p/ and /t/ can both be used to provide a set for the production of the unreleased /k/.

Set, using previously learned behaviors to facilitate the teaching of a related new behavior, can help at every stage of speech acquisition. In the following chapters, the use of set and the prerequisite behaviors in teaching each sound pattern will be specified. Here, the purpose is to provide sufficient examples of its use to demonstrate its pervasive force in the speech teaching process. This will be further illustrated by the following consideration of the development of consonants.

set in the production of consonants

Hearing aids, tactile devices or cochlear implants may not, on their own or together with speechreading, permit consonants to be spontaneously acquired by certain children. Once such children are producing vowels, however, consonant acquisition can be rapidly promoted. The first step in this process is for the teacher or clinician to help the child develop a core repertoire of sounds that have different manners of production. The second step is to elicit each of the remaining sounds of like manner through the provision of set (ensuring as this is done that all speech patterns are systematically developed and used phonologically). The simplest core sounds to begin the process are those that can be most readily heard, seen and/or felt by the child. These are the sounds that are produced at the front of the mouth. The order imposed by this procedure, and followed in the discussion below, is close, but not identical, to that followed by normally hearing children in their acquisition of controlled consonant production. Some slight variations in order might occur with some hearing-impaired children (e.g. sh before /s/ on account of the relatively greater acoustic salience of sh.

The plosives or stops can be developed best from /b/ in the order /b/, /d/, and /g/. The /b/ can be developed simply by providing any vowel as the set and interrupting its production by closing and opening the lips to produce the repeated syllable ub, ub, ub, ub. Central vowels may be preferred in the development of these sounds because they lead to more marked ballistic movement of the tongue with the /d/ and the /g/. Once production of the /b/ sound is established, it provides the set for the /d/, in the sequence ub, ub, ub, ud, ud, ud. This set, produced by the repetition of syllables containing the /b/, indicates to the child that the sound the teacher or clinician wants is a voiced plosive of the same type produced (as is evident from the speechread component) with the blade of the tongue instead of the lips.

The /g/ is evoked using a set provided by both previously acquired plosives. The simplest way to obtain the /g/ sound if children do not develop it spontaneously is to provide them with a set consisting of a series of syllables containing the /b/ and /d/, asking the child to try to say some of the /d/ sounds with a finger held over the front of the tongue. The effort to produce a /d/ in this impossible situation will usually result in them raising the back of the tongue and producing the /g/. Once the voiced plosives are produced in this way, their conscious production in other vowel contexts and unconscious inclusion in spontaneous spoken language will require systematic development of the sounds. Clearly, both the released and unreleased /p/, /t/, and /k/ can be developed in that order with the same sort of use being made of set. However, other methods of providing set can be used when sufficient information is available through one or other of the available devices discussed in Chapter 4.

The nasal sounds can best be developed in the order /m/, /n/, and ng. The /m/ is developed, like the /b/, through a set provided by vowels and awareness of voicing. To elicit /m/, one only has to close the lips during vowel production and continue to voice (unlike eliciting the /b/ by interrupting both vowel and voice). Again, using the central vowels tends to facilitate the production of these sounds. It is important to ensure that the oral breath stream of the vowel is restored each time the mouth opens on the release of /m/, otherwise nasalized vowels may occur. A chain of several syllables, such as um, um, um, on one breath and in various vowel contexts will lead to competent production of the /m/ sound. The initial placing of the /m/ in syllable final position avoids the risk of intrusive plosion (/m/ followed by /b/ as in /m^{ba}/). The continuity of voicing, if it needs to be brought to conscious awareness by touch, should be established by feeling the vibration on the lips, chin, or chest. Vibration on the nose can be felt, but feeling the nose tends to lead to an exaggerated production.

Once the /m/ is produced clearly with several vowels, a protracted /m/ can be used to provide the set for the /n/. After producing a long ummmmmmmmm sound and having the child imitate it, produce a similarly long sound but smile with the tongue tip resting lightly between the teeth half way through its production, and the /n/ will emerge in the sequence ummmmnnn. From this, it is a simple step to producing unununun or words like "no." As with the plosive /g/, a velar sound, the ng can be elicited by providing a set with the /m/ and /n/ syllables. If necessary, one can ask the child to produce a sound like /n/ with a finger over the blade of the tongue at the end of such a set, and this will usually result in the ng.

Fricative sounds are created through turbulence in the breath stream. Fricative turbulence is greater for unvoiced than voiced fricatives because voicing absorbs energy from the breath stream. The breath stream of voiceless fricatives is, therefore, easier to feel, and this is a good reason for teaching unvoiced fricatives first; that is, /f/, unvoiced th, /s/, and sh before /v/, voiced th, /z/, and zh. Fricatives are best developed first in syllable-final and word-final positions so that they can be clearly differentiated from plosives.

Because /f/ and /th/ are the most visible fricatives, they (and their tangible breath streams) contain the most salient features for the provision of a fricative set. Any whispered vowel provides the required set for tangible breath stream. Having children imitate the visible lip-teeth contact while maintaining a tangible breath flow (initiated with the whispered vowel) will lead to the production of /f/. Having them imitate the visible contact of tongue and teeth while maintaining tangible breath flow will lead to the production of th. The production of these sounds without tension or exaggeration provides the important foundation for their speedy repetition without intrusive plosion. Repetition of these sounds on one breath (e.g. /afafafafaf/) in different unvoiced and voiced vowel contexts is required to develop the motor skills and the oro-sensory patterns required for their use in providing an adequate set for other consonants, and for their inclusion in communicative speech.

To use the th as a set for the production of /s/ and sh, have a child draw the tongue slowly back over the top, or alternatively the bottom, teeth while maintaining breath stream, and the /s/ will usually appear. Again, such a sound should be rehearsed in chains of repeated syllables or words on one breath (e.g. us us us us us) and in various vowel contexts, so that the oro-sensory patterns are unconsciously established as articulatory coding referents. This done, the sh can be derived from a set provided by the th and the /s/ by repeating the tongue retraction process, but having the child take it back just a bit further. Once established, the unvoiced consonants in repeated strings of syllables or words, such as *off off off off off*, provide a set for their voiced cognates (sounds with the same manner and place of production). For example, one only has to instruct the child to sustain voicing throughout such an utterance and it becomes *of of of of of*, a series from which other syllables and words containing /v/ can be developed. (It has already been suggested that such a strategy is particularly effective in eliciting the /z/ from the /s/.) Finally, with respect to fricatives, the whispering of any vowel provides a set for /h/ because this sound may be regarded simply as the whispered form of the vowel that follows it.

The above discussion illustrates how efficiently a target pattern can be elicited through the provision of a set, a provision that involves reference to two previously learned behaviors (one or more sounds) that have characteristics in common with the target pattern. The use of a set in the teaching of speech will be developed further in relation to other manners of consonant production and other stages of speech development in later chapters. Any previously learned behavior and any sense modality can be used to provide a set, as the following section illustrates.

set and modality

Set can be provided in any one of the three sense modalities. In the examples involving different children, provided above, vision and touch were both used in providing the set, first to develop the unreleased /p/, and second, to move from that to the two other sounds that share the same manner of production, but are made in different places in the vocal tract, namely the /t/ and the /k/. Such a strategy would have been quite unnecessary if the similarities and differences between the three speech patterns could have been otherwise perceived. In some cases, multi-channel cochlear implants or tactile devices used as aids to speechreading might permit all three of the unreleased stops to develop without such intervention. However, multi-channel devices are not equally effective with all children. Even when all electrodes are providing optimal stimulation, alveolar and velar sounds sharing the same manner of production are frequently confused by those who wear such instruments.

To illustrate the interaction of set and sense modality, let us look at the way Mary, a clinician providing itinerant support for several hearing-impaired children, helped two children, David and Ethel, to produce a /k/.

David is an eight-year-old boy who was born with profound hearing impairment across the speech frequency range, an impairment that has

248 FOUNDATIONS OF SPOKEN LANGUAGE

worsened over the years. He has had no measurable hearing for four years. He attended oral parent-infant and pre-school programs, and is now attending a special class attached to a regular school where he is integrated for several subjects. He has acquired an extensive vocabulary, and fluent, though faulty, speech communication skills. He has been wearing a multi-channel cochlear implant for two years. Ethel is a seven-year-old girl who survived meningitis that left her with no useful residual hearing at age two. She received a multi-channel tactile device at age four. Her history in other respects is like David's.

Rather than use /p/ (pattern A) and /t/ (pattern B) to create the set for eliciting the /k/ (target C), Mary decided that with these children she would use speechreading to supplement the information provided by the children's multi-channel instruments. The strategy was essentially the same for both. The known patterns from which she decided to work were the nasal sounds and the plosive burst of /p/. *First*, Mary checked to see that the children could discriminate and produce all three nasal sounds, the /m/, the /n/, and the ng. They could. *Second*, she asked them to say the /m/, and then add the sound /p/ to the end of it (as in the word *lamp*). As both the nasal and the plosive burst could be detected and dis-criminated, neither child had difficulty with the task. *Third*, she asked the children to repeat amp amp amp ensuring that both the nasal and the plosive burst were clearly present. *Fourth*, she asked them to do the same thing again, but to add three new syllables, namely ant ant ant. She thus firmly established the nasal + plosive burst at the same place of produc-tion as the set. *Fifth*, and finally, Mary asked the children to say am-p, an-t, and then ang-k (as in anchor), and both produced the desired /k/ without difficulty. There is clearly a motor component involved in this strategy. In fact, motor components are often an important part of the provision of set, and they remain important throughout the subsequent development of speech production skills.

automaticity

Automaticity in spoken language is reached when no conscious effort is given to its reception or production, and when attention in talking is not on *how* to say something, but on *what* is to be said. Just as those who are beginning to read may have to analyze each sentence and break down words in order to "sound them out," so may children initially need to follow similar analytic processes in order to master the elements of communication. But just as skilled readers mainly go straight to the meaning of what they read from the text, so must those who communicate fluently be able, for the most part, to go straight to the meaning of what others say as they talk. That point is reached by normally hearing individuals only after many years of experience in communicating through speech, experience that begins in early childhood. It is illogical to think that hearing-impaired children can reach automatic levels of communication with less. They must be provided with abundant opportunities to learn and to use spoken language, not just in special lessons, but in most of the situations they encounter.

Conscious attention and automaticity are two extremes on a continuum. Between these extremes lie several fairly distinct stages. These stages are readily illustrated by the process of speech production. At first, all speech is novel. Next, it becomes somewhat familiar. Then it becomes practiced. Later, it is produced with skill. Finally it becomes automatic. At the first stage, one can produce a speech pattern correctly if one tries hard enough. At the final stage one can produce it incorrectly only with effort. Brain scans show that when one attempts to do something that is novel, a great deal of the brain is involved with the activity, and that much less energy is used by the brain in dealing with something that has been practiced to a level of automaticity. This is why people can carry on doing something that is automatic to them when they are also required to attend to something else.

When any skill, perceptive or productive, has reached automaticity, four basic elements characterize its performance: accuracy, speed, economy of effort, and flexibility. Accuracy and speed are self explanatory. Economy of effort means speaking with as little effort as the task requires - not exaggerating, and not using muscles or making movements unless they contribute to the speaking task. Flexibility means being able to use the speech patterns in all sorts of contexts - loudly, quietly, slowly, quickly, in stressed and unstressed words, and with a variety of intonation patterns - contexts that enhance the intelligibility and normalcy of spoken language. These elements are acquired at the same time as each component of the skill. Increments in performance do not occur unless accuracy underlies practice. Nor does speed of performance increase unless the task is accurately, consistently, and frequently practiced. Economy of effort can be observed in the acquisition of every skill. As automaticity is approached, redundant mental or physical effort is progressively decreased until only the essential intellectual and/or motor components are involved in the exercise of the skill. Finally, no skill is automatic unless it can be carried out with flexibility; that is, in a variety of ways, and under a variety of conditions. Speaking, for example, can be done through shouting, whispering, talking in quiet, talking in noise, talking in confidence, or talking in public.

All four of the basic elements of performance must be attended to in the development of a child's spoken language. Many of the deficits commonly found in the speech of hearing-impaired individuals can be traced to professionals' unawareness of the importance of accuracy, speed, economy of effort and flexibility. All four elements can be developed mainly through activities that are meaningful and fun, rather than through drills that tend to be boring. The necessary (spaced) practice can be arranged at home and in school without long teaching periods being specifically devoted to it.

generalization and carry-over

Generalization is said to occur when a particular aspect of knowledge or skill is seen to relate or to apply to many other aspects of knowledge or skill. In order to generalize, then, one must perceive that particular elements are present in commonly occurring patterns, and from that perception deduce that they should also occur in less familiar patterns of the same sort. Thus, generalization can be said to have occurred when a child comes to understand how to use *many* and *much* correctly in various situations (e.g.,"There are too many potatoes," "That's too much milk," "I have too many spoons," "Don't give me so much salt, please," "How many sheep can you see?," and "How much sugar do you want?"). Awareness that *many* applies to all unit nouns, and *much* applies to all mass nouns is vitally important for clarity of conceptualization. (Readers who do not know what unit and mass nouns are, are hereby challenged to look at the particular examples above and generalize from them). Much, if not most, of what we know of language and the world at large, we have deduced, generalized, and then tested for validity in the course of our daily living. We would know relatively little if every single fact that is important to us had had to be formally taught.

The terms *generalization* and *carry-over* are often regarded as having the same meaning. It is useful, however, to make a distinction between them so that generalization refers to the process of extending a child's phonetic or phonologic skills in teaching, and carry-over refers to the child's transfer of formally taught speech skills from the classroom or clinic into a variety of real-life communicative situations. Generalization has mainly to do with extension of the context affecting the acquisition of sounds, words and sentence structures, and carry-over, the extension of the social and communicative contexts that feature all aspects of discourse. Such a distinction serves to clarify the different nature of the two processes, and the types of strategies that can be adopted to promote effective teaching and learning. Consider the following examples.

When a child first learns to produce a /k/ in one vowel context - for example, with ah - he or she may be quite unable to produce the sound with the ee, because the tongue has to make contact with the palate further forward in the mouth for ee than for ah. By having the child repeat the first consonant and vowel in the words *car car car, cat cat cat, Ken Ken Ken, cake cake cake , kick kick kick*, and finally *key key key*, each as quickly as possible, economy of effort will ensure that the point of tongue contact will be gradually shifted forward, so that the /k/ will be *generalized* by this strategy from the central vowel ah to all of the front vowels. A similar strategy can be used to generalize the production of the /k/ to the back vowels, including oo. The same sort of generalization process can be utilized in obtaining production of other sounds, such as /r/, /l/, /s/, and sh, in all vowel contexts, moving from the production of sounds in syllables to sounds in words, learning regular verb tenses, learning word order, and mastering a multitude of grammatical rules underlying sentence structures (see Chapter 6). Generalization of this type occurs when children are learning to produce sounds and spoken language patterns that are really *new* to them.

Strategies to enhance carry-over do not involve the teaching of new speech sounds and language patterns, but the promotion of the social and communicative use of those that are already somewhat *familiar*. The strategies to foster such carry-over include:

- mending meaning - "I'm sorry, I didn't get (or understand) that."
- requesting repetition - "Tell me that again please."
- specifying difficulty - "I didn't get what happened to Jim."

- using ellipsis (seeking completion) - "You and Jim went to see ____?"
- using questions - "So then what happened?" or "How did Jim like that?", and "What do you think Peter will do about that?" Note: Don't over-use questions that can be answered with a simple "yes."
- modelling + imitation - "Oh! you mean xxx xx xxxx. You tell me that."
- modelling + reflection of child's utterance - Child: "Pe uh te you hum oh wimme." Adult: "Oh yes! Peter said *you come home with me!*"
- encouraging continuation: "Really!", "Uh huh!", "Wow!"
- praising efforts - "My, you said that well! I understood every word!"
- demanding social elements - "Tell me what people say when ...."
- using directions - "Go to the store and ask Mr. Brown for some more chalk, please. Say: *"Please Mr. Brown, may I have some more chalk for our class."*
- using linguistic prompts - "You should use more breath (talk louder)."
- using non-verbal prompts - holding one's fingers in front of one's mouth to prompt the child to increase the breath stream, or on one's chest to indicate that the child should lower voice pitch, and so on.

Carry-over strategies must be used with caution. An adult's intervention in a child's communicative efforts should inspire further effort. It should provide immediate and specific positive reinforcement for correct spoken language use, indicate (hopefully genuine) interest in what is being said, promote a child's self-confidence and self-responsibility in his or her spoken language, and be sufficiently challenging to engender a child's best efforts. One must not be so accepting that a child makes no effort to improve, or so demanding that the child makes no attempt to talk.

Some of the examples of carry-over strategies listed above can be perceived by children as negative, or even demeaning, while others may offer enormous encouragement, stimulate a child to think, and result in pleasurable interchange. But any strategy can lose its effectiveness when repeated too frequently, so none should be habitually used. Correction should be kept to a minimum in the context of communication. When it is necessary to interrupt a conversation in order to understand what a child says, then attention is best directed towards identifying the source of the communicative breakdown, and repairing it quickly so that the underlying train of thought is not lost. The process of directing attention clearly to the source of a breakdown is highly informative; it helps children to learn socially acceptable repair strategies, suggests ways to avoid future problems of the same sort, promotes a sense of self-responsibility and a desire to be understood, and encourages continued efforts to communicate. If a child is using appropriate sensory aids, and has been taught well, many of the spoken language skills developed through the use of formal strategies should be spontaneously carried over - providing of course, that he or she spends enough high-quality time in a speech communication environment. Further teaching can be planned to enhance those aspects of previous teaching that are not spontaneously transferred from lessons to life.

There may be several reasons for a child's failure to generalize (or carry over) particular things that are being taught. The child may not be sufficiently intelligent but, more usually, the topic is of little or no interest, the subject matter is not sufficiently meaningful, the topic is too unfamiliar for the child to be able to perceive a pattern in it, the subject matter is too complex for the child, or the context of teaching is not sufficiently similar to the context in which everyday use is expected. Of course, we can help children to generalize by making a topic interesting enough to think about, giving it meaning, presenting it in sufficiently simple terms, ensuring that enough is known for them to perceive underlying patterns, and creating perceptible similarities between learning in school and living at home.

Carry-over is promoted by making sure that spoken language skills are acquired under a variety of conditions, in different places, at all times of the day, and through children's numerous social contacts with people - peers and adults other than their parents, teachers, and/or clinicians. It is not unusual for very young children - particularly those who rely heavily on visual information - to require their mothers or their teachers to "translate" what others say to them or they say to others. Such dependence may be flattering to the translator, but it should be gradually reduced - the children should be expected to communicate directly with more and more people as they grow. When one sets out to promote carry-over, it is just as important to ensure a child's optimal personal and social development as it is to provide whatever teaching is essential for the development of relevant skills.

Children who are at the stage in which generalization occurs spontaneously often make mistakes, and thus discover different rules or exceptions to rules. For example, when they realize that the regular past tense of verbs is signalled by ed, as in the words *picked* and *hugged*, they may say *digged* instead of *dug* or *thinked* instead of *thought* - even if they have used these verbs correctly at an earlier stage. Such mistakes are important evidence of generalization. Children usually become aware that they have (over) generalized a newly perceived rule without specific help from adults. If adults cannot resist an attempt to "correct" such errors, they should not draw children's attention to them, but just make doubly sure that sufficient meaningful natural language is addressed to them and to others in the family, and that their hearing aids - or other sensory aids - are in good order.

Generalization and carry-over are essential components, then, of any spoken language pattern. Once a child has had sufficient exposure to become aware that certain question forms are associated with particular intonation patterns, similar questions are then asked with that particular sort of intonation. When a child has had enough experiences of the adjective preceding the noun, as in a *big dog* or a *small spoon*, the deduction that all adjectives precede nouns can be made. That adjectives of size always precede adjectives of color as in *the big black dog* or *the little yellow ball* is perceived and generalized later. Only when a child does not have enough experience in the course of everyday communication is it necessary to teach that adjectives always precede nouns in a given order, namely number, kind, size, color and material. Experienced language users know, without having been taught, that "two clean large white cotton handkerchiefs" is acceptable, and "large clean two cotton white handkerchiefs" is not.

In developing the language skills of hearing-impaired children, we can leave it to them to take the initiative and to generalize, but only if we can be sure that they are receiving sufficient information through their hearing aids, cochlear implants or tactile devices to do so. However, if the integrity of their speech reception systems with the instruments they are wearing is poor, and the signals they are receiving are too degraded for them to acquire particular aspects of spoken language spontaneously, then we should set out not only to teach spoken language patterns, but also to help them generalize and carry over patterns they learn by providing carefully structured situations that highlight them.

In speech teaching, once a particular pattern has been evoked, the whole focus of its development is on generalization and carry-over. Once vocalization is established, its use should be generalized to such functions as attracting attention. As soon as different voice patterns are elicited, their use should be generalized to conveying different moods and eventually providing the prosodic features of utterances. When vowels can be produced, their use must be generalized to become the base of approximations to adult forms of speech. The production of every consonant sound, as soon as each can be said, must also be generalized to all vowel contexts, placed in words, used in sentences, and encouraged in discourse. The generalization of consonant blends allows children not only to produce new words, but to add morphemes, such as the possessive and plural endings, and a host of other prefixes and suffixes to known words.

It is rare for children who need formal speech teaching to develop high levels of spontaneous generalization and carry-over in the early stages of spoken language acquisition, because their range of experience with speech communication is too limited for them to be able to perceive its implicit patterning. Clinicians and teachers must, therefore, see the development of a speech pattern and the promotion of its generalization and carry-over as facets of the same task, one that has hope of bearing fruit only when the teachers and clinicians accept the challenge of making their spoken language work interesting and effective by promoting an atmosphere that closely reflects the characteristics of communication in everyday, real-life situations.

everyday communication

There are many good reasons why hearing-impaired children should learn to talk. It is what nine hundred and ninety-nine people in every thousand do well, so being able to communicate by speech enables hearing-impaired individuals to feel that they belong to society at large; it permits them to communicate with others in the family who can hear; it provides opportunities to have a wide variety of friends; it opens up many educational options that would otherwise be closed; and it offers opportunities for the school graduate to select from an abundant range of occupations. This list is by no means complete.

Speech communication must be practiced as such if it is to become effective. Clinicians and teachers are wasting their own and the child's time if they do not ensure that the speech they teach is used in the meaningful situations provided by everyday life. No systematic plan, no type of speech evaluation, no hearing aid, cochlear implant or tactile device, no application of the principles underlying set, no amount of work towards automaticity, will develop spoken language to a sufficiently high level unless speech communication is carried over from lessons into everyday life. The use of spoken language cannot be regarded simply as a complex skill; it must also be perceived as a system through which hearing-impaired children can learn, and can have access to the abundance of good things associated with living a full life.

recommended further reading

Further reading on the importance of the issues discussed above is available in Bess, Freeman and Sinclair (1981), Boothroyd (1982), Bunch (1987), Calvert and Silverman (1983), Cole and Gregory (1986), Lauter (1985), Markides (1983), Mencher and Gerber (1981), and Stovell (1982), and many other texts. The system has been most comprehensively described in the original text by Ling (1976), and its application referenced in many journals including *The Volta Review*, *The American Annals of the Deaf*, *The Teacher of the Deaf*, the *Journal of Speech and Hearing Disorders*, and the *Journal of Speech and Hearing Research*. See References pp. 433 ff.

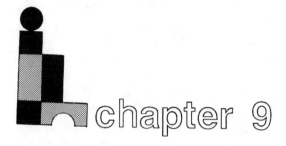

chapter 9

development of speech: breathing, vocalization, and voice patterns

introduction

The purpose of this chapter, and those immediately following, is to describe a variety of strategies that can be used to elicit speech patterns, and suggest how they may be integrated into spoken language communication. The target patterns will be presented in the same order as the developmental model described by Ling (1976) and in Chapter 8 of this text. The present chapter will focus on breathing, vocalization, and voice patterns (intensity, duration, and pitch). The following chapters will be concerned with the production of vowels and diphthongs, the development of consonants by manner of production, place of production, and voicing, as well as the acquisition of initial and final blends.

Four principles require emphasis in all work to develop spoken language skills. First, regardless of the sense modality or modalities used, speech reception must precede speech production. Second, the provision of abundant experience of meaningful speech patterns is the essential preliminary step in promoting all aspects of speech communication. Third, a child's perceptual-oral skills can be developed optimally, only when the instruments used as aids in the transmission of speech have been appropriately selected, and when they are kept in first-rate working order. Fourth, attention must be given to the development of a child's self-monitoring (feedback) skills if acceptable patterns of spoken language are to result.

The informal strategies described in the following pages are most applicable to the systematic development of speech skills in young children. The formal strategies are more appropriate for older children who need remedial help (see Chapter 7). Most of the formal strategies can be adopted - or adapted - for remedial work with adults, for the principles underlying them are valid for all ages. Materials that may be helpful will be suggested and, where appropriate, any contexts that are known to facilitate the production of a target will be mentioned. Because positive reinforcement should be provided at every stage of a speech pattern's development, it will not receive special and repeated mention or recommendation as a procedure. Finally, the comments and suggestions relating to the phonological use of speech that are made in this chapter are not necessarily applicable to all children, because language learning must be geared more to an individual's needs and interests than to a professional's or parent's plan.

speech errors

All sorts of errors are to be found in speech produced by hearing-impaired individuals, particularly among those who did not receive the benefits that modern technology and systematic speech development strategies can bestow during early childhood. Among the most common are: failure to regulate the breath stream for speaking; poor voice control that leads to harsh, arrhythmic, monotonous, weak, high-pitched, or breathy speech; failure to coordinate voicing and articulation; prolongation, neutralization and nazalization of vowels; as well as distortion and omission of various (particularly word-final) consonants. At least half of these problems result from inadequate control of breath, vocalization, and voice patterns - the fundamentals of all speech production. None of these speech errors is inevitable. Many profoundly hearing-impaired individuals, some of whom are totally deaf, speak with no serious impediment to intelligibility.

If the causes of error can be reliably determined, then procedures can be devised that will prevent their occurrence. The developmental strategies suggested in this, and in the following chapters are, in fact, such procedures. But if they are to work, they must be appropriately applied. Currently, many weaknesses in hearing-impaired individuals' spoken language skills can be attributed, not to the procedures themselves, but to our common failure as professional workers to use them effectively in developmental work. Prevention is better than remediation.

Spoken language is a very natural phenomenon, and reasons can be found for any aspect of it developing abnormally. The obvious underlying cause of the bulk of hearing-impaired individuals' speech faults is inadequate perception and feedback - insufficient awareness of speech patterns and how they are produced. Auditory perception of vocalization and voice patterns depends on how well the harmonics of voice, and changes in their intensity, duration, and frequency can be detected. Cues on vocalization are particularly strong, therefore, over the frequency regions that contain the most powerful harmonics. This is the frequency range below 1000 Hz. The audiogram shown as Figure 9-1 is that of a boy called Sean who, in spite of his profound hearing impairment, has good voice quality, and is able to sing in tune.

The audiogram presented as Figure 9-1 shows the CLEAR zone with bands of shading becoming darker as the acoustic cues on vocalization and voice patterns (carried by the harmonics of voice) become weaker. Note that Sean has aided responses (A – A) that fall well inside the optimal zone for the detection of vocalization and voice patterns.

developmental and remedial work

Developmental and remedial work in spoken language are distinctly different. In developmental work the objective is to promote the growth of spoken language through broadly normal stages of acquisition, and by this means prevent omissions and distortions of patterns that would otherwise (and commonly do) prevail. Both formal teaching and informal learning are basic to developmental work. In contrast, remedial work tends to require an individual's conscious attention, and hence the application of formal teaching strategies. Remedial work is essentially geared to the correction of faults that have been allowed to occur and persist because a developmental program has not been followed, or has not been monitored sufficiently well.

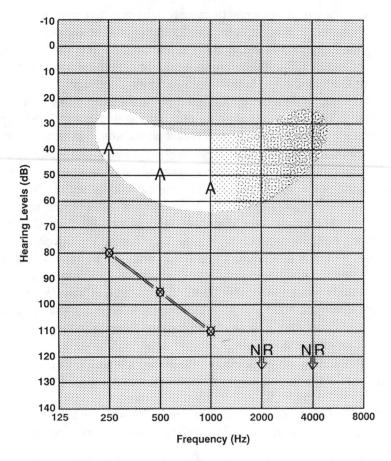

figure 9-1. An audiogram of a profoundly hearing-impaired boy named Sean. Note that his aided audiogram provides substantial amplification at 250 Hz. Because Sean has no hearing beyond 1000 Hz, there is no fear of upward spread of masking that could affect high-frequency acoustic cues. The increasing amount of shading in the CLEAR zone depicts the reduction of cues on voice and vocalization as frequency increases.

Remedial training also involves replacing old, ineffective habits with new and more adequate ones. Dealing with the formation of new habits is by far the most difficult aspect of remedial training. While carry-over into everyday speech communication may sometimes occur spontaneously among children in developmental programs, it is rarely achieved by more mature children or adults in remedial training programs unless a substantial amount of effort is directed towards establishing new communicative habits.

Research, advances in technology, and experience in the application of both over the past few decades, have permitted the development of new approaches to speech production, speech reception, and spoken language among hearing-impaired individuals. As a result, armed with knowledge and instrumentation that is superior to any previously available, professionals can, as previous chapters in this text show, now provide excellent opportunities for the acquisition of all aspects of speech communication. The productive use of emerging technology is not limited to developmentally oriented programs. It can also be used to remedy the major faults in speech found among older hearing-impaired children and adults -those for whom comparable opportunities were not previously available.

the importance of motivation

Neither young children in developmental programs, nor adolescents and adults in remedial programs, will make the effort to use spoken language unless they are motivated to do so. Most hearing-impaired adolescents and adults have either acquired effective spoken language skills, or require a great deal of externally generated incentive to acquire or improve them. Children, too, must be motivated to learn, and a wide variety of incentives may also be needed to promote their speech development.

Adolescents and adults who are candidates for remedial speech training (the professionals' potential clients) have usually been exposed to failure in some - perhaps many - aspects of spoken language acquisition over several years. Some have also experienced frustration, boredom, anger, and resentment in the course of their learning. Many, through experiences or persuasion, have developed very negative attitudes towards spoken language. Remedial training with such people is challenging, but it can also be lots of fun, and very successful, if two conditions are fulfilled: the professional must be highly competent, and the potential client must be strongly motivated. Competence on the part of the professional can only come about through a thorough knowledge of the theoretical issues, and reflective evaluation of sufficient practical experience. What are some of the motivating forces that lead adolescents

262 FOUNDATIONS OF SPOKEN LANGUAGE

and adults to enroll for remedial speech training? Do similar forces promote learning in children?

Motivation to improve speech communication skills can stem from both negative and positive feelings, experiences, and perceptions. Consider some negative forces and what they can contribute. Inability to interact through speech communication may deny a person - adult or child - certain social privileges. Such a situation, though not deliberately aversive, may be interpreted by him or her as punitive. Shame at being less fluent in spoken language than one's peers can be similarly motivating. Anxiety about the possible range of activities - perhaps jobs in the case of adults - that may be open to someone who speaks less than perfectly, or unintelligibly, may create the drive to do better. All of these motivating forces are essentially negative, and derive from fear. They may help a child to work hard at school, or lead an adult to seek professional help. Not all adults who are motivated to seek such help may, therefore, feel good about doing so. (Their view may be that the professionals who worked with them the first time round didn't do too good a job, and they may not understand that modern techniques can be more effective.) Motivation that derives from negative experiences can certainly provide the drive to learn, but positive forces are more likely to help individuals master new skills with the enthusiasm that is truly needed for most tasks - and particularly those on which previous failure has been experienced.

The most positive motivating force is success. Wilde was almost correct when he stated that nothing succeeds like it. But *being* successful is not as motivating as *feeling* successful. Just as when working developmentally with young children (see Chapters 7 and 8), one must ensure that older children and adults experience success as they enter and exit speech-training sessions. The first and last parts of a learning activity are those that are best remembered, and they will color an individual's attitudes to whatever happens in following sessions.

To provide an individual - adult or child - with a feeling of success, not just at the beginning and end of sessions, but all the way through them, remember to evaluate performance, and to provide feedback on the results of all trials. Individuals with hearing impairment who are learning to talk do not, as a rule, know which aspects of their utterances are acceptable and which are not. They must be told both clearly and consistently, so that they can begin to incorporate the proprioceptive (self-generated) sensations they experience as they talk into their concepts of correctly produced speech patterns. To be fair to adults and to older children, in recognition of their maturity, and to encourage self responsibility for the quality of their spoken language, they should know, and accept from the outset, the long- and short-term goals that are proposed for them on the basis of initial and ongoing evaluation. Achievement of known goals is in itself an incentive, and awareness of the number and nature of the goals to be achieved provides a realistic framework within which they themselves can also judge their work and achievements.

Those who know how well they are achieving clearly defined objectives are the most likely to become motivated by experiencing pleasure from the task itself. Such motivation is not the same sort as that derived from the pleasure that they will experience in communicating more effectively in everyday life. The two forms of motivation - intrinsic and extrinsic to the learning task - can be mutually enhancing. To optimize such effects, those concerned must not only have well thought out strategies to accomplish their training objectives, but well-planned procedures for ensuring that the results of training are carried over into everyday life. Having a hearing member of a student's family, or a hearing friend, share in the training sessions, so that what is learned can be insightfully practised at various times between lessons, can both assist in carry-over and provide motivation. There is considerably more incentive a person to succeed when others care enough to spend their time encouraging that person's efforts.

Adults' and children's experiences of using their improving communication skills in everyday life will be the most meaningful outcome of the training you provide. But the motivation provided by meaningfulness need not be limited to experiences outside training. The phonologic aspects of teaching should be deliberately geared to enhancing aspects of communication that are important to a student in everyday life. Additionally, it is important for teachers and clinicians to discover the range and nature of their student's interests, and to gear a significant proportion of a speech-training program to them. Professionals and family members should also be prepared to generate new interests through vivid and appealing presentation of new materials. Interests generated in this way can also be turned to advantage in speech training.

A range of consequences associated with success or failure in a speech communication training program can also spur an individual's efforts. Success can win approval of family, friends, workmates or playmates, and teacher. It can sometimes lead to relationships that would not otherwise develop. For an adult, it can ensure continuation of the present job, or lead to obtaining a better one. For a child it can lead to academic promotion or a prize, to being selected as the best speaker in the group, and to the continuation of training. Failure could prevent such benefits. To give too much importance to the consequences of the developmental or remedial work can lead to a state of over-anxiousness; giving too little, can destroy motivation. Careful thought must be given to achieving a balance, so that students do their best to succeed. Finally, clinicians and teachers must discover what motivational factors can be best be emphasized with particular students, for what motivates one person will not necessarily motivate another.

unisensory experience

Adults and children who need formal speech teaching are likely to have difficulty in acquiring control of breathing, vocalization, and voice patterns if they are expected to rely entirely on any one sense modality for speech reception. Even so, carefully planned unisensory experience in a selected modality is likely to be beneficial under certain circumstances. For example, the majority of profoundly hearing-impaired individuals who use appropriate hearing aids can identify the rhythms of speech through audition, but not through speechreading. Hence the exclusion of vision for part of the teaching aimed at improving the rhythm of their spoken language can help focus attention on the cues received through aided hearing (or through some other sense modality if other sensory aids are used). Such training can, if carried out in a responsible manner, lead to the refinement of many speech reception skills, and to the production of utterances with appropriate timing.

Errors that commonly occur when no unisensory experience has been provided include the responses of profoundly hearing-impaired individuals to the questions "How are you?" and "How old are you?" They often confuse these questions (one with three syllables, the other with four), and provide the wrong answer because they focus primarily, if not exclusively, on vision, and fail to integrate the auditory or other sensory information that is available to them. Similar individuals who have received appropriate unisensory auditory experience from an early age rarely confuse such rhythmically different utterances. Those who wear either a cochlear implant or a tactile device may also benefit from unisensory speech reception through whatever sensory aids they wear.

They may also find themselves unable to tell how many syllables there are in a word or other utterance if they rely habitually and heavily on speechreading. With appropriate unisensory training, most hearing-impaired individuals capable of receiving sufficient information about the acoustic patterns of speech can learn to perceive and produce the natural tunes and rhythms of speech. All prosodic patterns should, therefore, be developed in meaningful speech with appropriate emphasis on unisensory processing.

breath control

common problems and their causes

Breath supply in the speech of normally hearing people is governed mainly by the nature of an utterance. In general, the longer the segment of spoken language planned, the deeper the breath that must be taken. The segments to be supported on a breath may be as brief as a short phrase, or as long as a highly complex sentence, depending on the nature of the suprasegmental structure that best helps to carry the meaning of the intended utterance. An adequate breath stream is, therefore, essential to every aspect of normally spoken language. The main errors related to breath stream in older hearing-impaired speakers include producing fewer than the normal number of syllables on a breath, and expending more than a normal amount of breath on each syllable. The cause of these errors is not inadequate auditory feedback, for the acoustic component of breathing is negligible, and sufficient information on the amount of air in the lungs at any given time is available through proprioception - sensation provided by the receptors located in the body. They stem from the habit of initiating speech at or below lung-resting levels, and failure to associate appropriate breathing with the form and content of spoken language.

When speakers begin talking at lung resting levels, they fail to take advantage of the relaxation of the chest walls that sustains speech when it is produced on a sufficient volume of breath. Instead of taking in enough air and expelling the breath through controlled relaxation, those who begin to speak at lung resting level have to actively force the breath stream out of the lungs. Such forcing tends to result in tension that

266 FOUNDATIONS OF SPOKEN LANGUAGE

spreads through the whole speech mechanism. To illustrate this phenomenon, let readers reproduce the problem by initiating speech at lung-resting level - the point around which breathing can be sustained for long periods with very small amounts of air being inhaled or exhaled. *First* adjust your own breathing to lung resting level, and *next* start reading a passage or making a long statement about something, and continue doing this until your breath can no longer sustain speech. The outcome will have shown you that:

1. the first words sounded normal, but later words did not;
2. to speak as the breath supply runs out involves increasing effort;
3. such effort spreads tension throughout the whole vocal tract;
4. your utterance takes on some qualities of so called *deaf speech*.

Now repeat the procedure, starting with a lung volume well above resting level. You will find that all words sound normal, that the major effort involved is in taking in sufficient breath, and that strong sensations are generated in releasing breath during speech (sensations that can be used by hearing-impaired people as feedback cues for breath control).

objectives in developmental and remedial work

The objectives in both developmental and remedial work on speech breathing are to ensure that your pupil or client:

- initiates utterances at lung volumes well above resting level;
- expels the breath stream steadily throughout the utterance;
- becomes aware of the sensations associated with correct breathing
- takes in breath at appropriate points in the course of a message (either at the end of sentences or at points of juncture within them).
- is able to carry over breathing skills from lessons to life.

Breathing exercises on their own are not a great help in achieving the objectives specified above. This is because the intake and release of breath in speech must be closely related to the control of voicing, and to the prosodic (suprasegmental) structure of the utterances in a message. If taught to produce sounds, words, and short phrases without sufficient attention being paid to respiration, hearing-impaired children will learn to activate voicing by using no more than the amount of breath that is available in the lungs. Because low lung volumes are adequate for the production of such restricted amounts of verbal material, and longer utterances are not required from the beginning, the demand for greater lung volumes may not be experienced until longer sentences and complex language skills have evolved. By that time, the habit of beginning rather than ending their utterances at or near lung resting level will have been acquired. Too much concentration, then, on hearing-impaired children's production of short segments of spoken language, such as single speech sounds, or single words that demand little or no breath, will inhibit the development of an adequate breath support system, just as the production of long strings of speech sounds, the repetition and alternation of recently elicited syllables, and the encouragement of complete sentence patterns from the earliest stages of formal teaching will enhance it.

prerequisites

No complicated tests are required to determine whether an individual has enough lung capacity for speech. The prerequisites for speech breathing are present when an adult or child is normally active, can take a deep breath, and can expel it over three or four seconds.

informal strategies

The only informal learning strategy needed to promote normal breathing for speech is to ensure that most of a child's utterances are sufficiently extensive to require inhalation of air to volumes appropriately greater than lung-resting level. Just as informal learning can lead to the natural emergence of breath control, so can formal teaching lead to the prevention of future problems or the remediation of difficulties that have been allowed to occur.

formal strategies

Consciousness of breath can be developed through games like blow football, where books at each end of the table form goal posts, and the object of the game is to blow a table tennis ball into an opponent's goal. Such games can serve to develop verbal concepts that may be useful in later speech work, such as *to take a deep breath*, and *to breathe through the mouth*, but games or exercises that do not also involve voice control appear to be of little use in developing breathing for speech.

There is no need for formal speech breathing exercises as such in the course of providing a developmentally based program. Attention to speech breathing skills in the course of formal teaching should be focussed on gearing breath requirements to the accomplishment of increasingly higher levels of vocal development. Thus, at the earliest stages of speech, speech breathing should be related to the support of vocalization; at the next stage, integrated with whatever formal teaching a child may require to develop control of intensity, duration, and voice frequency, and their application in communicative speech; at the next stage, in the support of vowel production, and the use of vocalizations, vowels, and any spontaneously acquired consonants in the approximation of more mature forms of discourse; and in subsequent stages, extended in the development of consonants and consonant blends, and in the child's use of emerging spoken language in everyday communication.

Formal strategies for the control of speech breathing are often needed for older children and adults who have developed a habit of starting an utterance on insufficient breath. Some such individuals take in a great quantity of breath when asked to do so in preparation for talking, but then release most of it before beginning to speak at their habitual lung-resting levels. To determine whether this is the case with your client, simply ask him or her to take in enough breath to vocalize over several seconds. Provide a model to ensure that your requirement is understood. People with this problem often feel uncomfortable with a lot of air in their chests (perhaps more than they need) prior to talking, just as most normally speaking people would be distressed if they had to expel most of their breath before beginning to talk.

For clients with this problem, work at expanding the breath supply in gradual steps. The procedure will be illustrated with George, a young man of twenty, who has severe hearing impairment, many speech faults, and has only recently been fitted with a new hearing aid. At each step in training, ensure that George (or any other hearing-impaired person with habitual speech breathing problems) knows and shares your objectives, uses appropriate hearing aids (or other sensory aids), is provided with knowledge of correctness on each trial, and is made aware of the tactile and kinesthetic patterns created by his own utterances when they are produced with appropriate breath control. The consistent use of appropriate hearing aids or other sensory aids is considered by many professionals working with more mature clients to be evidence of a commitment that must be made before such remedial training is begun.

Begin remedial training with George by taking the following steps: *First*, ask him to vocalize as he normally does. (Stop the vocalization as soon as abnormal tension begins to occur. If his voice is produced with over-much laryngeal tension, have him repeat the trial while feeling the vibration of voicing on his chest. If the utterance is attempted without enough breath, have him create and feel the breath stream. Provide models if necessary.) *Second*, ask him for a slightly longer vocalization. (Watch to ensure that he takes in more breath to do this. If he does not, then explain and model how to breathe above lung resting level. Do not exaggerate by raising your shoulders when providing the model. If George raises his shoulders, encourage diaphragmatic rather than rib-cage breathing simply by having him fold his arms behind his back.) *Third*, time the duration of his vocalization. Practise extending it gradually until a conversational level voice of reasonably even intensity can be produced for 10-12 seconds. *Fourth*, repeat the first three steps, but have him produce a forced whisper (an /h/-like sound) rather than vocalization. (The larynx does not help to restrict breath flow to the same extent in whispered sounds as in voiced ones, so a goal of about five seconds' duration should be set for this task.) *Fifth*, have George produce a number of /ha/ syllables on one breath without stopping between them. Gradually increase the number until at least a dozen feels comfortable to him, and each is at an approximately similar intensity. *Sixth* have him repeat the fifth step with different vowels, syllables, or words, such as *he*, *ho*, *her*, *hay*, *hi*, and *how*.

When George has developed sufficient awareness of the sensations associated with the breathing patterns that permit achievement of all six steps outlined above, he should be in a position to begin using these patterns in the production of meaningful spoken language. The most appropriate utterances for this step in his training are those that relate to routine experiences in his everyday life, because they create the necessary similarities between what is learned in lessons and what is used in the contexts of living. Use sentences that George is likely to employ at any time during his waking hours, such as *It's time to get up*, *What time is it?*, *I'd like another cup of coffee please*, and *What sort of a day did you have?* As he masters these, and feels comfortable with actually using them in the course of living, his newly acquired breathing skills can be related to more complex sentences, such as *If you don't hurry up and eat you breakfast, you're probably going to miss the train*, as well as multi-sentence utterances.

There is always a possibility that the voice produced will at first be nasal. In this case, have George observe the movement of a piece of cotton or paper placed in an appropriately forceful oral breath stream, or have him feel it on his fingers. Dangling a tissue so that the bottom end of it is aligned with the lips at a distance of two or three inches, is particularly good for visualizing the effects of an adequate breath flow. This is because it can serve this purpose whether the utterance is a syllable, a word, a sentence, or continuous discourse. Wetting the finger tips makes them more sensitive to the breath stream. If the voice is initially nasal, using the above techniques gives George very positive and unambiguous goals to work for, goals that are much more effective than comments and directions, such as "You're sounding nasal. Don't let your breath come out through your nose. Make it come out of your mouth."

Breathy voice occurs when too much air is expended on the production of an utterance. This fault is usually due to failure to bring the vocal cords fully together during the act of voicing. Breathy voice is not a very important fault. While it may reduce audibility of a talker to some extent, it does not necessarily reduce intelligibility because, while not affecting vowel formant structure, a strong oral breath flow may lead to the enhanced production of various consonants, particularly plosives and fricatives. Furthermore, breathy voices tend to improve as talkers learn to relate their breathing to the demands of meaningful language use in an environment that features frequent use of speech.

If the reduction of breathiness is considered important for particular clients, it can usually be achieved through having them pull or lift something while vocalizing. When things are lifted, the vocal cords are brought and held together, an act that helps to stabilize the chest and support the shoulders. Exertion involving the shoulders thus tends to result in a smaller expenditure of breath. The repetition of this strategy, if it is successful, should permit the client to become aware of the sensations that accompany less breathy voicing.

Weak and breathy voices can, in certain cases, also be improved by increasing muscle tone within the larynx. This can be achieved by asking your clients to begin each of a series of arrhythmic vocalizations on one breath immediately you signal them to do so. In order to be ready to vocalize under these conditions, the vocal cords are brought together and, helped by the rib cage and diaphragm, serve to hold the breath back while awaiting the signal. Short bursts of vocalization then serve to ensure the coordination of the breath-voice system. This exercise should not be carried out frequently or with over-much vigor because, if abused, it can lead to the formation of vocal nodules and a harsh voice. The client should be alerted to sensations generated by bringing the vocal cords together, sensations that should offer a student guidelines on how to initiate vocalization in communicative speech.

vocalization

The basis for all vocalization is adequate breath supply and breath control. Inadequate breath stream and breath control often contribute to faulty vocal resonance, pharyngeal tension, weak voice, breathy voice, nasalization, and omission or distortion of consonants. The presence of a good breath stream allows children more easily to feel how they make the different speech patterns that constitute their spoken language. This, in turn, permits them to establish a well-differentiated articulatory code, essentially the mechanism that permits older children and adults who become totally deaf to continue talking intelligibly, if not normally, in the complete absence of auditory feedback. When children do not vocalize, it is usually because they are unable to hear or feel others' vocalizations adequately, and/or to receive sufficient sensory feedback of their own voices. In some cases it may also be that they are not talked to sufficiently. To bathe children in meaningful sound is as important to their development of vocalization and spoken language as keeping them clean and well nourished.

prerequisites.

The prerequisite behaviors for vocalization are all vegetative, life-support functions, such as use of the lungs for breathing, and the use of the lips, tongue, and jaw for sucking, chewing, and swallowing. The prerequisites for the spontaneous use of vocalization as a means of communication are the child's awareness of voice and speech as means of communication, and perception of the sensation of his or her own voice through auditory or other forms of sensory feedback. Before vocalization on demand can be established, a child must be able to vocalize involuntarily.

goals.

In this initial stage one's immediate goals for the child should be to:
1. secure spontaneous vocalizations; and
2. obtain vocalizations on demand or in response to one's own vocalization.

These goals are best achieved through informal learning, but they can also be developed through formal teaching. Vocalization on demand should be encouraged in all children, but it is truly essential only for those with whom formal speech development strategies are required. There is no need to insist on it as long as control of vocalization results from the use of informal strategies. Formal teaching to establish adequate control of vocalization is most frequently required for older children, those who need remedial work because the formal teaching of more advanced skills has been attempted before the appropriate use of breath and voice have been established, or because this stage of development has not been treated as an integral part of all later stages of spoken language acquisition.

In order to support the range of utterances that a child will eventually produce as spoken language, vocalization must be modified and refined at each successive stage of development. In short, attaining good quality vocalization must be a goal in teaching all vowels and consonants, and ensuring their appropriate use in discourse.

As vocalization cannot be directly detected through vision, the first step in establishing vocalization is to ensure that the child is able to detect it through audition (hearing aids or cochlear implants), touch, or tactile devices. It can be developed *informally* by interacting vocally with a child; by talking, singing, playing games, and engaging in activities with the child that require the abundant use of voice. Teaching vocalization skills *formally* usually involves numerous modelling and imitation behaviors that are supported by the use of operant procedures (reinforcement immediately following the use of voice), and the enhancement of feedback. The reinforcement can be any response or activity that encourages the child to repeat, interpret, or respond to vocalization in a contextually appropriate way. When formal strategies have been used to elicit vocalization, a return to the use of informal strategies will provide the necessary opportunities for its ongoing reinforcement in everyday situations. Unless the sensory aids used in formal teaching sessions are also worn at all other times, spontaneous carry-over from formal teaching to real life cannot be expected.

informal strategies.

All children vocalize during their first year of life. This is one reason that professionals regard it as important to recognize the presence of hearing difficulties early in a child's first year. Providing hearing-impaired children with appropriate hearing aids (or other devices) during this first year permits them to detect their own and their caregivers' voices. When they can do this they will, almost inevitably, vocalize increasingly often, and make a greater and greater variety of sounds. Humming while rocking a child to sleep can develop an awareness and love of vocalization. Early vocalizations can also be encouraged and extended by engaging the baby interactively through vocalization and eye contact. Caregivers' imitations of the vocal sequences initiated by the child are particularly important in building babies' awareness of speech patterns as a means of communication, and extending their speech reception and speech production skills.

Caregivers should use the relative immobility of young babies to advantage by coming close to them to communicate, thus ensuring optimal transmission of speech through the sensory aids selected for them. They should also use every possible opportunity to provide running commentaries on objects and events of interest to the child, to do this at close quarters, and to use normal speech levels (see Chapters 3 and 7). Abundant vocalization and babble in the early months of life provide children with an excellent basis for extending the quantity and the range of their speech patterns throughout the following years.

Older children vocalize either spontaneously or reflexively in the course of many activities, particularly in highly active play in which they are also emotionally involved. The quality of a child's vocalization closely reflects his or her feelings about ongoing events. The types of activities and play that yield most vocalizations should be noted and used as the basis of encouragement for further vocalization. At any stage during the early years, caregivers can vocalize in imitation of the noise made by, for example, a car, mmmmmmmm, an airplane, wheeeeeee, or a boat, bubububu, as they pass such toys to the children in response to their non-verbal requests for them. Consistent encouragement usually results in the children making similar sounds as they move the toys in play.

Caregivers' vocal and verbal responses to a child's vocalizations, and their commentaries about ongoing activities or objects of interest are the most powerful forces in encouraging the development of vocal patterns. It is important for them to be close, and to ensure reasonably quiet conditions when playing with or talking to their child, because every doubling of distance subtracts approximately 6 dB from the intensity of the speech signal, and noise that is as close, or closer, to their child may readily mask (obliterate) various components of their speech.

formal strategies.

Traditional ways of enhancing feedback of vocalization in those having difficulty with developing a good breath flow and a sufficiently strong voice, include having a child feel the vibrations produced by vocalization, first on the chest of the clinician or teacher, and next on his or her own. Vibrations created by voicing can also be readily felt by holding or touching a balloon or a drum. To use such a method when the child is already wearing a tactile device is a way of providing supplementary cues within the one sense modality. To use touch when the child is wearing hearing aids provides additional cues in a second modality. Traditional methods should not be scorned as old-fashioned. When such training is needed, it will be found to be effective. Once such strategies have been successful their use should be dropped, and the child taught to rely on the sense modalities that will be used for speech reception and feedback in everyday life. One of the most important feedback paths in speech production by profoundly hearing-impaired children is the oro-sensory information that is uniquely associated with the production of each sound - the tactile and kinesthetic sensations that are generated in the mouth as one talks. This form of feedback is essential not only for those who are hearing-impaired from birth, but also for young children who lose their hearing after having acquired spoken language (see Chapter 2).

Most modern ways to provide additional sensory information on vocalization involve the use of electronic devices that convert voice energy into a visual image or use it to operate an electrically powered toy. These devices can signal the presence of voicing, as well as reinforce the child for producing it. There is no limit to the number of such devices that can be created. Voice-operated relays can be used to make instruments turn wheels, make a monkey climb up a pole, set toy trains or cars in motion, illuminate a toy and so on. Instruments, such as oscilloscopes and television sets, can be used to provide interesting visual images for the duration of a vocalization. These devices have their place, but also their drawbacks. Children lose interest in inanimate things quickly, and their experience with visual devices does not relate closely to the everyday situations into which vocalization is to be carried over.

A simple way to enhance both vocalization and breath flow is to move towards a child (or move something towards the child) from ever-increasing distances as he or she vocalizes. As distance increases, deeper and deeper breaths have to be taken to sustain vocalization. Care in this particular strategy will result in excellent control of normally sounding voice patterns through tactile and kinesthetic feedback - the sensations the child creates and feels as he or she talks.

Avoid the development of abnormal modes of such feedback on vocalization. If hearing-impaired children do not receive adequate feedback through sensory aids, they often attempt to enhance the sensations they create as they vocalize by adopting abnormal modes of voice production. Such attempts may result in voices that are too high, too low, produced with pharyngeal tension, breathy, nasal, harsh, or even produced while taking in rather than releasing breath. To focus a child's attention on the larynx, particularly through touch, and to neglect breath flow requirements both tend to result in the development of such abnormalities. Attention is better paid to the effects of vocalization rather than to its source.

If there are marked voice abnormalities, the first thing to question is breath flow. The breath stream required to support normal speech is tangible. Nasal, tense, and harsh voices are less likely to occur if children are encouraged to use a sufficiently strong oral breath stream. Attention can be drawn to breath by having a child place a wetted finger or a light tissue in the breath stream. If one produces several syllables containing vowels that concentrate the breath stream, such as boobooboo, feeling or watching the effect of the breath stream on a tissue can help to establish an understanding that expenditure of breath is an intrinsic part of speech production. Once children have felt breath stream on their fingers, and/or lifted a tissue with their breath stream, they can, if necessary, be reminded to use sufficient breath by a visual prompt, such as placing one's fingers just in front of one's mouth as one listens to something they are saying.

If an abnormally high (falsetto) voice is produced, it can usually be brought within a normal range by having the child concentrate more on the information and feedback provided when more normal voice patterns are transmitted through appropriately selected sensory aids. (That such a voice problem has developed strongly suggests that such devices have not been consistently used.) Voice within the normal frequency range can usually be obtained by the simple tactile strategy of feeling vibration on the chest as voice is produced with the chin tucked in. If a normally pitched voice cannot be obtained with older pupils or adults in this way, the following strategy may be tried as a last resort.

First, ask the client to look up to the ceiling for a few seconds as soon as you signal him or her to do so. *Second*, when this request is understood, elicit any vowel and have the client sustain it for several seconds. *Third*, ask the client to vocalize in the same way, but to look quickly up to the ceiling as soon as you signal, and to maintain vocalization as he or she does so. This strategy should quickly lead to a lower voice as the client quickly looks up and maintains that head position. It works because falsetto voice is produced when the vocal cords are stretched and, on this account, vibrating over only part of their length. It is usually impossible to maintain such tension on the vocal cords when one suddenly faces upwards so, to permit the head to go back, the undesirable tension on the vocal cords is relaxed and a lower pitched voice is obtained.

Formal teaching to elicit vocalization is rarely necessary if informal strategies have been given an adequate chance to succeed. Formal work on vocalization is usually, therefore, much more concerned with ensuring its quality, and the support of vocalization through the development of adequate breath flow.

phonologic Use

Vocalization (control of breath and voice) is an essential basis for a wide range of skills in speech production. It supports the supraseg-mental aspects of speech (prosody), is present in vowel production (except in whispered speech), and is an essential feature of most voiced-voiceless distinctions in consonants and consonant blends. In a speech context it can convey many characteristics of a talker, such as age, sex, and mood but, on its own, vocalization can do little more than signal the presence of another person. It is, nevertheless, one of the most fundamental of speech skills, and its refinement is an integral part of all later stages of speech acquisition. The development of sufficient vocalization skills to support speech should not be a long drawn-out process. A few weeks of its encouragement through abundant interaction between an adult and a child should lead to the child's readiness to mold vocalizations into different voice patterns. The mouth movements that accompany a child's vocalization of pleasure, surprise, frustration, or some other emotion usually lead to the production of a wide range of vowels. Such mouth movements change the shape of the vocal tract and incidentally produce a range of different vowels as vocalization occurs. The adult's imitation (reflection) of such variations in vocalization, providing appropriate sensory aids are worn by the child, can encourage him or her to play with voice, and deliberately repeat the variety of sounds that were, initially, unintentionally made. It is through such processes that vocalizations are shaped into words which, when associated with objects and events, take on meaning, and eventually become used in communication through spoken language.

voice patterns, (duration, intensity, and fundamental frequency)

Vocal duration, intensity, and frequency all contribute to vocal stress, the emphasis on words in a sentence, as well as to the rhythm of sentences; in short, to the prosodic (suprasegmental) aspects of speech. They also provide cues on the voiced-voiceless distinctions among consonants (for example, /p/ vs. /b/; and /f/ vs. /v/), and help separate words in the continuous stream of sounds that constitute speech. There are no absolutes that govern duration, intensity, and the range of vocal frequency in spoken language. Within limits, one may talk slowly or quickly, loudly or quietly, and with or without a great deal of intonation, yet be perfectly intelligible. It is the relative rather than the absolute differences between these features of speech, and the way that they relate to the grammatical form and the meaning of an utterance, that are important. Thus, their refinement and combined use in meaningful utterances must receive attention at every stage of development.

The suprasegmental patterns (variations intensity, duration, and fundamental frequency) that occur in spoken language, then, are not random. In order to convey meaning as they do, their production has to follow certain rules. Appropriately produced prosody, the tunes and rhythms of speech, can be equally as meaningful as vowels, diphthongs, consonants, consonant blends, words, and sentences. Sometimes the prosody of a sentence can be even more meaningful than the words it contains. For example, tone of voice can tell us whether a comment has been said in all seriousness or in jest, and whether a remark should be interpreted as a compliment or as sarcasm. When we emphasize particular words in a sentence, or pause in an utterance, we can completely reverse its meaning. For example, "Don't! Take it away!" means exactly the opposite of "Don't take it away." These comments lead to some important points: the suprasegmental patterns are basic to speech intelligibility, and the rules they follow must be acquired along with all other aspects of spoken language. Just as children must take time to learn new words, and to use them in increasingly complex language, so must they have time and opportunity to refine their control of intensity, duration, and fundamental frequency, and be helped to assimilate the rules governing prosody.

Most hearing-impaired children, when provided with appropriate hearing aids and sufficient auditory experience can hear enough of the speech signal to acquire natural sounding, well-inflected voices, because sufficient (though not all) auditory cues on prosody occur in the frequency range below 1000 Hz. (The importance of this frequency range to profoundly hearing-impaired children is indicated in Figure 9-1.) Most multi-channel cochlear implants and many multi-channel tactile devices are designed to transmit information on prosody, but whether particular individuals can perceive them or not must be determined in the course of ongoing training. Single-channel devices of all types are usually able to provide children with enough cues on vocal duration and intensity for the development of rhythmic patterns, but may not transmit enough frequency information to permit control of fundamental frequency to be spontaneously acquired. The likelihood of the spontaneous acquisition of good prosody is increased by the close proximity of children and caregivers who use natural prosody, because proximity enhances the speech signal - particularly in the presence of noise - and thus provides optimal conditions for speech communication regardless of the type of instrument used to compensate for hearing impairment. In short, regardless of hearing levels, it should rarely be necessary to develop vocal duration, intensity or frequency through formal methods if appropriate sensory aids have been worn from an early age, or shortly after the onset of hearing impairment.

prerequisites

Vocalization and its prerequisites are essential underpinnings for the development of all voice patterns that vary in time, intensity, and frequency. Control of vocal duration and vocal intensity can be developed simultaneously, but it is an advantage to have a modicum of control over intensity in order to establish adequate control over vocal frequency. Unless control of vocal intensity is developed before formal teaching of voice pitch control is attempted, high pitch tends to be confused with a loud voice and low pitch with a quiet one.

goals

The goals at this stage are gross control over all three aspects: vocal duration, vocal intensity, and the fundamental frequency of voice. Refinement of control is to be achieved as the production of each of the vowels, consonants, and blends are subsequently mastered. Continuing refinement of voice patterns is an ever-present goal as more and more advanced speech skills are acquired. Such refinement will permit the duration of sounds and gaps in voicing to cue the differentiation of /s/ and /z/, as well as /p/ and /b/, and similar voiced-voiceless pairs. It will also permit the development of the suprasegmental patterns that underlie stress in sentences, signal the structure and semantic properties of an utterance, express notions and emotions in ways that are pragmatically appropriate, and govern turn-taking in conversations.

Failure to acquire acceptable prosody - particularly through control and appropriate use of vocal frequency (voice pitch) - is one of the most frequent of problems in the acquisition of speech by hearing-impaired children. It usually indicates that the information they are receiving about their own and others' speech patterns - either directly or through whatever devices they use to enhance their speech reception - is seriously deficient. Thus, poor prosody is usually observed when speechreading is over-emphasized (no prosodic features can be reliably perceived through vision), when residual hearing is extremely limited, when hearing aids are not appropriate, or when cochlear implants or tactile devices are used but do not provide sufficient cues on vocal frequency.

Many professionals come to rely on visual indicators of some sort to teach basic control of voice pitch. However, skills learned through their use are hard to generalize, and such devices cannot be used in everyday communication. Instruments that can provide training only in situations contrived by the teacher or clinician can permit the child to gather but scant knowledge of how prosody is used by normal talkers in real-life communication. Such instruments are, therefore, much less appropriate than sensory aids that can be worn all day and every day. Visual indicators have a place in teaching children to modify voice pitch but, even then, direct touch can be more effective, because it more strongly focuses the child's attention on the tactile and kinesthetic sensations that are involved in the production of sounds of different pitch.

informal strategies.

Vocal duration is most readily brought under control through a child's abundant use of vocalization. The durational aspects of the speech of others, and feedback of the child's own vocal duration can be perceived through either hearing or touch providing that appropriate devices are worn. Informal strategies are best based on communicative events, vocal play, and the types of games caregivers' can use to elicit any vocalization (see p. 273).

Control of *vocal Intensity* and *voice frequency* also emerge as use of voice is encouraged through verbal interaction, play, and stories. Stories, such as *Jack the Giant Killer* and *The Three Bears* in which loud and quiet, as well as high and low voices are contrasted, are a very effective means of alerting children to the different ways of using voice. When caregivers pretend to sleep, and then "jump with fright" as soon as the children have used a loud enough voice to "wake" them, quickly yields voices of loud intensity. It is a simple game that all children like to play.

Real-life situations in which loud and quiet comments or instructions with characteristic intonation patterns are given to children "helping" in the kitchen provide excellent examples of different voice patterns that can be associated with everyday language (e.g. *Don't touch!* or *Oh dear!* [loud with falling pitch] as compared with *You stir it* [quiet with falling pitch], or *Would you like some?* [quiet with rising pitch] or a whispered *Don't tell Jimmy. Let's surprise him!*) Caregivers' unabashed use of widely varying intonation patterns throughout the early years is recommended.

Variations in children's voices arise as a result of involuntary reactions to objects and events around them. Much as stretching the neck of a balloon when releasing air from it will raise the frequency of the sound it makes, increasing the tension of the vocal folds will cause them to vibrate at a higher frequency. Such increase in tension, not just in the vocal folds but throughout the body, often arises in response to surprise and fright, or in the course of an activity. A decrease in general tension will have the opposite effect. Such involuntary variations beg to be used.

Loud voices and laughter can be encouraged in very active games. Quiet voices and chuckles occur in more relaxed situations. Responding to children when they use appropriate voice levels and vocal frequency, stimulating abundant vocalization, encouraging variation in vocalizations, and praising pleasant and appropriate voice patterns will usually all lead to the control of voice production providing the child is appropriately aided, can effectively use a cochlear implant, or has a multi-channel tactile device that transmits information on F_0, as well as time and intensity.

The generalization problems associated with formal teaching can usually be avoided by promoting the use of prosodic patterns through verbal interaction, Under such conditions, these patterns are learned and used where and how they need to be used - in interactive communication. Formal (and more traditional) teaching methods are required only when informal learning has not spontaneously occurred following extensive exposure to spoken language through the use of appropriate sensory aids, and when breathing does not adequately support voice patterns.

formal strategies

Visual prompts and cues, and natural (unaided) touch are frequently featured in formal work on the development of vocal duration, intensity, and frequency. Formal strategies usually require professionals or caregivers to provide models that children can then imitate, and about which they, in turn, can provide feedback. For example, a teacher may trace a path in the air with a finger, or on a paper with a pencil, as she vocalizes and, as the child imitates the vocalization, do the same to indicate how well the child is succeeding. The provision of feedback on the correctness of a child's conscious attempts to imitate an adult is a feature that distinguishes formal from informal work on voice patterns because, when adequate indirect feedback is available to the children in the course of everyday life, they can, in the main, be expected to acquire such patterns spontaneously.

Activities to stimulate *control of vocal duration* that involve vision are not difficult to invent. Some that have been found useful for increasing the duration of voicing include walking towards a child from increasing distances as he or she vocalizes, slowly pulling out a carpenter's tape from its container as the child is voicing to "measure" the length of the vocalization, counting the number of pieces of different colored wools that can be taken from a box or the number of beads that can be threaded on a string as children vocalize, and counting how many syllables can be said on one breath. Such strategies permit children to compete with their previous performance levels, or with those of other children.

Activities involving touch include drawing a finger down the length of a child's arm to indicate the duration of voicing required, or circling the palm of the child's hand with a finger as many times as possible during a vocalization. Short duration sounds can be signalled visually or by hand taps, as can chains of sounds that contain items of both long and short duration. Having the children voice long or short syllables to set the mode for making toy animals or adults move towards them as they vocalize can result in hilarious situations in which children revel in making caregivers walk to babababa, limp to bibaabibaabibaa, or skip to baabibibaabibibaa.

Control of vocal intensity can usually be initiated through natural touch by such strategies as having children feel the differences between loud voice, quiet voice, and whispering on the speakers' and on their own chests. Two somewhat less direct procedures are having them press lightly or heavily on one's hands, and having them associate the lifting of light objects with a whisper, those of medium weight with a conversational level voice, and those that are heavy with a loud voice. A popular formal strategy to increase vocal intensity is having them voice as they participate in a tug of war with caregivers or other children. The larynx serves a non-speech purpose related to lifting and pulling. The vocal cords close tightly together to help prevent breath escaping from the chest cavity, and so help to support the shoulders in such activities.

Strong voices can, therefore, often be obtained in games like tug-of-war and arm-wrestling.

A visual strategy that may help to ameliorate voices that are too quiet or breathy is to have the child vocalize quickly after waiting for one to signal onset with one's finger. The anticipation of voicing will usually bring the vocal cords together, and that, together with breath that is released after several pent-up seconds of waiting for the signal, will also produce the conditions for strong voicing. This strategy should not be used too frequently, as it can result in vocal nodules and subsequent hoarseness. In general, laughter and boisterous outdoor play will result in loud and frequency-varying vocalizations, restrained indoor activities, in quiet, more monotonous voices, and passivity with little or no vocalization. It can, therefore, be very helpful to promote a range of activities, and to bring a child's attention to the voice patterns that result as the various activities are pursued. Such a variety of situations also provide excellent opportunities to positively reinforce the use of patterns initially developed through formal teaching.

Whispering can be promoted from panting and, if necessary, panting can be developed from blowing. The breath stream during panting can be directed to the back of a child's hands. If voice intrudes in the panting, the child should be trained to feel, and to report "yes" or "no" to the presence or absence of vibration on the chest when the clinician or teacher says either a series of clearly voiced ah syllables, or an unvoiced set of whispered /ha/ syllables. Once a child can produce whispered syllables without consonants, then a series of whispered syllables initiated with either unvoiced plosives or unvoiced fricatives, such as fafafafa or papapapa, will help to establish the act of whispering. When this strategy is used, and whispering is later required but not produced, the adults' production of these syllables against the back of their hands will usually serve as an adequate prompt for the child, and result in the correct imitation of the pattern.

Control of voice frequency is hard to teach without adequate direct feedback through audition and/or touch. Sensory information provided by residual audition and touch can be directly used by hearing-impaired children in the reception and production of low and high voice patterns, whereas a clinician's or teacher's visual hand signals provide only an indirect indication of vocal frequency. For these reasons, hearing aids and multi-channel cochlear implants provide such children with the most useful sensory information on how a low voice differs from a high voice.

These instruments can, therefore, be expected to yield faster progress in children's acquisition of voice-frequency control than the pointing of a finger down to indicate low, and up to indicate high. Electronic devices can be used to provide direct visual cues on voice frequency, but they are not strongly recommended (for reasons provided in Chapter 5). Fortunately, neither speech reception nor speech production requires very precise voice-frequency control. Intonation patterns can extend over as much as an octave (a doubling of the frequency of F_0), and as little as a tenth of that range.

The most effective formal procedures in helping to develop voice-frequency control are as follows: *First* teach discrimination between high- and low-pitched vocalizations using whatever devices the child normally wears in everyday life. Initially, this may be facilitated by using the vowel oo as the stimulus, because it contains more low-frequency information than the others and on this account is usually the most salient. Later, of course, a much wider range of stimuli should be employed. *Second*, require imitations of such voice patterns from the child while providing feedback on correctness on each effort. *Third*, require such imitations along with the child's judgements as to whether or not each trial was successful, judgements that must be confirmed or not as the case might be. *Fourth*, when these targets have each in turn been achieved, repeat the previous three steps using more than one stimulus at a time (e.g. low-high-low, high-high-low, etc.). *Fifth*, repeat these three steps yet again, but presenting continuous high-to-low and low-to-high, as well as continuous high-low-high and low-high-low patterns, rather than discrete low or high patterns as the stimuli. *Sixth*, and finally, when these steps are satisfactorily completed, further the process by introducing voice pitch into spoken language patterns. There is no substitute for working systematically to establish the use of appropriate intonation contours in all speech communication. Providing the child routinely wears a device or devices that transmit sufficient information on vocal frequency, these steps are not as burdensome as they might first appear. They are much more onerous (but not impossible) when input and feedback on voice patterns have to be provided in ways described below.

The development of intonation patterns among children who cannot hear them through hearing aids or by means of cochlear implants, or feel them through wearable multi-channel tactile devices, still requires the discrimination of different voice patterns through one or other of the available sense modalities. The senses that can be used are direct touch, vision, or a combination of the two. For children with impoverished reception of speech through the distance senses, the use of touch is preferable to the use of vision as the primary modality, because touch can provide the most precise and direct cues for both reception and production of voice frequency differences. However, when children need teaching through direct touch, their use of vision as a supplementary modality should usually be encouraged. The weakness of externally provided tactile and visual cues about voice frequency does not lie in the precision of information they can convey, for they can provide extremely accurate input and feedback on any speech pattern. Their frailty is due to their usefulness being limited to teaching situations. Only if a child's awareness of the internal sensations that accompany voice-frequency changes has been developed through formal teaching to the point where they can be automatically applied in spoken language contexts, can there be carry-over of such training into everyday communication.

The simplest and most direct use of touch in teaching differences in voice pitch is to evoke and contrast discrete (separate) vocalizations that are distinctly lower and distinctly higher than those the children usually produce. One can easily feel the vibrations that accompany vocalizations on some part of the body. Distinctly lower voices can usually be achieved by having children feel the vibrations of a low-pitched vowel on the chest. The teacher or clinician should first provide the model, and then have the child repeat the procedure. Distinctly higher voices can similarly be evoked by having them feel the vibrations of a high-pitched vowel on top of the head. These procedures appear to work for two reasons: first, this use of touch actually does pinpoint the locus of tangible vibration and second, the strategy tends to cause the child involuntarily to lower or raise the larynx towards the point where the hand is placed.

Once a child has learned to produce high- and low-pitched voice in these ways, it may be helpful to prompt further high-low voicing visually, by raising or lowering the hand. As a step towards the development of automaticity in voice control and its application in spoken language, the child should, once the high and low targets are achieved, be encouraged to seek feedback on voice pitch not through the fingers, but from the sensations that are directly created by the act of voicing.

Following the reliable production of discrete low- and high-pitched voice throughout whatever range of vowels a child can produce, a professional can usually obtain continuously changing pitch by asking the child to voice for several seconds or longer as she provides a series of prompts demanding alternately high- and low-pitched vocalizations. By moving her hand up and down as a child vocalizes continuously from low to high, and from high to low, she will obtain a pitch glide. Again, once this stage is reliably mastered, intonation should be integrated with simple and familiar language patterns.

A "last resort" tactile strategy is one involving feeling the rise and fall of the larynx - a strategy illustrated with Joel, an eight year old boy who is near-totally deaf. *First*, Joel is asked to feel your larynx as you swallow a sip of water. He does this by lightly resting his fingers on your throat. *Second*, the procedure is repeated as he feels his own throat and swallows a sip of water. *Third*, Joel feels your throat as you raise and lower your larynx without vocalizing. *Fourth*, you ask him to do the same. *Fifth*, you have him feel your throat as you raise your larynx and vocalize, and then lower your larynx and vocalize. *Sixth*, you have Joel do the same. Each step must meet with success before a child taken through the remaining steps of the procedure. This strategy, carried out carefully, rarely fails. It is to be avoided if a child can learn to control voice pitch by other means, because it can associate the production of intonation with too much tension, and thus lead to a voice with an unduly harsh or strident quality. If the strategy is used, attention should quickly be moved away from the throat to sensations on the chest or in the head.

phonologic use

To begin the final section in this chapter, it is as well to reiterate an important point; namely, that voice teaching procedures carried out in the clinic or classroom are notoriously difficult to carry over into everyday communication. This is particularly true when the use of hearing or other sensory aids that can be worn all day and every day is not fully incorporated into the formal teaching process.

Children who need formal teaching in order to acquire control of voice patterns that vary in intensity, frequency, and duration do not often spontaneously carry over such patterns from school to home. When such patterns are acquired formally, it is usually necessary to program the transfer of skills very carefully from classroom or clinic into everyday communication over a considerable period of time. Everyday greetings (Hi there!), questions (Would you like one?), and statements (I don't know!) offer excellent ways of getting children to first base in the phonologic use of voice pitch. Once control over voice pitch has been established in a few verbal contexts, it should be gradually extended to all aspects of all further spoken language development. Once it is elicited by one clinician or teacher, its use should be encouraged by all other adults as a matter of course. Once it is used in one context, in one place, in certain lessons, or at certain times, its use should be encouraged in many other places, during other lessons, and at all other times.

Parents can be exceptionally powerful forces in helping their child to develop phonologic use of formally taught speech patterns. While their role in formally eliciting new patterns should not be overly encouraged (it can conflict with normal parenting practices), they often have ideal opportunities to promote carry-over from training by providing model utterances for imitation and use in familiar situations. Their role can include encouraging the production of certain patterns informally through play, asking for clarification of a message, pointing out an error, suggesting how an utterance should be phrased, encouraging the child to act speaking parts in family plays, drawing the child's attention to their pleasure in hearing a well-produced utterance, and praising effective use of particular patterns when they are used in communication around the house or neighborhood. Positive and constructive reactions rather than critical comments are most likely to lead to effective carry-over. Too much criticism can lead to discouragement, a situation that must (and can) be avoided, though parents may need guidance to achieve an effective balance between appropriate praise and non-acceptance of a particular child's speech patterns.

There is a tendency to forget about suprasegmental patterns, particularly voice frequency, when working on segmental aspects of speech. Be aware of this and do not overlook them. Just as voice patterns of all sorts grow out of simple vocalizations and, at the same time, extend them, so must all other aspects of spoken language be based on voice patterns and, simultaneously, refine them.

Finally, many children are unnecessarily deprived of musical experiences because it is wrongly taken for granted that their hearing impairments prevent them from enjoying singing, and from playing musical instruments. Middle C on the piano is at the lower end of the frequency of speech (see Chapter 3). Thus, even children with no hearing beyond 1000 Hz can hear most notes on a piano. Not all children with profound hearing impairment can discriminate between notes that are close together on a keyboard, but most can learn to identify and sing different tunes with identifiable pitch characteristics and rhythms. Some cochlear implants and tactile devices, as well as most hearing aids, can provide children with enough spectral information to permit the majority of hearing-impaired children to have fun with musical instruments. Singing can have beneficial effects on all aspects of voice and speech development, particularly when music and singing are introduced at an early age.

suggestions for further reading

There are no books written specifically on strategies for developing the production of different voice patterns in the spoken language of hearing impaired children. However, several, such as those by Calvert and Silverman (1983), Haycock (1933), Lack (1955), and Ling (1976), all contain some discussion of the subject, and offer useful guidelines. Encouragement of pleasant voice patterns through informal strategies have been suggested by Cole and Gregory (1986), by Grant (1987), Ling (1984a), Ling and Ling (1978), and Stovall (1982), among others. Articles relating to voice patterns in hearing-impaired children appear from time to time in various journals such as the *Journal of Speech and Hearing Disorders* the *Journal of Speech and Hearing Research,* the *Journal of the Acoustical Society of America,* and articles relating to the teaching of some aspect of voice control occasionally appears in *The Volta Review.* There are many more articles reporting the presence of abnormal voices among hearing-impaired people than there are articles about the prevention or remediation of abnormal patterns. See References pp. 433 ff.

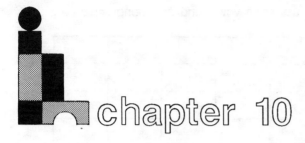

chapter 10

development of vowels and diphthongs

introduction

Although the vowels and diphthongs are represented by only five letters in written English, there are actually over a dozen of them in our spoken language. This may sometimes lead to confusion in the early stages of reading, because some words that sound different can be written in the same way. (For example, "The violin is usually *bowed*[1] rather than plucked" and "He *bowed*[2] to his partner.") A few lines of doggerel amusingly illustrate some possible confusions between pronunciation and the written form:

Beware of *heard* a dreadful word
That looks like *beard* but sounds like *bird*,
And *deaf*: It's said like *chef*, not *sheaf*
For Heaven's sake, please don't say *deef*.

Vowels and diphthongs carry more of the burden in speech reception and speech production than is generally realized. They serve to create the differences between words, as in *booed, buoyed, bowed*[1], *bowed*[2], *bored, bard, bud, bird, bad, bed, bade, bide, bid, beard*, and *bead*. In addition, they carry most of the information on prosody, and provide us with personal information about a speaker, and the intention of a message. Also (see Chapter 2), their transitions help us to differentiate words like *kip*, *kit*, and *kick*, and their relative durations also help us to recognize words ending in voiced and voiceless consonants as different - words, such as *cup* and *cub*.

Rather than discuss each vowel and diphthong separately, the

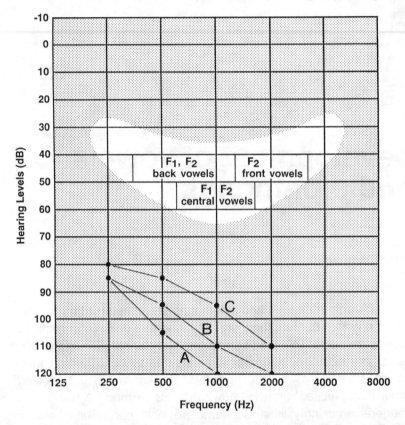

figure 10-1. The approximate frequency and intensity of F₁ and F₂ of the back and central vowels, and F₂ of the front vowels, depicted on an audiogram at the approximate hearing levels they would reach when produced at a conversational level by a talker speaking at a distance of about two yards.

material in this chapter will be presented in five parts as follows: the central vowels (for these are normally the first to emerge, and the easiest to produce); the back vowels (which contain abundant low frequency energy and are, on this account, readily mastered by any child with useful residual hearing); the front vowels (which require much more precise tongue placement than the others); the diphthongs (which require continuous movement between two vowels); and finally, the r-colored vowels and diphthongs.

The approximate frequency and intensity range of the vowels as one would hear them at a distance of about two yards, is depicted on the audiogram form presented as Figure 10-1. As this Figure indicates, F_1 and F_2 of the back and central vowels all occur within relatively narrow frequency bands. The range of F_1 of the various front vowels (not included) is the same as that of the back vowels (between about 300 and 1000 Hz). The frequency range of F_2 of the front vowels is from about 1250 to 3000 Hz. If aided audiograms were charted on Figure 10-1, they would suggest which types of vowels might be detected, and possibly identified, by hearing-impaired listeners, such as those whose unaided hearing levels (A,B,and C) are depicted in this Figure. Readers are invited to construct the aided audiograms that might be expected if children A,B, and C were provided with optimal binaural amplification.

choosing the type of strategy

Informal strategies offer the most direct route to the use of appropriate vowels and diphthongs in spoken language. Initially, therefore, they should always be chosen in preference to formal strategies, except for purposes of remediation. Formal strategies should not be introduced until informal learning procedures in the context of abundant verbal stimulation have been given a fair trial over a period of at least several months. Only if the full range of vowels is not then emerging in the child's spontaneous communication should one consider using formal strategies.

For either type of strategy to be successful, the prerequisite behaviors (vocalization, tongue, and lip control) must be present, the most appropriate sense modality for the perception of the target sounds must be selected so that the sensations associated with the patterns become familiar, and the child must be encouraged to perceive and produce these patterns in communicative situations. Immediate imitation is usually demanded in formal work, but not when informal strategies are used (see Chapter 7). The use of informal strategies to encourage the more extensive use of the various vowels when they have been acquired through formal teaching can ensure the carry-over of patterns into everyday speech communication.

encouragement of approximations

By the time children are in the process of refining their vowel systems, they have usually acquired several consonants, and are able to communicate through approximations to adult forms of words, sentences, and sometimes discourse. Their speech approximations may range from being completely intelligible to wholly unintelligible, or just partly so, depending on each child's verbal learning style, hearing levels, and past experience. It is important to encourage communication involving approximations, regardless of how difficult it may be to understand a child's utterances, for approximations are the essential underpinnings of the mature forms of spoken language that one is seeking to establish.

Speech communication should not, as a rule, be used as a vehicle for any form of speech correction. It is, of course, appropriate for caregivers and professionals to reflect children's poorly formulated utterances in correct English, both to provide a good model, and to signal their comprehension if they know what it is the children are trying to say. For example, a child might say, "ah hae fai bo." An adult, on the basis of cues provided by the situation, may correctly understand the utterance as the child's attempt to say " I can't find the ball." It would then be appropriate for the adult to reflect aloud "You can't find the ball." This response would encourage the child to keep on communicating. In contrast, a response that focuses on the child's speech, and ignores the content of the message (For example, "No, don't say ah hae, say I can't") could lead to the child's reluctance to improve his speech, or (more important) discourage further attempts at communication. Children's communicative utterances can, of course, be used as the basis for developing vowels, extending vocabulary, and expanding language when the message that the child is attempting to express is clarified by such intervention.

the integration of various skills

The previous chapter stressed the importance of encouraging approximations to mature forms of spoken language, while ensuring that children learned to exercise gross control over vocal intensity, duration, and frequency. If, as recommended, communication is made the end-goal of work on the development of vocalization, some vowels sounds will inevitably emerge as children attempt to talk. They have to, because it is impossible to open the mouth and vocalize without producing a vowel of some sort.

The more children are encouraged to vocalize, and to attempt speech communication, the greater the range of their emerging vowel system is likely to be. In developing a child's vowel system, therefore, one is not starting from zero. The primary purpose of this chapter is to propose strategies by which children can learn to control the production of vowels that they have already begun to use, and to extend their repertoire of vowels to meet the requirements of spoken English.

More than just the acquisition of vowels has to be accomplished at this stage of speech development. The previously acquired control of voice patterns must be integrated into, and refined by, the use of vowels in the children's emerging speech communication. For normal sounding speech to develop, their utterances must not only contain clear vowels; they must also have suprasegmental (prosodic) structure (see Chapter 2). Rhymes and songs are excellent means of refining and integrating suprasegmental aspects of speech as one is developing vowels.

Vowels and diphthongs are differentiated on the basis of their frequency components (their formants), and on their intensity and duration. Central vowels, such as ah, are louder than other (back or front) vowels (see below). Some vowels, like oo, ah, and ee, are also longer and louder than those in the words *cook, cut, cat,* and *kick* that are adjacent to them. When the earlier stages of development have been well covered, they should help a child to differentiate between the various vowels more readily. For example, the concepts of high and low, loud and quiet, as well as long and short will be familiar. This vocabulary may not have been learned, but the child should certainly have had experience in the sensory discrimination of these acoustic properties.

Children who have learned to perceive and to produce voice pitch changes are in a better position than those who have not to discriminate between the formant frequencies of vowels, and to produce them appropriately. If appropriate sensory aids have been selected, and are used (not just worn), the task of ensuring the acquisition of vowels and diphthongs should be a relatively simple one. It becomes a complex and much more difficult process when children are expected to develop them mainly or entirely through speechreading, because the tongue cannot be adequately visualized, and the effects of the tongue's position on the spectral (frequency) components of speech are available only in modalities other than vision (see Chapters 3 through 5).

In the following discussion of the different types of vowels, mention will frequently be made to the possible contributions that each sense modality can make to their acquisition. In addition to being on guard against over-emphasis on speechreading, professionals should not attempt to have children visualize tongue positions. Not only does this tend to encourage exaggeration, but it suggests to the child that some aspects of speech are static when, in fact, speech is a constantly changing activity. As indicated in Chapters 2 and 8, it is the coarticulation of consonants and vowels that provides formant transition cues that assist in the identification of consonants. If the vocal tract is not continuously and dynamically shaped by constant movements of the tongue, then these transitions, which are vital to speech intelligibility, will not be present. A goal that pervades this, and all later stages of speech acquisition is the development and refinement of vowels so that they assist appropriately in consonant identification.

prevention and remediation of vowel errors

Prolongation, neutralization, and nasalization of vowels by hearing-impaired talkers are problems that stem mainly from the inadequate perception of their own and others' speech patterns. They can also result from the habits of production that are caused by, or are allowed to develop in the course of, formal teaching. In general, these faults should not develop in children who have useful residual hearing up to and including 1000 Hz if they are fitted with appropriate hearing aids, and have the opportunity to communicate through speech as they develop their auditory learning skills. Hearing is usually sufficient to prevent the emergence of all three problems.

For those who have developed such problems, vowels should be placed, as soon as they are taught, in the context of consonant-vowel (CV) or vowel-consonant (VC) syllables, and strings of a dozen or more such syllables practised at *repetition* rates of not less than three per second. Vowels in CV or VC syllables should then be rehearsed through *alternation* in a similar manner, in order to develop accuracy and speed, and to ensure economy of effort (prevent exaggerated movements of the articulators). When strings of CV or VC syllables constructed from fricatives and plosives are practised at speed, the vowels within them cannot be nasalized, because the velopharyngeal port has to be closed in order to achieve sufficient oral breath stream for the adequate production of either type of consonant. Producing syllables at speed, and ensuring the presence of vowels in spoken language patterns that have normal rhythmic structures, should ensure that none of these faults develops. In contrast, the acceptance of isolated vowels, single syllables, or single words over weeks or months of speech development, will almost inevitably result in the development of these vowel errors. If they do occur, they should be treated as outlined above as soon as possible, because the longer they are allowed to persist, the more difficult they are to eradicate.

the central vowels

The central vowels include those contained in the words *father*, *shut*, *hat*, and a, as in *about*. These are the vowels that are most likely to emerge when the mouth is open, and the tongue occupies a relatively neutral position. (The vowel in the word *hat* is made with the center of the tongue raised slightly towards the hard palate). Usually, as one produces these vowels in the above order, they require less lowering of the jaw, their relative intensity declines, and their duration decreases. They are the vowels that typically occur in a child's non-linguistic vocalizations. Because the tongue does not appreciably constrict the vocal tract during their production, the central vowels - with the exception of the neutral vowel a, as in the word *again* - are usually several dB louder than all other vowels, and hence the easiest to hear or to feel.

prerequisites

The prerequisites for the controlled production of the central vowels include several different abilities: to take breath in quickly, and to release it slowly; to exercise gross control over vocal intensity (including whispering), vocal duration, and vocal frequency, to control tongue placement; to use residual hearing (if present), and other sense modalities (if required); to imitate visible body and mouth movements; and ability and willingness to concentrate on a task for at least a few minutes at a time.

goals

To evoke the four central vowels in numerous different words that can be used as basic vocabulary, and also as reference points for the extension of the child's vowel system; and to develop the use of vowels as the carriers of prosody and consonant cues in meaningful utterances.

informal strategies

One of the most effective informal strategies is to work from involuntarily produced speech patterns. Another is to play games in which particular vowels can be deliberately used. Central vowels are involuntarily produced in crying, so making a doll "cry" in a play situation often results in the imitation of the act by young children. Exclamations during play with the child, such as *ow!* when hurt, *ah-hah!* when something is discovered, *ugh!* in disgust, and *uh-uh!* meaning "No. Stop it!", are ways of rendering these vowels salient and inviting imitation of them.

Playing with toys, and talking about objects and events that interest the child, can always be associated in some way with the various vowels. Saying the vowel ah, for example, over several seconds as one moves a toy car from one spot to another, can encourage the child to vocalize in a similar fashion when moving similar playthings. The most opportune time to engage in such vocal play is when children's interest in their toys has already been stimulated, and when they are looking for an adult to share in their play. Shared play is usually a very effective situation in which to promote the production of speech patterns.

Vowel discrimination can also be encouraged in play. For example, the words *a car* and *a truck* (both having central vowels) can be contrasted, as can the sounds that animals make - ba for a sheep, moo for a cow, and so on.

Real, as well as toy animals can help, and numerous children have developed clear central vowels by repeatedly telling the family pet that it's a *bad puppy*, or *a fat cat*.

Many opportunities for using central vowels are offered by naming people in the children's families, e.g., *Mum*, *Papa*, *Grandpa*, and *Grandma*.

Rhymes, such as *Ba Ba Black Sheep*, and *Pat-a-cake Pat-a-cake*, can be sung - even if the child only contributes the vowels - and stories in which people sing (lalalala) or laugh (ha ha ha) can all contribute when the children are encouraged to participate actively. Informal strategies can as frequently be based on words as on sounds.

formal strategies

Because central vowels are produced in spontaneous vocalization, formal strategies that are used to evoke voice can also be used to elicit this range of vowel sounds. The F_1 and F_2 of these vowels all lie just below and just above 1000 Hz, so auditory reception and feedback during their production is possible for most hearing-impaired children. On this account, and because there is very little visual information on tongue position available from these vowels when they are normally produced, audition is the modality of choice for teaching them. There is little kinesthetic sensation arising from tongue movement in the production of these vowels, although the tongue is more forward in the mouth, and the lips are slightly more spread, for ae, as in *pat*, than for ah, as in *Pa*. Kinesthetic sensation, which provides information on the tongue and lip positions for these vowels, is best enhanced by contrasting back, mid, and front vowels without consonants. The presence of the bilabials /p/ or /b/ reduce the kinesthetic sensation associated with tongue movement. Sensory information essential for speech control must, of course, also be obtained through the repetition of syllables that involve consonants made with the tongue, such as *daedaedaedae* and *googoogoogoo*.

In view of the relative ease with which these vowels can be elicited, and the relatively small amount of tongue, lip, and jaw movements they involve in the absence of coarticulated consonants, little time should be required, and consequently scheduled, for the phonetic level rehearsal of central vowels.

Care should be taken to avoid exaggerated jaw movements in the early formal teaching of these sounds. Exaggeration is often promoted by the use of mirrors at this stage of speech development. Such use of vision is to be avoided, particularly because sufficient tactile cues are available for direct feedback. Wider than necessary jaw opening tends to lead to taking the tongue further back in the mouth than necessary in the production of all vowels, to the jaw-assisted production of alveolar consonants, and to the breakdown of natural speech rhythms. Rapid repetition of a half-dozen or more syllables, such as *bababa* or *baebaebae*, should result in the appropriate production of central vowels without exaggeration.

To ensure differentiation of, or close approximation to, these vowels, sufficient feedback on the correctness of their pronunciation in words must be provided by the teacher or clinician. This is particularly important when formal teaching is necessary. Such feedback permits a child to integrate information received from the clinician or teacher with the sensations that are created in the mouth as each of these sounds is produced.

phonologic use

It is always helpful in the early stages of development of any speech pattern to ensure that a child acquires a number of commonly used words that are not only useful in their own right as elements in everyday discourse, but can be used as reference points for correct pronunciation of words yet to be learned. Simple, monosyllabic words best serve as "key" vocabulary for this purpose.

The routine situations that pervade children's lives offer plenty of opportunities for them to learn a wide range of words that contain these vowels. They can, for example, be found in the following words and situations: *a cup, supper, all gone, not much, I want some,* and *pass the butter* (eating), *a bus, a car* (travelling), *a bath, wash under your arms* (toileting), *hurry up* (dressing), *what's that?* (questions), *What a lot!, that one* (exclamations), and so on. It is important not to restrict language to the range of words that contain central vowels and are, therefore, emphasized at this stage. Furthermore, emphasis should be provided in a natural way. For example, after playing with some toys one can ask the child in "put away" games: *Give me the.... dog* or *Pass me a... car*, pausing and raising vocal pitch on *the* (the only one) and *a* (one of several) to render these determiners more salient. To use the appropriate body posture and facial expressions along with such a pause is a natural way to indicate that one is making up one's mind which toy to ask for.

the back vowels

The vowels that occur in the words *too, could, low,* and *law* are known as back vowels. They are so-called because the back of the tongue is normally raised towards the soft palate during their production. They all involve a certain amount of lip rounding and lip protrusion, features that are most marked with oo, and least marked with aw. The various ways that the lips and tongue shape the vocal tract, result in these vowels having mainly low-frequency formants that are quite audible to children with no hearing beyond 1000 Hz.

Lip-rounding and lip-protrusion lowers the frequency of all resonances in the vocal tract. The back vowels can, therefore, be closely approximated by exaggerating their lip configurations, and moving the tongue minimally, if at all. Indeed, many deaf adults who have been taught mainly through speechreading have learned to achieve the pronunciation of these vowels in this way. Such a strategy leads to the marked neutralization effect that has come to be regarded as typical of "deaf speech". The reader can reproduce, and thus come to understand this effect by slowly saying the word *pool*, initiating the word with exaggerated lip rounding, and keeping the tongue in the neutral position until the tip is raised to produce the /l/. The result approximates *pewahl*. To avoid this common speech fault, teachers and clinicians must ensure that lip configurations are not exaggerated, and that the tongue is the organ primarily involved in the production of these vowels. Encouraging children to pay attention to the auditory components of these vowels, or to the information about them provided by cochlear implants or tactile devices, rather than to the highly visible lip patterns, will usually ensure that exaggerated patterns of production do not develop.

prerequisites

The back vowels have the same prerequisites as the central vowels but, in addition, children learning these vowels formally should have the ability to tense (push, pull, or squeeze playthings), or relax on request. This additional range of skills, generalized to speech, assists in obtaining high-back tongue placement, and the differentiation of long (tense) and short (lax) vowels. Lip-rounding and tongue-raising occur in sucking and swallowing, so if there are no difficulties in feeding, one may assume the presence of these prerequisites.

goals

The goals at this stage are to evoke these four vowels, to contrast them with the central vowels, and to use them in a basic vocabulary of different words on which the pronunciation of further words can be built, and with which the child can communicate.

informal strategies

Playing games like hide-and-seek, or pretending to scare someone with boo, are strategies that offer considerable fun through active learning. Saying ah in mock surprise when startled, exclaiming oo and withdrawing the hand quickly from hot water, or saying oooooh when shivering at the touch of something cold, are reactions that fascinate children and encourage imitation.

Attributing particular noises to animals, birds, and various toys (cows say *moo*, owls say *hoo hoo*, boats go *bobobobo*, etc.) is also an effective way of presenting back vowels to young children. Using these, and central vowels in words that occur frequently in everyday routine situations, as well as in play, also offers numerous opportunities for their repetition and imitation. Exclamations and questions, such as *Oh, look!*, *Who's that?*, *One for you, one for Mummy!*, *No!*, and numerous phrases, such as *Shut the door*, *on the floor*, and *on the path*, offer opportunities for caregivers and professionals to focus attention on the production of back vowels, as well as on the contrast of back and central vowels.

Because the back vowels have strong acoustic components under 1000 Hz, the sense modality of choice in their development is audition for all except totally or near-totally deaf children. Such children, when effectively fitted with multi-channel cochlear implants or multi-channel tactile devices, should be able to discriminate between central and back vowels, but may not be able to perceive differences among the back vowels themselves. Although some children who wear single-channel tactile aids are able to differentiate between vowels without the assistance of speechreading, such ability is unusual.

formal strategies

Formal teaching strategies for the back vowels are rarely necessary, because the low-frequency energy that characterizes them permits most hearing-impaired children to acquire them through the use of residual audition. Visual strategies are to be avoided if possible because of the emphasis that they place on lip movements - rather than tongue movements, which are obscured by the lips and teeth during normal production. If direct input and feedback are not available to a child through the use of hearing aids, cochlear implants, or tactile devices, then direct tactile cues, and feedback on correctness from the teacher or clinician will be required.

The necessary raising of the back of the tongue for the oo vowel can generally be stimulated best by having the child waggle one or two fingers in the mouth while saying oo. This produces a "Tarzan calling Jane" sound that a child can be encouraged to listen for, or otherwise perceive. An alternative tactile strategy is to have a child press his or her head back and up against the teacher's or clinician's hand for the vowel oo, and to relax the pressure for the vowel ah, in the series oo-ah-oo-ah-oo-ah. If the adult provides feedback on correctness as these vowels are produced, the children should be able, on the basis of the kinesthetic information generated as the tongue moves from vowel to vowel, to associate the correct tongue position with each. Because the tongue position is closely correlated with lip configuration, speechreading, if need be, can provide the necessary cues for teaching the vowels that lie between oo and ah (those in the words *Who would know more of art*). The lips assume less and less marked protrusion and rounding as the tongue assumes more central placement.

Any tendency to neutralize the back vowels as they emerge in spoken language can be overcome by *first* obtaining an oo vowel in isolation, *second*, requiring its maintenance for several seconds as one moves a finger horizontally along in front of the child as a visual indication of required duration, and *third*, repeating the previous step, but briefly dropping the finger from time to time, while the hand continues to move, as a prompt for the child's production of a selected consonant. Each time the finger is restored to its original horizontal track the vowel must also be restored to correct production. If it is not, the trial must be terminated. Initially, only one or two consonant prompts should be given on each trial, so that child's focus remains almost entirely on the production of the vowel. For example, in a five-second trial during the early stages of acquisition, the sequence would be *oooooopooooopooooo*. Later, more and more consonant prompts can be introduced until rapid repetition of a syllable results with the consonants accurately coarticulated throughout each trial. It is advisable to begin this strategy with consonants requiring no tongue involvement, such as /b/, /p/, or /m/. When trials with these consonants can be completed with accuracy, the alveolar consonants /t/, /d/, and /n/, and later, the velar consonants /k/ and /g/, can be introduced in like manner.

Formal teaching of a particular speech pattern is best concluded by using informal learning strategies relating to the same pattern, and finally by encouraging its production in as much of the child's everyday spoken language as possible, particularly in words and phrases that are frequently used. When teaching additional words with the same vowel, the vocabulary acquired earlier can be used as a reference point. For example, if the word *too* is already acquired, and accurately spoken, it can, through repetition, serve to orient the production of other words, such as *tool*, *pool*, and *cool*, through saying a sequence, such as *too too too tool*.

phonologic use

There are many commonly used words and phrases that incorporate back vowels, and also provide contrast between back and central vowels. The oo vowel is used in such early words as *boot*, *shoe*, *who*, *do*, and *school*, and in everyday phrases (with central vowels), such as *Who's that?*, *Oh! a new tooth!*, and so on. The short (lax) counterpart of oo is found in words and phrases like *book*, *look*, *took*, *cook*, *You pull, and Daddy'll push*, and in expressions like *whoops!*. The long vowel contained in the word *owe* also occurs in early verbs like *blow*, *know*, and *grow*, early nouns like *boat*, *coat*, *toes*, *nose*, and early phrases, such as *No, no more*, *Go to Mum*, and so on. The aw vowel is often modified by the presence of r-coloring in words like *door*, *more*, and *floor*. Children should nevertheless be encouraged to approximate such words, because refinement of pronunciation is a simple matter if approximations are not allowed to persist for an unduly long time.

the front vowels

The front vowels include those contained in the words *bed*, *bake*, *kick*, and *cheese*. These vowels are the most difficult for profoundly hearing-impaired children to acquire through audition alone, because the F_2 of each one lies in the octave band centered on 2000 Hz (see

Chapters 2 and 3). If the F_1 of these vowels is audible, and the F_2 is not, then these vowels can easily be confused with the back vowels when they are presented through audition alone, because back and front vowels have F_1 components in common (see Figure 2-1).

Visually, the front vowels are distinctly different from the others, because the lips are increasingly spread as one pronounces them in the order they are listed above. As with all other vowels, the lips and teeth mask the tongue position when the front vowels are produced in a normal manner. Since the tongue position for these vowels is crucially important for their intelligibility, the attention of children with no aided hearing responses beyond 1000 Hz should be directed primarily to audition, and secondarily to vision. For such children, an audible low formant with visible lip-rounding is sufficient to define the back vowels, and an audible low formant with visible lip-spreading can unambiguously define those produced at the front of the mouth. If, with such children, the auditory component is neglected in favor of the visual patterns (as it can be, for example, in programs that focus mainly on speechreading or Cued Speech), the front vowels can be identified reasonably well, but the acquisition of production skills will be impeded.

Most multi-channel cochlear implants and tactile devices provide some information on F_2 of all vowels, and if these instruments work satisfactorily for a child on all channels, they can provide enough information for discrimination between back, mid, and front vowels, and possibly enough cues for discrimination within each of these vowel groups. If such instruments are worn, then strategies to promote the informal learning of front vowels should be sufficient. If neither hearing aids nor such instruments provide the necessary cues, then direct tactile strategies can be adopted to promote their acquisition through formal teaching.

Some pervasive problems can be caused by thoughtless teaching procedures for the development of vowels. One of them is exaggeration of mouth movements on the false premise that it will enhance the acquisition of vowels through speechreading. Not only does it lead to inappropriate tongue placement, and unhelpful substitution of jaw and lip movement for the vocal tract shaping that should be accomplished by the tongue, it also makes it very hard for children to speechread anyone but their caregivers.

prerequisites.

Apart from the ability to elevate the blade of the tongue towards the hard palate and alveolar ridge, the prerequisites for the development of the front vowels are the same as those for the back vowels.

goals

To evoke the four front vowels, to contrast them with central and back vowels, to use them in a basic (key) vocabulary, and to encourage the production of words, sentences, and discourse containing these and previously learned vowels.

informal strategies

One informal strategy, suggested in the discussion relating to informal teaching in Chapter 7, is to develop the ee sound from an involuntary giggle, because most children can easily be persuaded to giggle and vocalize. Labelling the noise a toy airplane makes as eeee, saying wheeee as one is giving the child a big swing in the park or playground, exclaiming clearly as one handles objects (e.g.*it's wet*), and referring to common objects that contain these vowels, particularly those that consistently command children's interest (e.g., *a bed*, *a cake*, *a fish*, or *a tree*), will all serve to focus a child's attention on them. Encouraging a child to vocalize when he or she wants something, such as *ice cream*, can also work, but care has to be taken not to frustrate progress by demanding more spoken language than the child can give in such situations. When the phonologic targets are vowels, then one should be delighted if the vocalization and vowels are acceptable and few, if any, of the consonants are present or correct.

formal strategies

Although jaw opening and lip configurations play a significant part, the feature that dominates adequate vowel production is tongue position. Formal strategies are therefore directed primarily to tongue control. The simplest and most dynamic formal strategy is to have a child rhythmically and vigorously repeat the sequence oo-ah- ee-ah several times, so that the tongue, if it moves at all, tends to overshoot the central vowel positions, and thus extend its trajectory to encompass the full range of normal vowel production. Sensing this range through the oro-sensory feedback created by the tongue's motion allows a child to develop a strong awareness of the topography of the mouth, and the range of tongue movement that vowels require. Achievement of the rhythmic motion, and the raising of the tongue with the required tension for oo and ee, can often be assisted by swinging the arms backwards and forwards in time with the vowels, high for oo and ee, and low for ah.

The same sort of strategy can be used to obtain just the oo and ee vowels. Indeed, it is helpful to extend and establish the vowel range using both the two- and the three-vowel combinations. It is not helpful to use these strategies with the addition of consonants. As the reader can verify by repeating the sequences *ee-oo-ee-oo* and *bee-boo-bee-boo*, the involvement of the lips (or the tip of the tongue in *tee-too-tee-too*), which are more sensitive than the body of the tongue, masks the sensation of tongue movement that one is seeking to establish.

Having children push their hands vigorously against those of the clinician or teacher when attempting to say ee, and relaxing them for the production of ah, in a long rhythmic sequence of ee-ah syllables, can also establish the production of the ee vowel. The principle involved in this strategy is that all moveable parts of the body tend to be thrust forward against any resistance offered, and such thrust will bring the tongue forward for the correct production of ee. By the same token, the tongue position for the oo vowel can sometimes be obtained by joining hands with the clinician or teacher, and pulling and relaxing in a long rhythmic sequence of oo-ah syllables. Of course, adults using these strategies must provide feedback on correctness to the children as they teach, and gradually fade out the overall physical activity without losing the target pattern thus obtained.

A more direct strategy involving pushing is to have the child press two fingers of one hand against the upper lip, over the eye teeth, when attempting to say ee. The adult can, in demonstrating this strategy, fast press the child's fingers against her upper lip when she says ee, and in this way indicate the force that is required. This action tends to spread the tongue to an appropriate width, and bring the tongue, rather than the whole body, forward into the desired position.

A tactile strategy for evoking the ee vowel that has been used for hundreds of years, and is useful today for those who have no useful hearing or devices to complement speechreading, is to have a child feel the adult's tongue as a series of ah-ee syllables are produced, and then, with the corresponding finger on the other hand, feel his own tongue as he attempts to imitate. This strategy may be the least appealing for some adults to initiate, but it is probably the most direct and effective of all the tactile strategies in the formal teaching of the ee vowel. Clearly, cleanliness must be ensured to avoid choice, and hygiene is of concern, then surgical gloves can be used.

phonologic use

Many commonly used words contain front vowels. Like any other speech pattern that is receiving particular attention, they should be emphasized through the use of voice patterns within sentences, and in situations that are meaningful and interesting to children. If they are presented out of context, children cannot readily associate them with events or experiences that are significant, and they are therefore less likely to be remembered, or to become part of a child's active vocabulary.

Many different words containing front (or any other) vowels can be used when washing, when dressing, at meal times, during play, on outings, at bedtime, or on any other occasions that are repetitive. They include *bed*, *red*, *dress*, *head*, and *men*; *play*, *take*, *break*, *ran*, and *make*; *lip*, *skip*, *hit*, *give*, and *this*; and *feet*, *knee*, *we*, *key*, *see*, and *me*.

At this stage of vowel acquisition, children may be expected to have a range of central, back, and front vowels, as well as some approximations to adult sentence forms. Their speech should therefore be much clearer than before. At all stages of speech acquisition there are natural ways of emphasizing the target patterns phonologically. It is rarely necessary to reduce sentences, or to adopt abnormal language in the course of teaching any speech pattern. For example, to emphasize the ee vowel as the child is dressing or being dressed, one has only to select a word like *sleeve*, and then incorporate its use into the activity in sentences, such as *"Put your hand through the sleeve," "Your sleeve is inside out," "Let's find your long-sleeved shirt"* and *"Oh look! Your sleeve is dirty."* The strategy of linking spoken language to routine, repetitive activities not only provides children with a meaningful context that allows them to associate words with experience, but also provides caregivers with a constant reminder of the opportunities that exist for spoken language development throughout each day. Just as important, it provides hundreds, if not thousands, of opportunities to provide meaningful spoken language experience in the course of a year.

The three vowels of greatest importance are oo, ah, and ee, because they can serve as reference points for all other, intermediately placed vowels. Once these three vowels can be produced, the tongue's height, and position in the mouth, can be accurately deduced, and other vowels rarely need to be specifically taught because, in English, the posture and placement of the tongue is closely correlated with the configuration of the lips. The degree of lip rounding and lip protrusion is reduced as one moves through the vowels from oo to ah, and the lips become increasingly spread as one moves from ah to ee (see Figure 2-4, or the first paragraph of this chapter, if in doubt on the order of the intermediate vowels). Accordingly, no formal strategies for evoking the production of specific intermediate vowels need to be suggested.

the diphthongs

Two adjacent vowels spoken without pause create a diphthong. There are two very common diphthongs in English. They are contained in the words *how* and *eye*. A third, less common but important one is present in the word *toy*. There are others, but they are not universally used throughout the English-speaking world. For example, in some areas the words *low* and *say* are dipthongized, although they have been treated in this text as words continuing vowels. Some words containing diphthongs, such as *hair* and *ear*, are also often pronounced with r-coloring. Their development will receive attention in the following section. Because pronunciation differs from place to place, readers should be guided by local use in deciding whether particular words should be taught with vowels or diphthongs, and whether they should be given r-coloring.

prerequisites

The prerequisites for diphthongs include the correct production of their component vowels, and the ability to alternate various vowels clearly and without break on the same breath.

goals

To evoke and contrast the various English diphthongs, to use them in a basic vocabulary of different words, and to encourage the production of words, sentences, and discourse containing these diphthongs and previously learned vowels.

informal strategies

Once their component vowels have been established, diphthongs can usually be elicited simply by using them naturally under conditions that ensure their optimal perception. Profoundly hearing-impaired children with no audition beyond 1000 Hz may sometimes confuse the diphthongs present in words that rhyme with *eye* and *ow*. Although these diphthongs sound quite different to normally hearing listeners, they have similar acoustic properties for listeners who have no hearing beyond 1000 Hz. This is because, as shown in Figure 10-2, the F_1 trajectories of these two diphthongs are quite alike.

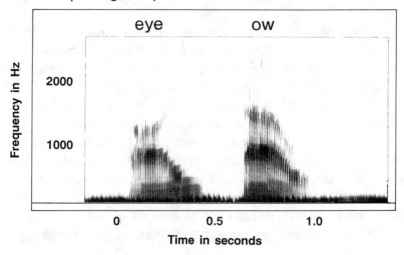

figure 10-2. A spectrogram showing the similarity between the F_1 trajectories of the diphthongs in the words *eye* and *ow* - words that sound very different indeed to the normal listener. Cover the frequencies above 1000 Hz, and then study the patterns that remain. The lower portions of the spectrograms indicate how easily one of these sounds could be mistaken for the other by a listener with no hearing beyond that frequency.

Hearing for F_2 of either component vowel should be sufficient to permit auditory discrimination between all diphthongs. Auditory- visual differentiation usually presents no problems even to profoundly hearing impaired children. Most multi-channel cochlear implants, if successfully fitted, and most multi-channel tactile devices will permit the identification of all diphthongs.

When the straightforward use of diphthongs in communicative situations does not permit a child to acquire them, it may help initially to lengthen them, so that their component vowels can be more easily perceived. For example, ow as a reaction to pain (real or pretended) can be expressed as aaaahoooow to indicate continued suffering, eye can be pronounced as aaaaheee when naming body parts, and toy can also be said slowly. To slow the pronunciation of these diphthongs should, of course, be simply an introductory measure and normal, or even rapid, production should quickly become the standard. Production of diph- thongs can easily be speeded up in play situations and in real life by saying a brief ow to signify sudden and short-term pain, and establishing it as a reflexive exclamation when such hurt is experienced.

The development of diphthongs first in a number of key words that are interesting and meaningful to children permits other words contain- ing the same sounds to be derived from them. It is clearly better to use words containing consonants that have already emerged through com- municative speech for this purpose. These are usually the visible ones, such as /p/, /b/, and /m/, and perhaps /t/, /d/, /n/, or /l/. Typical key words for young children are ow, house, and the cat's meeow; bye-bye, light, and mine; and, for the least used diphthong, boy and toy.

formal strategies

The simple expedient of having children alternate the component vowels will establish the motor skills required for the production of any diphthong. To give a child a clear idea of what is required, the professional can: First take each of the child's hands in her own, and evoke one of the component vowels while holding up the left hand, and the other component vowel while holding up the right. Second, say the component vowels in turn, and without pause, while simultaneously and rhythmically moving the hand with which each component vowels has been as- sociated. Third, once the child can alternate the component vowels in this way, speed up the process until the two vowels blend into the required diphthong. *Fourth*, when the diphthong is pronounced with ease, incorporate a word that the child can use, and *fifth*, have the child repeat the word without the use of touch.

The component vowels of the diphthongs are normally those of short duration, such as the i in *hit*, and the oo in *book*. However, because these vowels are difficult to sustain, the adjacent long vowel, such as the ee in sheep and the oo in *too*, can be used when strategies like the one described immediately above are found to be necessary. Rehearsal at increasing speed, and the rapidity with which the diphthongs are normally produced, together with appropriate feedback on correctness, will quickly ensure their acceptable pronunciation.

The underlying procedure presented above can, of course, be carried out using visual rather than tactile prompting. Each component vowel can first be associated with an object, such as a colored block, or a mark on a chalkboard, and then the second to fifth steps, above can be accomplished visually. The tactile prompt is usually the more efficient, because it better conveys the rhythm of the procedure to most children who need formal teaching. Additionally, such children also need to use their eyes to learn how to speechread the diphthongs as they are modeled by the teacher or clinician.

phonologic use

Diphthongs abound in early vocabulary. Frequently used nouns include *bike*, *kite*, *night*, and *light*; as well as *cow*, *house*, *sound*, *ground*, and *mouse*. Other types of words include *dry*, *high*, *like*, *bright*, *smile*, *I*, *my*, *mine*, *fine*, and *shine*, as well as *now*, *brown*, *out*, *about*, *around*, and *loud*. The *how* and *why* questions also employ these diphthongs.

Questions and answers can provide good opportunities for emphasizing diphthongs. For example, "Is this *mine*?," "*How* much.. many.. ? "and "Do you *like* it?"

If emphasis is required to ensure that children perceive and produce these diphthongs (or indeed any speech pattern), it is usually simpler, and more effective, to encourage their production in key words that are not nouns. There are several reasons for this. The selection of nouns may direct language towards things that do not interest a child, or engage his or her attention; naming things (e.g., Those are *mice*) may expand vocabulary, but does little to expand other language skills. The number of times that a particular noun containing the desired diphthong (or other speech pattern) is normally referred to, limits the number of opportunities for its presentation. How many opportunities are there, for example, to meaningfully draw a child's attention to the sky or to a *plough*? There are many more opportunities to use all other types of words because almost anything can be *dry*, *nice*, or something one would *like* to have now; and, moreover, it is quite difficult not to put words other than nouns in sentences and discourse. Such words are both more varied and more relevant to children's interests.

Once children have reached this stage of vowel and diphthong development, their approximations to adult forms of spoken language in everyday communication should feature good rhythm, some intonation, stress on key words, and mostly clear vowels.

the r-colored vowels and diphthongs

There are five vowels and diphthongs that are commonly pronounced with r-coloring. It is present in words like *bird*, *farm*, *cork*, *ear*, *bear*, and *mother*. In writing, the /r/ appears after the vowel, but it may not be pronounced at all in speech (as in England, Australia, and Boston), may be pronounced as a consonant (as in Scotland), or may be incorporated as r-coloring into the vowel (as in most places in North America).

When the vowel and the /r/ are pronounced together, the pronunciation of the vowel is significantly changed, because the /r/ component requires either the elevation of the back of the tongue or the retroflection (turning back) of the tip of the tongue. The /r/ sounds that result are vocalic (vowel contained) rather than consonantal (/r/ sounds like those that precede rather than follow vowels). The effect of r-coloring is to lower the frequency of all vowel formants. The differences between vowels that are r-colored, and those that are not, are quite fine, and they are not readily distinguished through any sense modality or combination of modalities if aided hearing extending beyond 1500 Hz is not available, or is not used. The perception and production of r- coloring by children with more than severe hearing impairment is, therefore, best achieved through linguistic context.

prerequisites

In addition to the skills inherent in the production of other vowels, the major prerequisite is the ability either to retroflex the tip of the tongue, or to raise the body of the tongue in such a way that the breath stream is diverted around it.

goals

To evoke the r-colored vowels, and to incorporate them into words, words in sentences, and everyday discourse.

informal strategies

If r-coloring does not emerge without specific intervention, informal learning of the r-colored vowels and diphthongs can best be promoted by first focusing children's attention on their pronunciation in words that can be stressed. Producing certain words with natural linguistic stress simply renders them easier to perceive through whatever device a child may be using. Such stress would occur in sentences, such as "That's the *right* way to do it!," "Now give me the *round* one!," and "That onion's *rotten*, isn't it." In words like *mother*, the final syllable cannot be stressed, and it is, therefore, one of the least perceptible sounds in running speech. Words such as this can be rendered more salient by using suprasegmental cues, such as intonation patterns and pauses.

The r-colored vowels and diphthongs may normally be pronounced with a small amount of lip rounding and lip protrusion. It is very important not to exaggerate such lip movements in focusing children's attention on these sounds, because it is the tongue in well articulated speech that produces the r-coloring, not the lips. It may even be helpful, in the long run, for the professional to de-emphasize the lip configurations while developing this range of sounds informally.

formal strategies

The development of r-colored vowels and diphthongs through formal strategies is best left until the consonantal /r/ has been acquired. They can then be taught through the repetition of syllables containing the consonantal /r/. This is most easily done in the context of the ah vowel, because the trajectory followed by the tongue - between the /r/ and the vowel - facilitates children's acquisition of the target sound by providing them with the greatest amount of kinesthetic information.

To begin the shaping procedure that constitutes this strategy, *first* have the child repeat /rararara/. *Second* have the child repeat these syllables rhythmically in tune with your raising a finger for the /r/, and lowering it for the vowel. *Third*, repeat the second step, but this time arrhythmically, interrupting the a̲h̲ vowel by raising and lowering your finger quickly and sporadically. *Fourth*, instead of lowering your finger quickly from the /r/ position, hold it there longer before dropping it to signal return to the production of the vowel. This will result in a vocalic rather than a consonantal /r/. *Fifth*, repeat step four, maintaining the /r/ position for much longer. *Sixth*, because you now have an r-colored vowel, your goal in this step is to see that it is used in a word. So repeat the fifth step, but instead of returning to the vowel from the /r/ position, ask the child to close the lips after the /r/ and produce an /m/. The result will be a clearly pronounced r-colored vowel in the word *arm*. Repetition of this word, its association with the arm as part of the body, and reinforcement of children's successful attempts to produce it, will ensure the desired production of the word from this point on Generalization to other words with the /ar/ component is simply a matter of adding or changing the surrounding consonants, for example, to create *farm* or *car*.

Generalization to other vowels may be attempted directly, for example by having the child say *far-far-far* — *for*, or repeating the steps described above with each vowel. Generalization from the tense and stressed i̲r̲ vowel, as in *bird*, to the lax and unstressed e̲r̲ vowel, in words like *mother*, *older*, *baker*, and *rather*, can be achieved simply by alternating the two syllables in such words, one loudly, the other quietly.

phonologic use

Early words with r-colored vowels include nouns, such as *bird*, *word*, *girl*, and *work*; *arm*, *farm*, *car*, and *yard*; *cork*, *door*, *horn*, and *floor*; *ear*, *tears*, and *fear*; *hair*, *bear*, *stairs*, and *prayers*; *sister*, *brother*, *under*, and *over*. Early words with r-coloring, other than nouns, include *first*, *burn*, *stir*, and *curl*, *hard* and *bark*; *for*, *tore*, *more*, and *snore*; *wear*, *tear*, *where*, and *there*; as well as *hear*, *near*, *clear*, and *we're*.

Any word can serve as a key for the pronunciation of other words but, for the reasons suggested in the preceding section, nouns are less likely to serve as helpfully as words of other types.

suggestions for further reading

The normal production of vowels has been well described in a text by Minifie, Hixon, and Williams (1973). There are few recent books or modern articles that deal with the teaching of vowels to hearing-impaired children. Calvert and Silverman (1983), Ewing and Ewing (1964), Haycock (1933), and Ling (1976) provide the most extensive information on the topic. See References, pp. 433 ff.

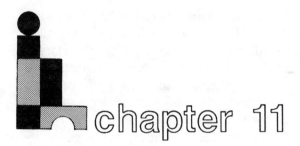

chapter 11

development of manner distinctions in consonant production

Consonants should be considered mainly as ways of releasing, arresting, and interrupting vowels. Only when they are coarticulated with vowels and other consonants do they truly become a part of the stream of sound that is speech. In general, the way that speech sounds relate (move to and from one another) is at least as important as the way they themselves are produced. Emphasis in this chapter is, therefore, on developing consonants and consonant blends as dynamic elements in the stream of speech. The terminology used, and the concepts of speech production embodied in this chapter were introduced in Chapter 2.

When a child can detect a target consonant, and discriminate between it and most others, informal rather than formal strategies should initially be chosen to develop its production. Whenever formal strategies are used to reach a target pattern, one should subsequently turn (or return) to the use of informal strategies so that the child can become more fully familiar with the use of that pattern in everyday speech. The greatest opportunities for familiarization with speech patterns exist, of course, in their use in everyday communication through spoken language.

The primary emphasis in this chapter is on front consonants and their manner of production. The next chapter is concerned with the development of alveolar and velar consonants. The voiced-voiceless distinction and the development of blends is treated in Chapter 14.

In each section of these chapters the various speech patterns are described, and the prerequisites for their successful detection through the different sense modalities discussed. Additionally, procedures for the development of consonants having different manners of production are outlined in ways that extend the information presented in Chapters 3 through 5. Informal learning and formal teaching strategies for the development of these consonants are contrasted (see Chapter 7), and some function words that can be used as "key" vocabulary in generalizing pronunciation to other words, and to different aspects of spoken language are suggested. Three levels of function words are provided for each sound. Level 1 words are those that are the easiest for children to conceptualize, and the earliest normally learned. Level 2 words are those of intermediate difficulty, and usually learned somewhat later. Level 3 words are the most advanced. As explained in Chapter 10, key words of this sort are to be preferred over nouns because they can be used more frequently and more meaningfully in everyday spoken language. Their use also stimulates the production of utterances of at least sentence length.

manners of consonant production

Consonants can be classified according to their *manner of production*; that is, according to whether sounds are stops (plosives), nasals, semivowels, fricatives, affricates or liquids. The sounds /b/, /m/, /w/, /f/, ch, and /l/ are phonemes differing in these manners of production. Manner cues are carried more by time and intensity than by spectral (frequency) cues, although frequency cues help to differentiate the liquids from the semi-vowels, and the fricatives and affricates from all other manners of production (see Chapter 3). Thus, all sensory aids that provide sufficient low-frequency information will permit discrimination between stops, nasals, and semivowels, through reference to their time and intensity patterns. Multi-channel tactile devices or cochlear implants should also permit fricatives and affricates to be detected, and their manner of production to be identified. In short, the cues that most sensory aids are able to provide when appropriately selected and adjusted can help the majority of hearing-impaired children to achieve high levels of performance in both the reception and production of consonants that differ in manner of production.

Speechreading, by itself, results in many confusions among consonants that differ in manner of production, although it can provide a moderately useful supplement to all types of sensory aids - hearing aids, tactile devices, and cochlear implants. When fitted appropriately with sensory aids, most hearing-impaired children respond well to informal learning strategies in their acquisition of consonants that differ in manner of production. In the application of formal strategies, one may include the use of various technological devices, such as nasal, plosive, or fricative indicators, but traditional strategies to develop manner distinctions are plentiful, as well as efficient. It should be emphasized that, once they can be produced, manner distinctions, like all other aspects of speech, must be used meaningfully in real-life communication.

the plosives /b/ and /p/.

The easiest consonant for hearing-impaired children to produce is the /b/. This sound, and its unvoiced counterpart /p/, are known as plosives (because they cause an explosive burst of air to occur as they are released), or as stops (because the vocal tract has to be stopped - that is, closed - in order to make them). In this section, the /b/ will be regarded as the primary target, because the simplest way to teach plosives is to treat them as ways to release, interrupt, and arrest vowels - sounds that have already been learned, and are also voiced. To insist on both voiced and unvoiced sounds at this stage introduces unnecessary complexity. Of course, if both the /b/ and the /p/ are acquired together spontaneously, the production of both should be positively reinforced and developed.

The *prerequisites* for evoking and developing /b/ consist of an extensive repertoire of vowels that are produced with good oral breath stream, and ability to interrupt the breath stream with the lips. The sounds cannot be acceptably made if breath is allowed to escape through the nose during lip closure. The /b/, as it releases, interrupts, and arrests the different vowels, has marked acoustic effects across the whole speech spectrum. It can, therefore, be detected by hearing-impaired children who wear appropriate hearing or other sensory aids.

Children with no hearing beyond 1000 Hz may find that they are unable to discriminate between the /b/, /d/, and /g/ through audition alone. They should experience no difficulty in identifying the /b/ through audition and vision. Through vision alone, the /b/ can be confused with the /p/ and the /m/. It is, therefore, important, when speechreading is the primary avenue for a child's reception of these sounds, to prevent such confusions by consistently supplementing visual cues with information from another sense modality. Once these different sounds have been developed to the point that a child can use them meaningfully in words, the very different sensations that occur as they are being made should permit their differentiation. The sensitivity of the lips in comparison with other parts of the vocal tract renders such information particularly strong, and this is a good reason for ensuring accurate production of bilabial sounds from the outset.

Informal strategies can lead to most hearing-impaired children producing /b/ spontaneously. However, its acquisition can, if necessary, be informally enhanced with young children in several ways. For example, one can pretend that a toy motor boat says bubububu as it is pushed across a bath tub, or associate the sound ba with sheep when playing with toy animals. One can also play games, such as *peek-a-boo*, blow out candles to boo, and sing nursery rhymes like *Ba Ba Black Sheep* and *Rub-A-Dub-Dub*. The consonant can also be used in sentences to name people, objects, and events, such as a *baby*, a *boy*, a *bag*, or *bedtime*, or in utterances of at least sentence length, containing particular function words (see below).

Formal strategies are more often needed to correct a poorly produced /b/ than to develop it from scratch. The usual problems with its production are its confusion with /m/, and implosion. Implosion occurs when there is insufficient breath stream to produce a burst, or when the burst is produced as the air is sucked into - rather than expelled from - the mouth as the lips are parted. If there is need to develop the /b/ formally, it should first be evoked in a chain of syllables interrupting different vowels (for example, ooobooboo). This strategy ensures that the sound is associated with the continuous breath stream provided by the established vowels, and that the appropriate pattern of lip closure occurs with each vowel. The breath stream may, if necessary, be felt with a wet finger resting lightly on, or held just in front of the lips (a wet finger is more sensitive to the air stream than a dry one), and the effect of the /b/ on the vowel should be perceived through the hearing aid or alternative sensory device. Once the /b/ is well produced in this way, it can be used in series of syllables releasing and arresting different vowels. Use of the sound in meaningful spoken language should quickly be encouraged.

The /b/ is much more common in initial than in medial or in final positions within words. However, teaching it in sequences of repeated syllables, such as /bibibibi/, is not just helping the child to master the /b/ in word-initial position; it is also ensuring that a child can use the sound to interrupt and to arrest vowels appropriately. This is because, in such a series *b + vowel* (word-initial as in *bee*), *vowel + b + vowel* (medial as in *rabbit*), and *vowel + b* (word-final as in *cub*) all occur. Plosive bursts often go unreleased in word-final position. Once the child has mastered the adequate production of a series of syllables that release and arrest the /b/, such as /babababa/, the next step is to develop the word-initial and word-final allophones (variants) of the sound as distinct entities so that unwanted intrusive voicing or plosion will not be allowed to occur in the word-final position. The effect of such faults, when they are permitted to develop, is indicated with asterisks in the sentence "Pass the hub* cap* please." When words like *hub* and *cap* are each pronounced with two syllables rather than one, the rhythm and the intelligibility of an utterance can be destroyed.

The /p/ is the unvoiced counterpart of the /b/, and the two sounds have similar effects across the speech spectrum. Like all plosives, the /p/ requires a short silent period ahead of its production to permit the build-up of breath pressure in the mouth in preparation for plosion. Its bursts, like the bursts of all unvoiced plosives, are stronger than those of any voiced plosive because the act of voicing does not hold back any of the breath stream. Whereas the /b/ releases the plosion and the vowel simultaneously in words, such as *bat* and *bill*, the /p/ plosion is released just a little time (about 20-30 msec) ahead of the vowel in words, such as *pat* and *pill*. Such a difference in voice onset time (VOT) applies among all voiced and voiceless plosives in English (see Chapter 14 for details on the distinction between /b/ and /p/). Children who have appropriate hearing aids, and hearing beyond 2000 Hz, should be able to identify /p/ as such. Those with no aided hearing beyond 1000 Hz, and those who have alternative sensory devices, should be able to recognize /p/ as an unvoiced plosive, but may confuse it with /t/ or /k/ without speechreading. Through speechreading alone the /p/ can be confused with /b/ and /m/.

As suggested above, the development of the /p/ as distinct from the /b/ is not crucial in the first stages of consonant acquisition. It is more important to develop other manner and place distinctions than to take up time with voicing differences, which are less important to understanding and intelligibility. The voicing distinction is one that involves control over delicate timing, control that will evolve as other teaching proceeds. It is such timing rather than whether the vocal cords vibrate or not that governs most of our perception of voiced-voiceless distinctions (see Chapter 2). The magnitude of the voice onset time lag will more readily become clear to children who have had the chance to develop and use voiceless fricatives to release, interrupt, and arrest vowels. Many children, given such experience, spontaneously develop /p-b/ discrimination and usage. For those who do not, the strategies that can be adopted will be described in Chapter 13.

Level 1 function words containing /b/ include be, big, both, and bad. Those containing /p/ include peep, push, and pop.

Level 2 function words with /b/ include but, back, because, by, before, behind, between, both, bent, below, beside, above, about, and beautiful. Those containing the /p/ include paddle, pink, poor, polite, peel, put, please, pretend, poke, and pass.

Level 3 function words containing /b/ abound in the language so this list could be bigger and better than the preceding ones, if not the biggest and best in the book. To list them all would keep a person ridiculously busy. Older children who are able may not object to finding some for themselves. The prefix be as in bedevil and becalm could provide some practice for older children at the appropriate stage of language development. Function words containing /p/ include pack, upon, appear, permit, pile, podgy, and impolite. It may be advisable to leave rehearsal of function words with /br/ and /pr/, such as proper and practice, and the numerous verbs that begin with /sp/, until blends have been spontaneously acquired or taught.

the nasal /m/

The /m/ is a nasal sound. It is created simply by vocalizing while the lips are closed and, at the same time, expelling the breath through the nose as in regular breathing. Accordingly it has the same prerequisites as the /b/, plus the ability to open and close the velo-pharyngeal port to initiate and terminate nasal airflow. The most salient feature of the /m/, and other nasal sounds, is a marked resonance around 300 Hz, which is known as the nasal murmur (see Figure 4-2). Other, but less intense, nasal formants are to be found at higher frequencies in the spectrum, but they will be audible only to those with aided hearing that extends beyond 1500 Hz. Most children can receive enough information to detect /m/ either through their hearing aids or through alternative devices. Unless speechreading is used to resolve the ambiguity, it may be confused with any other continuously voiced sound by users of single-channel implants. It may also be confused with /n/ and ng, the other nasal sounds, by those who have no aided hearing beyond 1000 Hz, and by others who wear alternative sensory aids. As already stated, /m/, /b/ and /p/ look alike on the lips.

Because the vowels oo and ee both have first formant (F_1) components that are about the same frequency as the nasal murmur, it is best to encourage the production of /m/ initially in the context of central vowels, such as those that occur in words like *arm* and *hum*. This renders the nasal quality distinct to most children who have more than a severe hearing impairment. Later, when the sensations that occur in the vocal tract as the sound is produced become familiar, its use can be generalized to the context of high back oo and high front ee vowels.

Another reason for initiating the formal teaching of /m/ in the context of the central vowels, is that there is less of a tendency for hearing-impaired children to nasalize central than other vowels, such as the ee and the oo. Following the /m/ with a good oral breath stream from the beginning helps to establish the nasal/oral contrast that is so important in English. There is a mechanical reason for ee and oo to become more readily nasalized than ah. The proximity of the tongue to the palate in the production of these sounds may, unless the velo-pharyngeal port is closed, result in so much restriction of the vocal tract that the air is driven out through the nose rather than through the mouth. Indeed, this is the very mechanism that underlies the production of the French nasal vowels. The ee and the oo do have stronger breath streams than the ah, however, and this feature can, with the strategies outlined below, also lead to appropriate velo-pharyngeal valving - directing the breath stream through the mouth or nose, as the occasion demands, by using the velum and pharynx appropriately.

Prerequisites for the development of the /m/ consist of many more skills than being able to produce it in isolation. Like most other consonants, it must serve to release, interrupt, and arrest vowels. Each of these uses requires different skills. At the beginning of words, the velo-pharyngeal port has to be already open (to direct the breath stream and the sound through the nose). In between vowels, it has to be quickly opened, and just as quickly closed. Closure must occur as soon as the /m/ is made, so that the vowels each side of it are not unduly nasalized. If a sentence ends with a word like *come*, the velo-pharyngeal port has just to be opened following the vowel. However, if there are other words that contain consonants following the word-final /m/, its length is usually modified to indicate whether the following sound is voiced or voiceless. One can hear how the /m/ changes before voiced and voiceless consonants by comparing the two words *camper* and *camber*.

Unless very careful attention is paid to velo-pharyngeal valving (the appropriate opening and closing of the velo-pharyngeal port) from the start, nasal consonants tend to be omitted, or vowels tend to be nasalized, in the speech of children who have more than a severe hearing impairment. This fault can be corrected, but it is better prevented. If nasal sounds are not immediately terminated after their production, then neither the fricatives nor the plosives that follow them can be produced with sufficient strength, if at all. This problem often causes much of unintelligibile speech that is to be heard among profoundly hearing-impaired children who have not received formal speech teaching of good quality.

Informal strategies for evoking any sound include listening for its involuntary production by a child, and then imitating it back to enhance its perception, and to encourage its further production. This procedure helps children to become aware of the relevant sensations when the pattern is produced by others, as well as by themselves. The /m/ occurs involuntarily in crying, and caregivers can reflect its production by using the sound (and the appropriate facial expression) to express empathy with the child's hurt (for example, <u>mmmmmm</u>! <u>mmmmmm</u>! you hurt your finger!). The /m/ is, of course frequently needed to call *mummy*. If *mummy* is mispronounced as *bubby*, then it is always better to use the term *mum* instead, as this requires less velo-pharyngeal valving skill, and helps to establish discrimination between the /m/ and the /b/. The sound can also be used to express tastiness (<u>umm</u>! *yummy!*), a learned response that can often be appropriately evoked. The /m/ can be associated with the noise made by a toy, such as the movement of a big truck (mmmmmmmmmmmm), or the noise made by an animal, such as a cow (mmmooo). (As mentioned above, the /m/ in the context of oo may lead to the vowel's nasalization unless a strong oral breath stream is present.)

Such informal strategies certainly encourage production of the sound, but their shortcoming is that they do not necessarily teach velo-pharyngeal valving, particularly the closing of the velo-pharangeal port following the /m/. Word-final fricatives are particularly useful in this regard, and a pet *mouse*, a dog called *muff*, and a doll called *Martha* can be advantageous. With everyday meals, as well as in play, reference to the *mouth*, and the call for *more*, can be frequent. Useful function words for the development of /m/ are suggested following some further notes on formal teaching.

Formal strategies for teaching the /m/ require its careful development through a variety of steps. *First* use the /m/ to interrupt central vowels that are produced with a well-established breath stream, as in the sequence aaammmaaaaaammmaaa. (Children should have no difficulty with this because vocalization on demand and the required vowel have been established, and no other sound but /m/ can result if voicing continues for a second or so once the lips are closed). *Second*, following its production in this context, one should have the children produce /m/ in syllable final position, as in aaam-aaam-aaam, so that both its continuous and its nasal properties are enhanced. This procedure ensures that it is not confused with the /b/, a sound that has neither property in common with it. *Third*, the first and second procedures should be repeated in the context of other vowels. No tension or exaggeration should be allowed to occur in this step if confusion with /b/ is to be avoided, and if the lips are to be closed in a manner consistent with the coarticulated production of each vowel. If there is a tendency to nasalize either the back or the front vowels when the /m/ arrests them, the child should be encouraged to concentrate mainly on their correct (oral) production - if necessary, using a wet finger to feel the oral breath stream they create. *Fourth*, when these steps have been accomplished without introducing plosion into the sequence, or nasality into the vowel (repeat the third step if either does occur), one should introduce sequences of smoothly executed syllables initiated with the /m/, such as maamaamaamaa. Such syllables, either in a sequence or singly, should not cause the child difficulty, because *ma* and *mama* syllables are contained in aaamaaamaaam sequences that have already been practised. When such formal teaching is followed by emphasis on informal strategies, and by the use of words containing /m/ in everyday discourse, the correct and habitual use of /m/ in speech communication should result in a matter of weeks rather than months.

In any of the formal teaching steps described above, it may be helpful for a child to place a finger on his or her lips to feel the vibration caused by the production of the /m/. However, this strategy should be avoided if possible, and rapidly discarded if used, because the objective is to focus the child's awareness on the internal, rather than the external, sensations produced by the sound. If a child requires extra tactile cues to accomplish production of /m/, the placing a finger placed lightly on the lips will yield better tactile sensation than placing them on the nose. The strategy also has the advantage that any inadvertent plosion can be felt on the finger when it is so placed. It can thus readily signal the unwanted production of the /b/. None of the four steps described above can be considered as having been mastered if the fingers continue to be used in any way to obtain tactile cues. Sensations from the mouth, not the hands, provide the type of tactile and kinesthetic feedback the child requires for speech production.

Level 1 function words include those related to personal identification and possession and are therefore very commonly used by children of any age. They include *me, my, I'm*, and *mine. More* and *come* also appear frequently.

Level 2 function words include *much, many, most, may*, and *must.*

Level 3 function words include *might, among, muddy, important, impossible*, and *impolite*. (To use the medial /mp/ blend early on in speech acquisition can be a useful way of developing velo-pharyngeal valving, because the /p/ immediately following the /m/ cannot be produced unless the breath stream is quickly directed towards building up the necessary pressure in the mouth to produce a plosive.) Clearly, the *im* prefix offers plenty of opportunities when working with older children to integrate speech with a minor, but important, aspect of language.

the semi-vowel /w/

The /w/ is a semi-vowel that is used to release or interrupt vowels. In writing, the /w/ occurs at the end of words, such as *now*, but in speech it never arrests other sounds. The /w/ starts near the oo vowel position and moves without pause to the following vowel.

Prerequisites for this sound include the ability to round the lips somewhat more tensely than for the oo and previously mentioned consonants. This is a fairly easy sound for most children to detect and identify through aided hearing, and also through most multi-channel sensory aids. This is because it has only slightly less intensity than the adjacent vowels, and because it also changes in intensity and frequency as it is produced, its F_1 locus is in the low-frequency range, and, as consonants go (and they usually go quickly), it is quite a long sound. It is sometimes confused with /r/ through speechreading because of the tendency towards lip rounding in the production of /r/ with some vowels.

Informal strategies will usually ensure the development of the /w/. There appear to be no involuntary exclamations or utterances that one can use to promote the informal learning of the /w/. However, learned exclamations can be used to emphasize this particular sound. These include *what!* and *wow!*. Animal noises include the *bow-wow* of the toy or real dog. Noises produced by children as they make their toy cars go round corners include woooow and wheee!. Everyday life offers many possible situations for giving the /w/ some emphasis in such injunctions as *wait!*, questions beginning with *what* and *where*, common verbs such as *walk*, *wave*, and *wash*, and frequently encountered nouns, such as *woman*, *water*, and *wind*.

Formal strategies involve the alternation of two vowels while varying their length. Imagine teaching the sound to Sally, a near-totally deaf child who has a single-channel-cochlear implant, and relies heavily on speechreading. *First*, have Sally produce the oo vowel while holding and pressing gently on her left hand. *Second*, have her produce ah while holding and pressing gently on her right hand. *Third*, have her alternate the two vowels several times on one breath, beginning with the oo, while conveying, through hand pressure, that equal length should be given to each. *Fourth*, have Sally again alternate a long series of the two vowels, beginning with oo, but this time convey, by means of similar hand cues, that the oo should be made shorter than the ah. *Fifth*, once Sally is comfortable in making the vowel oo much shorter than the ah, continue the shaping procedure until the oo portion of the series is so short that the /w/ rather than the oo is heard. *Sixth*, repeat the above procedures as necessary using the /w/ to release different vowels. From this point, informal strategies should be followed to emphasize the sound in ways that are meaningful to her in everyday life.

Use of the sound in words appropriate to the children's level of achievement should be sufficient to permit them to use the /w/ to interrupt a vowel sequence (as in *away*). If not, then following the acquisition of the sound in word initial position, it can be developed by alternating the first part of the word with the part of it beginning with the /w/.

Of course, cues on the relative duration of sounds can be provided through vision, rather than through vision and touch as outlined above if the clinician or teacher prefers that. An amusing strategy of this sort is for the teacher or clinician to walk as the child vocalizes, putting a foot down each time the vowel is changed; and next, having the child make one sound long and the other short, so that the adult has to limp in order to keep in time with the child. Getting a child to play this game may require providing him or her with a model - a simple thing to do. The strategies as suggested tend to be compelling, and to achieve their purpose quickly. The use of prompts and cues should, of course, be abandoned as soon as the child has achieved the target pattern, and the sound rehearsed without prompts or cues so that, initially supported by teachers feedback of correctness, the child can come to associate the internal sensations created by the sound with the sound itself. Following such rehearsal, the /w/ can be encouraged by using the following words appropriately in communicative situations that involve utterances of at least sentence length.

Level 1 function words include *one, we, what, was, will, won't, away, where, with, were, awake, well, white, wet,* and *windy.*

Level 2 function words include *why, when, which, well, without, wide, worse, weak, wicked,* and *wonderful.*

Level 3 function words include *weather, while, would, worried, wealthy, worth, worthless,* and *wise* plus words with the er and est endings that can be added to several of the above to form comparatives and superlatives.

The /w/ occurs frequently in blends, such as /tw/ (as in *twice*), /sw/ as in *switch*, and /kw/ as in *quick*. The reader is advised to study the second part of Chapter 14 in relation to the development of blends, and use of words containing blended consonants.

the fricative /h/.

The /h/ is a glottal fricative. It is characterized by a turbulent breath flow known as aspiration. There are several /h/ allophones (forms of /h/), each rather like a forced whisper in the form of the vowel that follows it. Unlike other consonants, the /h/ tends just to release vowels, not to interrupt them (aha! is an exception), and never arrest them. If children can hear, or otherwise perceive vowels produced with a forced whisper, they can be expected to detect and discriminate the /h/. The /h/ cannot be perceived visually because its speechread form is identical to that of the subsequent vowel. Thus, *hair* and *hold* look exactly like *air* and *old* respectively. On this account it may be missed, but it is not, as a rule, visually confused with any other consonant.

Prerequisites for production of the /h/ include being able to bring the vocal cords partly together (adduct them) to produce a forced whisper and, at the same time, shape the vocal tract for the production of the vowel that is to follow the sound.

Informal strategies for learning the /h/ can include imitating and reinforcing an involuntary sigh, or promoting its use in laughter (ha-ha-ha and ho-ho-ho). The words *house* and *home* are frequently used in play, and in real-life situations. The /h/ is also frequently used in the greetings *hi* and *hello*, as well as in commonly asked questions, such as *who, how, how many*, and *how much*. The /h/ abounds in everyday verbs and nouns like *hit, hip, hill, head, hen, hop, heap*, and *hope*. This list is not long enough to provide exhaustive coverage, but it does indicate what an enormous range of sentences can be constructed to enhance the reception and use of this pattern.

Formal strategies, required for children who cannot hear or other-wise detect the /h/, are best initiated *first* with high intensity panting. This strategy, if necessary, permits children to feel the breath stream on the fingers, and is often sufficient to yield an unvoiced hahahaha. If produced in this way, the /h/ can, as a *second* step, be slowed and used to serve as /h/ in the release of a number of different vowels - such as those that occur in the words *who, hi, how*, and *hey*. Such immediate generalization is essential to convey the nature of the /h/ to the child through example rather than explanation. Note that panting can quickly lead to hyperven-tilation (too much oxygen), and thus cause children to become giddy or faint. This strategy should not, therefore, be given more than a brief trial.

A second strategy to teach the /h/ to children who can hear whispered vowels, but who have not acquired the sound spontaneously or through informal strategies, is for the clinician or teacher to employ the following series of steps: *First*, draw a finger lightly down a child's arm from the elbow to the wrist while saying a vowel and using a normal voice. *Second*, have the child imitate the vowel as the finger is, again, lightly traced along the same part of the arm. *Third*, repeat the first two steps, using whispered vowels, while the finger traces a path higher up the arm, from the shoulder to the elbow. When these steps have been mastered, the *fourth* step is for the teacher or clinician to lightly draw a finger down the full length of the child's arm, from the shoulder to the wrist, starting with the production of a whispered vowel, and changing to a normally voiced vowel as the finger reaches the elbow. The *fifth* and final step in the strategy, is to speed up the process. This should (amusingly) result in well produced syllables, such as ha-ha-ha, ho-ho-ho and hee-hee-hee. If either the consonant or the vowel is missing from the syllable, the child can be asked for it, and reminded of it by pointing to the part of the arm associated with either the voiceless or the voiced vowel. The process of associating voicelessness with the upper arm, and voicing with the lower part of the arm, is a useful strategy because it can also be used to differentiate between all the voiced-voiceless pairs of consonants in English.

A third formal strategy, one to use should all else fail, is *first* to have the children blow either on their hands, so that they can feel the breath stream, or on a piece of paper or cotton, so that they can see it move. The noise created by normal blowing is akin to a whispered oo, so *second*, continue by having the children produce a long, whispered oo. Practice of this second step will usually lead to the right amount of glottal involvement - the production of a forced whisper. Once this is accomplished, the *third* step is to have them produce chains of two whispered syllables on the one breath, such as oo-ah-oo-ah-oo-ah. The *fourth* step is then to have the child complete either of the other formal strategies outlined above.

Level 1 function words include *her, he, him, his, hers, has, had, have, who, high, hot, hop,* and *happy.*

Level 2 function words include *whose, hold, hard, heavy, hungry, healthy, half,* and *hear.*

Level 3 function words include *hundreds, hollow, handsome, healthier, healthiest, harmful, harmless, holy, haste,* and *hasty.* There is no shortage of function words beginning with /h/ and the lists here provided can be extended with little effort.

the fricatives /f/ and /v/.

The *prerequisites* for /f/ and /v/ are the abilities to adjust the jaw and retract the lower lip. Other prerequisites are those that pertain to the production of speech patterns developed at earlier stages.

As with other voiced and voiceless fricatives, their crucial feature is the turbulent breath flow that results in high-frequency energy. The /f/ is not, therefore, audible to children with little or no hearing beyond 2000 Hz. Although the /v/ can be detected through audition by most hearing-impaired children on account of its low-frequency voicing, it cannot be identified specifically as a fricative, and may even be confused with nasals by those whose aided hearing does not extend beyond 1000 Hz. Children who can hear part of the fricative turbulence may tend to confuse the /f/ and /v/ with other fricatives. Children who speechread rarely confuse the /f/ and the /v/ with other sounds because they are the only labio-dental sounds in English. However, the two sounds cannot be visually differentiated. The reception of /f/ and /v/ poses similar problems to those for any voiced-voiceless pair of fricatives. The reader is, therefore, referred to discussion of other fricative pairs (see discussion on th in the next section and the notes on the voiced-voiceless distinction in Chapters 2 and 14).

The turbulence of fricatives is stronger in the voiceless member of the pair. As readers may recall, this is because some of the energy contained in the breath stream is diverted to the larynx in the act of voicing. Thus, /f/ can be more easily felt on the fingers than /v/. This fact is important when formal teaching strategies are required to teach these sounds. The turbulence of /f/ is also easier to detect than that of /v/ through single- or through multi-channel cochlear implants and multi-channel tactile devices. For these reasons, and because refinement of the children's skills in the control of breath stream and timing can be promoted by teaching unvoiced fricatives at the same early stage as voiced plosives, teaching the /f/ first may be considered as the preferred procedure. The /v/ may develop with use, and without specific teaching, once the /f/ is acquired because the presence of the extra voicing cue can be readily perceived by most children through aided hearing, or through an alternative sensory device. If not, it may safely be left until the more important manner and place distinctions have been developed.

Fricatives are important, not only in their own right, but also because they provide an essential feature contrast with other manners of production, particularly the nasals. Fricatives cannot be made except with an oral breath stream, and hence their alternation with nasals in chains of syllables, such as fa-ma-fa-ma-fa-ma, and their use at the beginning of words like *thumb* and *muff*, and at the end of words like *mouth* and *knife*, helps to promote children's mastery of velo-pharyngeal valving - directing the breath stream through either the mouth or the nose, which is the basic mechanism underlying the distinction between nasal and non-nasal sounds.

Informal strategies for developing the /f/ must be drawn mainly from play and everyday interactions, because there are few occasions when the sound is produced involuntarily by either adults or children. Sometimes a prolonged fffffffffff is repeatedly produced as one releases breath after intense exertion, and because of this we find the words *huff* and *puff* in our language. These same words can be introduced in stories, such as "The Three Little Pigs", and the sound is used extensively in "Jack the Giant Killer" by the Giant who says *fee-fie-foe-fum* as he looks for Jack. It can be emphasized through *finger* play, and play with toy animals or pets (the dog says *woof*). It can also be introduced in other activities, such as making a tower of blocks *fall* down, and in commentaries about things that are *full* as compared with empty in real-life situations.

Formal strategies for developing the /f/ are usually required for children who have aided hearing that does not extend into the high frequencies. To avoid it being produced with plosion, it should initially be developed from syllable-final or word-final position. Hearing-impaired children who cannot develop it simply through aided hearing, or through the use of sensory aids, must use more than one sense to achieve this target pattern; vision, to see how the speech organs (the teeth and the lips) are placed, and touch, to feel the breath stream. There is a danger that the lower lip will be folded under the top teeth in a grossly exaggerated manner if children are too often asked to make the /f/ or /v/ in isolation. Such exaggeration impedes the acquisition and use of the sound with accuracy, speed, economy of effort, and flexibility in spoken language. It also tends to encourage the (faulty) release of /f/ as a plosive. To prevent such faults, it is important to ensure that the child is provided with a correct model from the outset - one in which the lower lip is not retracted. If this fault has already been allowed to develop, one can apply a simple remedial strategy, such as having the child place a finger lightly over the bottom lip to ensure its correct position, but the following visual-tactile strategy, to be used with a profoundly hearing-impaired child called Mary-Lou, can be used both in developing or correcting the /f/ without introducing the risk of intrusive plosion - providing that each step is achieved and practised without exaggeration.

First, ask Mary-Lou to wet a finger and then, holding that finger close to your mouth in such a way that she can both see your mouth and feel your breath stream, say off-off-off. Second, ask her to hold her wetted finger in front of her own mouth and do the same thing. If all the previously described target patterns have been developed as recommended, this simple strategy should immediately result in her production of the word-final /f/. Third, generalize the use of the sound in word-final position with other vowels, as in if-if-if and oof-oof-oof. Fourth, have Mary-Lou rehearse the /f/ in chains of syllables initiated with the /f/ sound. This step is best begun with the oo vowel (foo-foo-foo-foo) because, with the lips rounded, there is less chance of intrusive plosion occurring. If plosion does occur, have her alternate steps three and four and, at the same time, ensure that she introduces no undue tension, or any other form of exaggeration. From this point, informal learning and phonologic use should be promoted.

The /v/ is the voiced counterpart of the /f/. Once the /f/ has been developed, one often finds that the /v/ is spontaneously produced. The voicing component of the /v/ is not as important as its fricative component, so it is not a crucial matter if the /v/ is produced as an /f/ or an /f/ is produced as a /v/ until further consonants differing in manner and place features have been acquired. In everyday speech, the word-initial /f/ occurs more frequently than the word-final /f/. The reverse is true of the /v/.

Level 1 function words containing the /f/ target include off, fast, funny, fall, fat, and full. Those containing the /v/ target include I've, of, very, over, love, and lovely.

Level 2 function words containing the /f/ target include if, often, after, front (as in "in front of"), for, from, first, fine, frighten, and afraid. Those containing the /v/ target include every, everybody, everywhere, live, alive, and living.

Level 3 function words containing the /f/ include fewer, and fewest, as well as other comparatives and superlatives. They also include false, *relief, failure, fair, fond, foolish,* and *famous.* Those containing the /v/ target include *lively, valid, invalid, vacant, verbose, vocal,* and *review.*

the voiced and unvoiced th

The *prerequisites* for this sound are the same as for previously presented consonants. Acquired skills must include ability to the place the tip of the tongue between the teeth.

The unvoiced th (as in *think*) consists of a wide band of low intensity, high frequency energy that extends from about 3,000 to about 15,000 Hz. The voiced th (as in *the*) has a similar range of high frequency energy but, in addition, has a low-frequency voicing component. Children with aided hearing levels of better than 30 dB that extend beyond 3,000 Hz should, therefore, be able to detect some of the high frequency components of the sound, as should those who have cochlear implants or multi-channel tactile devices. The sound is very similar to other fricatives. Such children may not, therefore, be able to discriminate between this and any other pair of fricatives without speechreading. (In communicative speech, of course, context may provide sufficient cues to permit identification without discrimination.) Children with aided hearing that does not extend beyond 1,000 Hz will be able to detect only the voiced component. The voiced and the unvoiced th are readily confused by speechreaders, but the two sounds are visually distinct from all others. Under auditory-visual conditions, therefore, both of these sounds can be correctly identified and produced once the presence of a fricative component is known. Children with aided hearing that does not extend beyond 1,000 Hz may discriminate between them on the following basis:

th tongue position plus low-frequency energy = voiced th;

th tongue position and silence = unvoiced th.

This sort of discrimination may be helpful in speech reception, but the child's knowledge of language and familiarity with words that contain the th sounds are essential to it.

Children who cannot detect high frequency energy do not spontaneously acquire the correct pronunciation of the th sounds. While the inter-dental tongue position is evident to them, the fricative turbulence is not. Because they can see the tongue position, but not hear the full range of the sound, they tend to substitute a plosive. Such a fault should not be allowed to become habitual, because the unvoiced th provides an important base for the development of other fricatives, and the voiced th is one of the most frequently used consonants in English.

Normally hearing children often substitute the /d/ for the voiced th during their early years, and such substitution should be accepted when it is produced by young hearing-impaired children, providing that speech acquisition is otherwise proceeding normally, and other fricatives are being produced. However, should the /d/ substitution persists over several months, particularly among those who have needed some formal teaching at earlier stages, acceptable production of both the th sounds and other fricatives may have to be promoted through the use of further formal strategies.

Informal strategies for developing the th sounds involve only the use of words in which they appear, either during play, or in other real-life situations. The sounds rarely, if ever, appear in involuntary vocalization. Great care must be taken to ensure that the tongue-tip protrusion is not exaggerated when encouraging a child to produce the sound, which appears in words, such as *mouth, tooth, thumb, think, thank,* and *therapy,* and in the function words listed below.

Formal strategies should initially be aimed at the development of the unvoiced th, so that the association of fricative turbulence with the inter-dental tongue position is established, and so that the unvoiced th is available as a reference for generalization to the voiced th, and for the development of other fricatives. The voiced th should develop with little or no teaching once its unvoiced counterpart has been acquired, because the additional presence of voicing should be detectable through aided hearing or any of the alternative sensory aids, and because voicing will tend to be assimilated into the sound through its frequent use in spoken language. Prepositional phrases, such as *on the door, in the bath* and *over the wall* spoken with an appropriate rhythm usually ensure th becomes voiced in such contexts.

Let us now see how the th sound can be taught to Joe, a child with no residual hearing, by means of a formal strategy involving vision and touch. *First,* take Joe's wetted finger and, holding it near your mouth, say a vowel followed by the unvoiced th as in *ooth* or *uth.* This permits the child to see the tongue position, as well as to detect both the cessation of voicing and the continuation of the breath stream as the th is produced. (The oo vowel tends to facilitate the production of the unvoiced th because the breath stream is more concentrated for this vowel than for others. It thus enhances the child's awareness of breath flow. The th is placed at the end of the syllable so that its continuant properties are enhanced, and the risk of it being confused with a plosive is reduced.) *Second*, have Joe imitate the sound while holding his finger in front of his own mouth. As he does this, ensure that there is no exaggeration in the placement of the tongue tip. (If this is not successful, elicit the unvoiced th in isolation as in the steps above, and then repeat these steps with the vowel preceding the target sound.) *Third*, have him repeat chains of several syllables or words ending in the unvoiced th, such as *tooth tooth tooth* or *teeth teeth teeth*, on one breath. (Ensure that the required fricative turbulence is produced on each trial.) *Fourth* repeat the third step using a variety of vowels. *Fifth*, focus on Joe's reception and production of words containing th in running speech, constantly noting whether some (but not excessive) fricative turbulence is present when he uses the sound. If it is not, put aside some time for more practice on the steps described above.

Level 1 function words that are said with the unvoiced th include *thanks, thin, thick, throw, threw, three*, and *thirsty*. Those said with the voiced th include *the, this, that, there, they*, and *with*. The frequency of occurrence of these words is exceptionally high.

Level 2 function words with unvoiced th include *thank, through, think, third*, and *thirty*. Those with the voiced th include *these, those, them, their, theirs, than, other*, and *bother*.

Level 3 function words with the unvoiced th include *thaw, thread, thunder*, and *thump*. Those with the voiced th include *either, wither, therefore*, and *thus*.

the liquid /l/.

The /l/ is classified as a lateral sound as well as a liquid because, in making the sound, the airflow from the lungs is directed around the sides of the tongue rather than over the top of it.

The *prerequisites* for production of the /l/ are the narrowing and raising of the tongue, and these movements are present in chewing, as well as in the production of the vowels and consonants that are previously discussed. The tongue is narrower in the production of back vowels than in other vowels, so the required airflow round the tongue tends to be facilitated in the context of oo and aw vowels. Exaggeration that leads to protrusion of the tongue used to be encouraged by some teachers who developed the /l/ through visual teaching strategies, but such exaggeration is not only detrimental to its reception and production in everyday speech; it is also absolutely unnecessary when speechreading is supported by the use of appropriate sensory aids.

The /l/ is a mid-frequency sound that is voiced except in blends, such as /pl/, /sl/, and /fl/ that are initiated with unvoiced consonants. In such contexts its voicelessness is due to assimilation - the effect that one consonant has on another when they are coarticulated. The /l/ can be detected by children whose aided hearing does not extend beyond 1,000 Hz, and by children who wear any type of cochlear implant or tactile device. However, aided hearing beyond 2,000 Hz, or the use of a multi-channel cochlear implant or multi-channel tactile device, increases the chances of the discrimination and identification of /l/. It can be confused with other alveolar consonants, such as /d/, /t/, /n/, and /s/ through speechreading, but if a child's speechreading is supplemented by an appropriate sensory aid, such confusions can be avoided.

 Informal strategies that promote learning of the /l/ include singing a tune to the syllable /la/ rather than to words, and using the sound in play with toy animals, such as a *lion* and a *lamb*. It can also be used as one names parts of the body in the course of bathing - the *leg*, the *lips*, the *little* finger or *little* toe - or in commands to children, such as *Tell me*, *Pull the* —, *Smell the* —, *Roll the ball*, *Tell*—, *Listen to*—, *Look at*—, and *Help me* —. One of the most frequent words used with children is *love*. The /l/ should also be used as frequently as possible in function words (see below).

 Formal strategies focus primarily on direct touch. One time-honored technique is to smear honey just behind a child's upper teeth, on the alveolar ridge, and have them lick it off with the tongue tip while vocalizing. Another is to have a child place the tip of a finger on the teacher's alveolar ridge to feel her tongue tip moving up and down as she says a series of syllables, such as looloolooloo, and then to have the child repeat the procedure using another finger tip to feel his or her own tongue doing the same thing. A further strategy is to have the children vocalize as they touch the alveolar ridge with the tip of the tongue and the tip of the little finger, and then say oo as they take the finger away.

 Once the /l/ has been evoked by any of these strategies it should be repeated in chains of syllables without any extraneous tactile cues of the types mentioned above, first in the context of back vowels, as in *lawlawlaw*, next with central vowels, as in *lalala*, and finally in the context of front vowels. The medial /l/, as in the word *allow*, will automatically be developed through the repetition of several syllables on one breath, and the alternation of several syllables containing different vowels, such as *low-lea-low-lea*. The word initial /l/ should be encouraged in words, such as *like, love, leaf, light,* and *lemon,* and in discourse, as soon as the sound has been evoked.

Once the word-initial /l/ has been rehearsed, the word-final, or dark /l/, should be developed. The series of steps suggested will be illustrated in teaching Sharon, a girl with useful hearing up to 1500 Hz. *First,* have her say a vowel of several seconds duration, while you move your finger in a straight line in front of her to indicate how long the sound should be. *Second,* have her interrupt a vowel of the same length with the /l/ each time you raise your finger and return to the vowel as you drop your finger to continue its original path. *Third,* Repeat the procedure, but stop at the end of each syllable as the /l/ is produced. *Fourth,* use the final /l/ in words, such as *ball, tall, fall, bell, well* and *bowl.* Finally, encourage the use of all words containing /l/ (except, possibly some blends) in speech communication.

Level 1 function words include *little, low, loud, long, ill,* and *I'll.*

Level 2 function words include *like, along, only, else, last, lazy, late, light, large, loose, cool, lucky,* and *early.*

Level 3 function words include *later, less, least, alone, likely,* and the host of adverbs that end in *ly.* Adjectives that end in *al,* such as *critical* or *crucial,* and those that end in *ful,* such as *thoughtful* and *beautiful,* also provide opportunities to relate speech and language learning.

application of strategies

The informal strategies described above should result in the production of the target sound in words in a matter of weeks, providing that all the prerequisites for the production of the pattern are present. The application of informal strategies is rarely complete, however, because once the sound is produced it must continually be integrated (with appropriate suprasegmental patterns and vowels) into new words, and into everyday discourse. At the same time that new words containing a given target are being acquired, new targets are being mastered and, as their integration into words proceeds, one must ensure that the contrasts and similarities between the various speech sounds become evident to the children. The process of acquisition is complete only when a child's spoken language is free from inappropriately produced sounds, and is completely intelligible.

Formal strategies, when applied with children who have the prerequisite skills can (and should) evoke a sound within minutes or less. However, it must constantly be borne in mind that to elicit a sound is but to begin the process of development. Sound patterns may be considered as acquired only when they are used in fluent and meaningful discourse.

suggestions for further reading

The books dealing most specifically with the types of formal teaching described in this chapter include those by Calvert and Silverman (1983), and Ling (1976). More suggestions on words and sentences that can be used for the rehearsal of various plosives and fricatives are provided in a series of books designed for use with adolescents by Subtelny and Lieberth (1985). See References, pp. 433 ff.

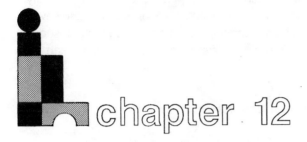

development of
place distinctions (1):
the alveolar consonants

place of consonant production

The term *place of consonant production* refers to the location of
the speech organs as they create a particular sound in the stream of
speech. Thus /p/, a phoneme made with the lips, is regarded as a front
consonant. The /k/, a phoneme made with the back of the tongue
touching the velum, is regarded as a back consonant. The /t/ is made
with the blade of the tongue touching the alveolar ridge, and occupies a
position midway between the /p/ and the /k/. The differences between
consonants made in the back, middle, or front of the vocal tract (place
distinctions) strongly influence intelligibility, and thus are among the most
important in the production and the perception of speech (see Chapters
2 and 3).

The position that the speech organs occupy when a sound is
produced has a marked influence on its frequency. It also affects the
frequency of adjacent vowels and consonants. Just as the space left in

339

a bottle resonates at a higher and higher frequency as it fills up drip by drip, so do the spaces in the mouth resonate according to their shape and size. (Say the sh and the /s/ without pausing between them, for example, and note how much higher the frequency becomes as the tongue moves forward in the mouth for the /s/.) Under reasonably good visual conditions, speechreading usually permits children to identify place of production of consonants with high levels of accuracy. However, identification of place of consonant production through other sense modalities requires that frequency differences (spectral cues) can be perceived.

perception of place distinctions

Auditory perception of the spectral cues on place of consonant production requires high-frequency hearing. Children with residual hearing that does not extend up to or beyond 1500 Hz are able to make few, if any, place distinctions through audition. Auditory discrimination of cues on place of consonant production improves as hearing extends upwards within the frequency range 1500 to 4000 Hz (see Figure 12-1). Cues on place of consonant production occur at relatively low intensity levels. They are, therefore, easily masked by noise. Such masking can be exacerbated by too much low-frequency amplification. Additionally, acoustic cues on place of production are brief, and are mainly contained in the transitional energy created as one sound moves to another. Children with insufficient aided hearing for frequencies higher than about 1500 Hz cannot, therefore, acquire the ability to perceive or make place distinctions unless they use both hearing and vision (see Chapter 5). Single channel tactile aids may, through frequency transposition, make some high sounds tangible, and single-channel implants may make them detectable, but neither type of device will permit reliable discrimination between consonants that vary in place. Successfully fitted multi-channel cochlear implants, and well-adjusted multi-channel tactile devices are, however, both capable of providing coded information on frequency that may permit moderately good place identification.

How place distinctions are best perceived will largely determine what types of strategies are best used to develop them. Informal strategies in the acquisition of place distinctions can be only as effective as the transmission of information permits. When no hearing is present beyond 1000 Hz, auditory-visual or instrument-visual strategies will succeed where the use of a single modality may fail. Formal strategies that involve both touch and vision are traditional, but effective. The basis of effective perceptual-oral skills is the optimal use of a child's sense modalities in both the reception and production of speech. What is effective for one child, may not be for another; and a given sense modality that may best help a hearing-impaired child acquire certain speech patterns, may help little in his or her acquisition of others. For this reason,

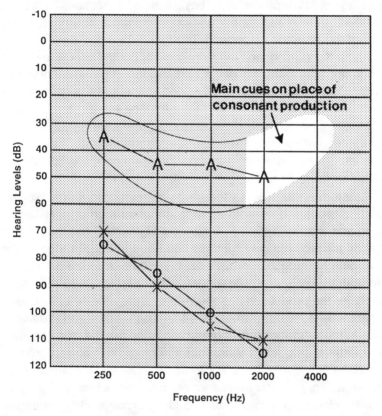

Frequency (Hz)

figure 12-1. An audiogram showing the frequency band within the CLEAR zone in which the main cues on place of consonant production occur in conversational level speech from a distance of two yards, and the unaided and aided thresholds of Jim, a profoundly hearing-impaired child who through aided audition alone, could discriminate between some consonants differing only in place. Most severely hearing-impaired children (those with less restricted aided audition in the high-frequency range) can be expected to perceive most place distinctions through the use of hearing under good acoustic conditions.

various strategies involving the different sense modalities are presented in the following discussion of consonants in relation to their place of production.

In this, and in the next chapter, the voiced-voiceless distinction that differentiates members of a cognate pair (a pair that shares the same manner and place), such as /d/ and /t/, or /s/ and /z/, are not specifically considered. Discussion of these distinctions are treated in Chapter 14. At this stage of development, when basic manner distinctions have been established, speech intelligibility and communication are more readily enhanced by mastery of place distinctions. Voicing distinctions are largely based on timing, and the refinement of control over voice onset and duration can often be developed incidentally in the course of acquiring the place distinctions. If a voiced member of a cognate pair is produced instead of the unvoiced target (or vice-versa), then it should be accepted as a distinctly different sound, positively reinforced, and nurtured into habitually correct use in spoken language. The child's production of the original target sound should, nevertheless, continue to be an immediate goal.

Most formal strategies for teaching place distinctions in consonant production are based on vision and touch rather than on audition, or audition and vision. This is, of course, to be expected, because formal strategies are required only if a child has failed to acquire a particular speech pattern through informal learning. However, formal visual and tactile strategies provide a child with very little direct feedback of the type required for the production of speech in everyday life. It is, therefore, important when formal strategies have been used to elicit and to develop sounds, to follow up such procedures by ensuring that the child becomes familiar with the articulatory sensations associated with correct produc-tion, and that these sensations are, as far as possible, supplemented by whatever auditory, auditory-visual, or other form of sensory aided per-ception the child can use in everyday life. Once formal teaching strategies have been used to elicit given sound patterns, it can be helpful to employ some of the informal learning strategies suggested, in order to promote their further development.

anticipatory set

Concepts underlying set were extensively explored in Chapter 8. Nevertheless, some more examples of set will be provided here, because set is a particularly important tool in the production of place distinctions. The essence of set is expectation arising from a given context. Contextual cues exist at all levels of language use. In normal conversation, the first few words will provide expectation that a certain range of words and sentences will occur as the utterance proceeds. When the expectation proves to be correct, listeners know that they have, in fact, inferred what was likely to be said from what had already been expressed. Being able to predict through inference is very helpful in listening under poor acoustic conditions. Skilled teachers include the provision of set in order to stimulate learning in every subject they present.

When, in teaching, one deliberately employs a selected context to increase the chances of obtaining a desired response, one is creating a set. If this strategy is to be successful, the teacher must, in some way, imply what is required so strongly that the listener cannot help but infer the nature of the correct response. By first evoking sounds that are made at or near the front of the mouth, such as /p/, and then relating them to the teaching of sounds that have the same manner of production that are made further and further back in the mouth, such as /t/ and /k/, one can exploit the compelling force that anticipatory set provides. Using the symbol → to mean "provides a set for," a few examples of set within different manners of production are shown in the sequences that follow. More examples will be provided as particular sounds are discussed.

Plosives:　voice + /b/ → /d/; and /b/ + /d/ → /g/.
　　　　　　no voice + /p/ → /t/; and /p/ + /t/ → /k/.
Nasals:　　voice + /m/ → /n/; and /m/ + /n/ → ng.
Fricatives: no voice + th → /s/; and th + /s/ → sh.
Laterals:　voice + /l/ → /r/.

Using the ng as a target among the nasals as an example, the child is first asked to produce the /m/ (behavior A), then the /n/ (behavior B), and finally to produce an /n/-like sound with the tongue tip held down. The result is ng the (the target behavior C). Because both behaviors A and B had an increasing number of features in common with the target behavior (voicing + nasality for /m/, then voicing + nasality + tongue contact for /n/), the type of sound that the child expected to make had to include at least these features. The only sound that could satisfy the conditions was the ng. The use of set makes more demands on teachers and clinicians than on children, since it is the professionals who have to organize and obtain the sequences of behaviors that will almost inevitably lead to the required outcome. When a child does not succeed on a particular trial, it is highly likely that the adult has failed in some way to provide an adequate set. Sequences will be suggested that usually provide a sufficiently strong set for all sounds discussed in the following sections. When the sets suggested do not work (and on rare occasions they may fail) a more extended set (perhaps behaviors A + B + C + D → target) may have to be introduced.

the plosives /d/ and /t/

The *prerequisites* for /d/ and /t/ are the ability to produce /b/ and /p/, and the ability to raise the blade of the tongue to the alveolar ridge - as many people do when sucking through a straw.

There are many different ways that /d/ and /t/ can be produced in English. They can release a vowel, as in /ta/, in which case the plosive burst will be at its strongest, and they can release another consonant such as /r/, in which case the plosive burst is directed around the tongue, so that it gives a fricative quality to the two consonants (see Chapter 14). They can also serve to stop a vowel without a release, as at the end of the first words in the utterances *bad boy* and *at work*, and to stop a vowel in the middle of words, like *kitten* and *middle*, depending on how one prefers to pronounce them. With front vowels, the tongue tip may touch the teeth, but with back vowels it is unlikely to do so. If children tend to make the sounds too far forward in the mouth, the habit can be changed by having them rapidly rehearse the sounds with back vowels; if too far back, one can adopt the reverse procedure. Adults concerned with a child's speech must develop and maintain critical listening skills to determine when such forms of intervention are needed.

Audition is the most appropriate sense modality to use when a child's residual hearing extends beyond 3000 Hz, because both the F_2 transitions and the plosive bursts occur in the frequency range 2000 Hz plus or minus a half-octave (see Figure 3-7). If audition does not extend beyond 1500 Hz, the plosive or stop quality can usually be detected as a suddenly occurring release of (or gaps in) energy; but the sounds themselves, without speechreading, cannot be identified through such low-frequency residual hearing. Some children wearing multi-channel cochlear implants or tactile devices can discriminate between the /d/ and the /b/, and the /p/ and the /t/, but single-channel devices of either type are unlikely to permit such discrimination without speechreading.

Informal strategies include development of the /d/ through the adult's imitation of the baby's reflex babble. In the later part of the first year, /adadada/ is a common form of babble, particularly as children cut their front teeth. These speech patterns can also be developed informally through using the sounds in play (for example, /didididi/ as the sound of a boat being pushed around in the bath), and naming people in the family (for example, *dada* or *daddy*). The sounds can also be emphasized by using them in rhymes that exist, or that one creates, such as *tick-tock says the clock, Humpty-Dumpty, Hey diddle diddle*, and *Peter, Peter, Pumpkin Eater*, and in common expressions in everyday life, such as *"Don't touch!," "Put it down!," "tip it out!," "Let's wash your toes,"* and *"Oh dear!."* These sounds occur very frequently in everyday language (see Chapter 6).

Formal strategies used to develop these sounds are most effective when they include the use of set. The /d/ is easier than /t/ for most children to master, because the voicing provides a strong cue on its manner of production. Begin by having the child voice a long ah vowel to establish voicing, then have him or her say /babababababa/ to establish the notion of periodic interruption of the vowel. Finally, follow this immediately with /dadadada/. If this strategy does not work, have the child repeat the procedure with the tongue tip just visible between the lips. Readers who find this suggestion surprising, are reminded that an interdental /d/ does exist in English. It is produced in words beginning with /d/ that follow a th. The adjoining words *with Dad*, and *worth doing*, provide examples. When this strategy is successful, repeat the procedures yet again, but with the child's tongue tip behind the teeth, and in the context of the vowel ee, as in /didididi/. Then have the child attempt it while smiling all the time. This procedure accentuates the tactile and kinesthetic sensations associated with tongue tip involvement. It is almost impossible not to produce a /d/ with this strategy. Using the ee vowel and a smile also prevents excessive jaw movement, a fault that can result if extensive unsupervised practice of the sound is permitted in the context of ah vowels.

As with most sounds, the /d/ and /t/ should be taught in the context of a string of syllables to ensure that they are carried by an appropriate breath stream. If there is any tendency towards excessive jaw movement in making these sounds, call attention to it in a positive way, and prevent it by having the child hold a pencil or similar object lightly between the teeth when saying various vowels released with /d/. If the pencil falls, then more than the necessary amount of jaw opening is being used to assist the tongue in stopping the breath flow. Keeping the pencil in place for the duration of a series of syllables, such as /dadadada/, will quite adequately provide a child with the concept that, in making the /d/ and /t/, it is primarily tongue movement, not jaw movement, that creates these sounds. This concept is particularly helpful in the formal teaching of the /k/ at a later stage.

Another formal strategy is to have the child place a finger tip between the teeth, and press against it each time the /d/ occurs in a string of /didididi/ syllables. Once the /d/ can be produced with ease in a string of syllables of this sort, the unreleased (syllable-final or word-final) /d/ pattern can be established by asking the child to release the syllables as the teacher or clinician drops a finger (much as a conductor gives the beat to the orchestra). Asking the child to release the syllable in such a procedure will result in the production of *did, did, did*, rather than /didididi/, and rehearsal of this and other words will soon enable the child to use the unreleased /d/ in saying sentences, such as *I'd like one* and *I want that ball*, with the natural rhythm unbroken by intrusive voicing.

The formal teaching of /t/ can similarly be based on the prior production of /p/. However, as mentioned above, it is not as important to teach /t-d/ discriminations through formal work at an early stage as it is to develop other place of production contrasts (below). Children who have appropriate hearing aids, and useful hearing beyond 2000 Hz, and those with other multi-channel sensory aids, should be able to differentiate between /d/ and /t/ once the /d/ has been formally taught, providing that they then have sufficient experience of spoken language.

Level 1 function words containing /d/ include *down, do, don't, under, dry, dirty*, and *different*. Those containing the /t/ include *top, to, tidy, tired*, and *tall*. *Short, it, out, at*, and *hot* are all examples of words in which the final consonant may be unreleased.

Level 2 function words with /d/ include *does, doesn't, dark*, and *deaf*. Those containing the /t/ include *to, too, tight, tiptoe*, and *terrible*. Both the /d/ and the /t/ are met in their released and unreleased forms very frequently, of course, in the past tense of all regular verbs.

Level 3 function words containing /d/ include *dear* and *difficult*, as well as all words with the prefixes *dis* and *de*. Those containing /t/ include *until, towards, tough*, and *tender*.

the nasal /n/

The /n/ in vowel contexts is made by directing the breath through the nose and vocalizing while the blade of the tongue is resting on the alveolar ridge. If one breathes in and out through the nose with the mouth open, the tongue is quite likely be in position for the production of an /n/. As with most consonants, the tongue position for /n/ varies according to what sounds precede and follow it. The most extreme forward position for this sound in running speech is with the tongue tip between the teeth - a position that is quite common when the /n/ is followed by the th, as in the prepositional phrases *in the bath* and *on the wall*. If hearing-impaired children do not acquire an interdental /n/, or do not learn to slide the tongue forward in preparation for the th as an /n/ is being produced, intrusive voicing is likely to occur, so that *on the path* is then said as *on a the path*.

The *prerequisites* for making the /n/ include those for making the /m/, and ability to raise the blade of the tongue to the alveolar ridge. The prerequisites for using it linguistically include being able to open the velopharyngeal port in time to make the sound and to close it immediately before moving on to a vowel or oral consonant. This skill prevents the production of nasal sounding utterances. The proper timing of such velopharyngeal valving is essential to the production of clear speech.

The /n/ occurs in all positions in words, and it can become a syllable in its own right in words like *mitten* when the /t/ in unreleased. The /n/, in common with other nasals, has a major formant (the nasal murmur) around 300 Hz, and this differentiates it from all other consonants except the other nasals (the /m/ and ng). It can be identified through audition by most of those with hearing up to and beyond 3000 Hz in many speech contexts, providing they have hearing aids that provide sufficient amplification above 2000 Hz, and by many with multi-channel tactile devices or multi-channel cochlear implants. The sound can be differentiated from other nasals through speechreading, but not reliably so through single-channel sensory aids, or through a limited range of low-frequency hearing.

Informal learning strategies include developing the /n/ from its involuntary use in either laughing or crying. The quiet type of laughter that is accompanied by a smile is often just an /n/. Similarly, the quiet type of crying that is interrupted with a sniff, and is accompanied by a facial grimace often results in an /n/. (A sniff can only be produced when the lips are parted, if the tongue is in contact at some point along the palate.) Encouraging the child to act these behaviors will often result in the production of the sound. Once made, the /n/ should be practised, and later be carried over into speech contexts. The sound can often be associated with the noise made by toy motor cycles, airplanes, or tractors. It is also the sort of noise that can be used to describe the sound created by a kitchen appliance.

Many of the words used in everyday communication can be used to focus on the /n/ sound. These include *no, now, want, can*, and *when* (as in the questions *Can I?* and *When can I?*). Like most other alveolar sounds, /n/ is very common in English (see key vocabulary, below).

Formal teaching of /n/ is required only by those who need visual cues to help them differentiate this sound from other nasals, and by those who confuse it with the high back and high front vowels (oo and ee) - those that, in most talkers' speech, also have low-frequency energy around 300 Hz. Maximum acoustic contrast between the /n/ and the vowels is provided by formally teaching it in the context of a central vowel, such as the ah. These, however, are the vowels associated with the greatest amount of jaw opening, and unless one moves quickly to elicit the sound in other vowel contexts, exaggeration is likely to be encouraged. In developing this sound, care should be taken to ensure that the jaw does not assist in making tongue contact with the alveolar ridge: the jaw should not move during the production of a group of repeated syllables. Formal teaching strategies should at least ensure the child's perception of the low-frequency nasal murmur through aided audition, or some other form of sensory aiding. When the higher frequency components of the sound cannot be perceived through input from a hearing aid, cochlear implant, or tactile device, formal teaching should also include identification of the sound through the use of speechreading as a supplement.

Set can be provided by relating the target to the previously acquired /m/. *First*, produce a long /m/ and have the child imitate it. *Second*, start making the long /m/, and then, with the child watching, part the lips in a smile. This usually results in the production of /n/. If it does not, then show the child where to place the tip of the tongue (just behind the upper teeth), and repeat the steps outlined above, allowing the child to feel the tongue tip with the finger between the teeth if necessary. (This strategy not only helps tongue placement, but indicates that there is no oral breath stream.) At most only a few tries are usually required to produce the /n/ in this way.

Another effective alternative strategy for producing the /n/ also involves using the /m/ to provide a set. *First*, obtain the /m/ to establish a set for continuity of voicing and nasality; *second*, have the child repeat the /m/, this time with the tongue tip just visible between the lips; *third*, repeat the procedure and have the child smile. This strategy results in the interdental /n/ that often precedes the th (see above). To have the child produce the lingua- alveolar /n/, the *fourth* move is to have the child slide the tongue back over the top teeth. Each of these steps can usually be achieved through visual imitation.

Ensuring maximal feedback on production of this (or any other) sound through other senses should be emphasized following the use of such strongly visual strategies. Once children have made the /n/ through reference to the /m/ several times, they can be asked to terminate each trial with the word *no*, smoothly saying mmm-nn-no. One should immediately encourage them to play with the sound by asking questions that require the answer "no". This can be great fun if the questions are sufficiently ridiculous, like "Are you an elephant?" or (to a girl) "Are you a little boy?", and so on. The giggling that occurs with such an approach can be helpful in establishing production of the sound in a relaxed manner. Once children have mastered this step, the sound should be rehearsed in syllable-final and word-final positions with all vowels. If sufficient time has not been given to the acquisition of the /n/ following vowels, it may be produced partly or entirely as a plosive - as /nd/ or just /d/ - particularly in an initial (vowel-releasing) position. The substitution of the /d/ for the /n/ is extremely widespread among those who have acquired their speech principally through vision. This includes children with useful residual hearing whose hearing aids have not provided sufficient amplification in the frequency band centered on 250 Hz (see Chapters 3 and 4). Phonetic level practice, first with the /n/ in word-final position, and later with the /n/ in word-initial position with all vowels, is usually required to overcome habitual faults involving intrusive plosion.

Level 1 function words include *no, not, and, on, in, under, now, naughty, nice, noisy, funny,* and *one.* The conjunction *and* is often produced simply as /n/ in phrases such as *bread 'n butter, fish 'n chips,* and *young 'n pretty.*

Level 2 function words include an, any, nothing, another, not many, not much, near, nobody, never, any, anybody, enough, narrow, nasty, neat, and only.

Level 3 function words include until, nearly, anywhere, need, instead, neither, one another, honest, interesting, and industrious. There are many other function-type applications of /n/, as in adding negation to a verb (for example, wasn't, didn't, and couldn't), and in prefixes, such as in and un (for example, insufficient and unfortunate). The /n/ also occurs frequently (and can, therefore, be practised) in the ion ending of nouns formed from verb roots, such as attention, concentration, and interruption.

the fricatives /s/ and /z/.

The prerequisites for successful production of the /s/ and /z/ are a good oral breath stream, fine control over the duration of voicing, and ability to adjust the tongue rapidly, and in such a way that a groove is created down its center towards its tip. An important, and often over-looked prerequisite is that the child should have a concept of fricative production gained from using other fricatives that require less precise control of the speech organs, such as the /f/ and /v/, and the voiced and unvoiced th.

The /s/ and /z/ are among the most frequently used sounds in English. Even so, the /s/ is more frequently written than spoken, for in words like is and has, the /s/ is pronounced as a /z/. However, when the /z/ is written, it is never pronounced as an /s/. These two sounds carry an enormous morphemic load in English. They signal plurals (cups, horses), possessives (Bob's bike, Tom's shoe), third person (he runs, she walks), auxiliaries (He's walking), and many other features in the language. They also occur frequently in blends. Their acquisition at a reasonably early age does much to enhance the quality of a young child's speech, but many normally hearing children are not able to produce them in all contexts even by age five or six.

Mastery of these sounds, particularly the /s/, may be elusive even for young normally hearing children, because many, while substituting it for the sh (so that words like ship and shoe become sip and soo), are unable at this stage to pronounce it in words like some and sit. Substitutions of the plosives /t/ and /d/ are common in the speech of hearing-impaired children, whereas the lisp that often occurs as a substitute for the /s/ before normally hearing children have mastered the sound, is rarely observed in the speech of hearing-impaired children. The reason for the predominance of plosive substitutions for /s/ among hearing-impaired children (e.g., *he ted* instead of *he said*) appears to be that they have either not developed a sufficiently strong oral breath stream, or have not acquired adequate concepts of frication. Thus even the sounds, such as /f/ and /v/, as well as voiced and unvoiced th, may be produced with some plosion. Attempts to develop /s/ and /z/ before automaticity has been achieved in the use of other fricatives is not recommended.

The /s/ and /z/ not only require finer motor control than any other sound for their correct production, but their acoustic characteristics are such that they are among the most difficult sounds for hearing-impaired children to perceive. For these reasons, these sounds are usually the first to become distorted in the speech of individuals who suffer severe hearing loss after having acquired spoken language. The fricative turbulence of these sounds creates a hissing noise that spreads across the frequency range from about 3,500 Hz to well over 15,000 Hz, depending on vowel context. The /z/ differs from the /s/ in three ways; it is voiced, and thus contains a range of harmonics (see Chapter 2), it has less intense turbulence (because the breath stream is impeded by voicing), and it tends to be somewhat shorter than the /s/. Whether the /s/ or the /z/ is heard in normal running speech may depend less on whether the sound is voiced or unvoiced than on the relative durations of the /s/ and the preceding phoneme (see Chapter 14).

The high-frequency components of the /s/ and /z/ can be detected through audition only by those whose range of hearing extends well beyond 3,000 Hz, and whose unaided hearing levels at and above this frequency are not in excess of 85 dB. Sufficient amplification to render these components detectable to severely hearing-impaired children requires the combination of well-selected hearing aids, and suitably flared earmolds (see Chapter 4). If these acoustic components are not detectable by those with low-frequency residual hearing, then silence will take the place of the /s/, and they will hear just the voicing component of the /z/. Most single-channel tactile devices provide little or no useful information for the detection of the /s/, whereas single-channel cochlear implants can provide useful information on its presence and its duration. Both multi-channel tactile devices and multi-channel cochlear implants are capable of transmitting sufficient information to permit the detection of the high-frequency fricative energy in these sounds. The discrimination of fricatives from other manners of production can also be achieved by children when these sensory aids are optimally fitted. However, discrimination between these and other fricative pairs is unlikely to be achieved spontaneously without the additional information supplied by speechreading.

Informal learning of the /s/ and /z/ is difficult to promote among children who have little or no high-frequency hearing. The sounds are rarely produced involuntarily. The /s/ is occasionally produced by children as they are sleeping in a certain position and, at the same time, breathing heavily through the mouth. Informal learning opportunities for the development of the /s/ from its involuntary production are, therefore, limited to having children pretend to be sleeping in such a way. The most important strategies to promote informal learning are those that are based on ensuring optimal reception of the fricative components, and ensuring that the child receives sufficient experience of the sound, sometimes in contexts that render the /s/ or /z/ more salient. Examples of such contexts include exclamations ending in these sounds, such as "Oh, there are two cars!" and "That one's Daddy's!" Plurals and possessives lend themselves well to this sort of treatment and, to a lesser extent, so do third person irregular verbs (He does! She is! It was!). Opportunities for such natural emphasis occur while caregivers and children are playing with toys, looking at picture books, or engaged in various everyday activities of another sort. Nursery rhymes, such as *Simple Simon, See-Saw Marjorie Daw, Sing a Song of Sixpence, Fuzzy Wuzzy Was a Bear*, tongue twisters involving /s/, and various songs (including the national anthems of English-speaking countries) contain lots of /s/ and /z/ sounds, and can be used to promote their perception and production.

Profoundly hearing-impaired children rarely acquire just one of these sounds spontaneously. Depending on how well they perceive them, informal learning tends to result in the acquisition of both or neither.

Formal teaching strategies for the development of /s/ and /z/ are best undertaken in the context of front vowels, because the tongue is most widely spread in their production. These vowels, therefore, tend to facilitate the creation of a groove over the blade of the tongue, and the flow of breath through the groove, rather than around the tongue. Lateral /s/ sounds, caused by the breath stream travelling around, or over a wide area of the tongue (not through a groove), are least likely to occur in the context of front vowels. Additionally, the front vowels bring the body of the tongue to a forward position, and this helps to create the restricted space that the production of the /s/ and /z/ requires between the alveolar ridge and the blade of the tongue. Once these sounds can be produced in this context their production should, of course, be generalized to include their coarticulation with both central and back vowels.

It is preferable to develop the /s/ before the /z/ when teaching these sounds formally, even though the /z/ occurs more frequently than /s/ in everyday speech. This is because the /s/ is easier to teach than the /z/ on account of its having a stronger breath stream - a feature that permits its turbulence to be more easily detected through hearing or touch. To produce /s/ instead of /z/ as the plural of words like *dogs*, *tabs* and *lads* will not affect their intelligibility, and voicing may be naturally carried over into such sounds from the preceding phoneme (a process known as *assimilation*). The characteristic turbulence of these sounds is, in part, created by driving the breath stream onto the front teeth. It follows, then, that formal teaching of these sounds should not be undertaken during the period when children have lost their first teeth and are waiting for their permanent teeth to arrive. It can be undertaken earlier, providing children have developed a substantial body of spoken language without approximations to these sounds emerging.

The first formal strategy that should be attempted with children who have sufficient high-frequency hearing to detect the fricative energy of the /s/ is to request a direct imitation of the sound through listening alone. All too frequently, teachers and clinicians jump into using visual and tactile strategies without first attempting to encourage the child to listen. Auditory strategies have the advantage, for children who can benefit from them, of providing an appropriate feedback channel through which they can monitor their own productions of the sound. It may be necessary for the professional to come closer than usual to the child (and thus increase the intensity of the sound at the child's ears by reducing distance), to use a speech-training aid, or work through an FM unit in order to ensure that the /s/ can be heard. This may be all that is required to initiate a natural production of the sound, and to ensure that an adequate feedback loop is established. Children's mouths are, as a rule, considerably nearer to the microphone of their hearing aids than are the mouths of most talkers around them. Hence their own speech is usually louder to them than that of others. It may be necessary for the teacher or clinician to cover the mouth when using this strategy so that the child's attention is exclusively focused on what is to be heard. Obviously, it would be a waste of time to use such a strategy with a child who has no hearing over 1000 Hz. While an isolated /s/ may not be detected by a child with no hearing beyond 2000 Hz, its effect on adjacent sounds may be detected if they fall within a child's auditory range.

Before attempting to teach the /s/ through listening alone, it is essential to determine whether children can detect the sound through their own personal hearing aids as they produce it. This is usually feasible if the child's unaided hearing levels are not in excess of about 85 dB at 4000 Hz, and if the earmolds and hearing aids are not only appropriate, but functioning correctly. Children who are unable to detect their own /s/ productions through their personal hearing aids, even when these instruments are functioning optimally, must rely on the tactile and kinesthetic patterns that are created in the mouth to provide them with feedback as the sound is produced. Such feedback should, of course, always be of concern, regardless of hearing levels and what speech pattern is being developed, but it should be of particular concern in the production of /s/ and /z/ - sounds that require such fine adjustments of the tongue.

Once a child with residual hearing that extends beyond 1500 Hz has learned to produce an /s/, and is beginning to use it in everyday spoken language, it may be possible for that child to deduce its presence in running speech without being able to detect its turbulent energy. In such a case, the child's ability to do this would relate to his or her perception of formant transitions and durational cues. Unisensory training can help such children maximize their perception of such cues.

Of course, not all children are fortunate enough to be able to learn to produce an /s/, or integrate the sound into everyday language through auditory strategies. For those who cannot, more formal teaching strategies can be used.

Formal strategies that use anticipatory set are usually the most successful for teaching the production of /s/. They involve relating the production of the /s/ to the unvoiced th sound that has already been developed (when the system described in Chapter 8 has been followed). As always, one begins by using whatever sense modality (or modalities) provide the greatest amount of information on the sound for the particular child who is to learn to make it. Let us illustrate this procedure by describing how you might teach /s/ to Anne, a profoundly hearing-impaired eight-year-old girl with no hearing above 750 Hz, a child who uses a multi-channel electro-tactile aid to supplement what she receives through her hearing aids.

First ask Anne to produce an unvoiced th, as in the word *thumb*. She has already learned to produce this sound, and can make it without difficulty. *Second*, check to determine whether she can perceive the high-frequency turbulence. You find that she can detect it through the electrode placed on her pinky (little finger). By these maneuvers you have suggested that the target will be unvoiced, and a fricative that she can detect in a similar fashion. *Third*, you take and hold her hand lightly between your fingers, and then ask her to pull it slowly back while pressing up on your fingers. She doesn't understand, so you teach her the concept "pull it back" by taking her wrist and encouraging her to do it. *Fourth*, after further trials, when she understands the idea, and pulls her hand back while pressing up against your fingers without assistance, you ask her to produce a long unvoiced th. *Fifth* you tell her to watch as you make a long unvoiced th, pull your tongue back over your top teeth, and draw her attention to what she feels through her tactile device. *Finally*, ask Anne to imitate what you have just done. If she has: (A) made the th; (B) understood the concept of "pull back and press up" and carried it out; (C) continued to detect the fricative turbulence throughout the trial, and (D) taken her tongue back far enough, you will have elicited the /s/. Once the sound has been elicited, be ready to have the child practice it in a variety of phonetic and phonologic level contexts.

The strategy of using set, together with tongue retraction from the th position, can be employed regardless of which sense modality is being used to provide detection of the sound. Working from a known to an unknown sound can provide more than a facilitating context; it can also provide a point of reference that the child can use in further trials. If Anne had had just a hearing aid and benefit of only low-frequency information, she would not have been able to detect the high-frequency fricative energy as described above; but she could have been taught to perceive it as a firm, cool, and continuous breath flow on a wet finger. If she had had sufficient high-frequency hearing to detect the fricative energy when it was produced close to the ear, then audition would have been used as the selected sense modality.

The /s/ is sometimes more readily produced by a child with the tongue tip down. If the above strategy fails, therefore, the procedures outlined above for Anne can be followed, but the tongue tip should be drawn back over the bottom teeth rather than over the top teeth. Regardless of how the /s/ is elicited, the child's attention must be immediately drawn to the sensation created by the production of the sound. If sufficient audition is present, then listening to the sound, as well as attending to the tactile and kinesthetic sensations associated with its production, should be emphasized. If alternative sensory aids are used, then attention should similarly be drawn to the patterns they provide for the child when a sound is correctly produced.

It is a sound policy to select the strategy that has the best chance of succeeding. The least direct strategies involving the provision of set are often the most efficient in the long run, because they usually yield the desired result in the shortest time - and the child receives a lot of encouragement through being able to succeed, and feel successful, at each of the steps in the strategy.

One very direct formal strategy for eliciting the /s/ is to have a child whisper the ee vowel, and then, without moving the tongue, gradually close the jaw, all the time feeling the continuation of breath flow.

A similar strategy is to have the child expel the breath stream through a straw that is first inserted, and then gradually drawn out of the mouth. This strategy is designed to provide the child with the concept of directing the breath stream through a narrow groove over the blade of the tongue. This strategy is most likely to work effectively in the context of front vowels. When the /s/ is elicited in the context of one vowel its production must, of course, be generalized to all other vowels, and carried over into words and everyday discourse.

In another, similar, strategy the child is asked to insert his or her little finger just over the front of the tongue during the production of an ee vowel, and then gradually draw it out while maintaining a fairly strong breath flow onto the tip of the finger. This strategy has the advantage of providing more tactile sensation than the use of a straw. If this strategy does not work, it can be augmented by the teacher or clinician taking another of the child's fingers, and drawing it over her own tongue while producing an eeesss syllable. All of the above strategies can be used effectively in correcting an /s/ sound that is pronounced with lateral breath flow.

Once the /s/ has been obtained in front vowel contexts, its production should be generalized to other vowel contexts, and then to use in syllables, words, sentences, and discourse. To achieve such generalization, have the child rehearse it in syllable-final position first with all of the front vowels, next with all of the central vowels, and finally with all of the back vowels. Sufficient rehearsal of the /s/, first in final position in repeated syllables involving each of the vowels, usually establishes the concept of its requiring a continuous breath stream, and thus prevents the intrusive /t/ that tends to occur when the sound is too quickly used to release rather than arrest vowels. Such intrusive plosion results in a child saying *Stue* instead of *Sue*, and *stee* instead of *see*.

Level 1 function words containing the /s/ and /z/ include *us, inside, outside, some, sunny, sick, sad, soft, sorry*, and *sore*. There are also the common auxiliaries *has, is, was*, and *does*. Although spelled with the /s/ they are, of course, pronounced with a /z/.

Level 2 function words containing the /s/ and /z/ include *same, somebody, sometimes, so, as, as - as, his, hers, yours, theirs, ours, its, myself, yourself, himself, itself, herself, sour*, and *easy*.

Level 3 function words containing /s/ and /z/ include *still, once, several, since, ourselves, yourselves, certain, simple, sensible*, and *satisfied*. In addition, the prefix *dis*, as in *dissatisfied, disappear*, and *disappointed*, provides extensive opportunity to practice /s/ production in a spoken language context.

suggestions for further reading

The most extensive treatment of the material presented in this chapter is to be found in Ling (1976). Some suggestions for speech practice materials suitable for work with adolescent children and young adults is provided by Subtelny and Lieberth (1985). See References, pp. 433 ff.

chapter 13

development of place distinctions (2): the palatal and velar consonants

introduction

Throughout this book, the reader's attention has been drawn, first to the perceptual aspects of speech communication, and subsequently to what is involved in the production of sound patterns. The same procedure is followed in the present chapter, because speech is more than the production of sounds; it is, as previously shown, a complex of perceptual-oral skills.

Acoustic cues relating to place distinctions in consonant production are, as stated in the previous chapter, to be found mainly in the frequency range beyond 1500 Hz. Auditory differentiation of consonants according to their place (as compared with their manner) of production, therefore, requires hearing beyond that frequency. Children who have no little or no hearing for sounds above 1500 Hz would require other types of sensory aids, such as cochlear implants or tactile devices, if acoustic cues on place of production are to be made available them. The acoustic cues relating to the identification of palatal and velar consonants, like those for alveolar consonants, also lie above 1500 Hz, but they differ from those of alveolar consonants in certain respects. The velar plosives /g/ and /k/ in the context of front vowels are characterized by transient energy above 3000 Hz, but in the context of back vowels, a considerable amount of low-frequency energy is present in the plosive bursts. The palatal fricatives sh and zh, are characterized by acoustic energy extending from under 2000 Hz to well above the normal audiometric range. The affricates ch and j have much the same frequency range as the sh and j, but are released from alveolar stops and, as a result, have much sharper onset. The consonantal /r/ is differentiated from the /l/ by F_3 rather than by F_2 transitions in the frequency range 1500 - 3000 Hz. More details on the acoustic properties of the various sounds are provided as each pattern is discussed. The selection and use of appropriate devices and procedures that permit a child to detect such acoustic properties is a prerequisite for teaching these and all other sounds.

The further back in the mouth consonants are made, the less tactile sensation there is associated with them. Thus, for example, production of /k/ and /g/ result in less sensation than the production of /t/ and /d/. To ensure that sufficient specific sensation relating to articulation is experienced by hearing-impaired children as they are acquiring palatal and velar sounds, particular attention should be paid to contrasting them with alveolar sounds having the same manner of production. In promoting their informal learning, this can be achieved by deliberately using the words listed for each sound pattern. In formal teaching, contrast most readily results through the alternation of syllables or words containing alveolar consonants with others containing palatal or velar sounds.

Although the palatal and velar sounds discussed below have traditionally been considered as among the most difficult for hearing-impaired children to learn, they should not prove to be so if present-day resources and knowledge are used to advantage. Indeed, the use of appropriate devices for transmitting acoustic information and the insightful use of set should combine to make the process of acquisition much easier than ever before. Anticipatory set is an exceptionally strong tool for eliciting palatal and alveolar consonants, because at least two well-established speech patterns sharing manner of production can be employed to specify the nature of the target sound (see Chapters 8 and 12).

the fricatives sh and zh

The *prerequisites* for the successful production of the sh (as in *ash*) and the zh (as in *treasure*) are similar to those for the /s/ and /z/ above. These sounds, however, can be made with less precise tongue placement and shaping. The sh, because it also has greater intensity and lower frequency, is often acquired at an earlier stage than the /s/ by many hearing-impaired children.

In the production of sh and zh, the tongue has to be elevated towards the palate rather than towards the alveolar ridge, and it does not need to be grooved. The tongue's position in the production of these sounds is very similar to that required for production of the vowel in the words *bed* and *said*, but the jaw is less widely opened. Because the gap between the tongue and the palate through which the breath stream flows is wider for the sh than for the /s/, and the sh has a longer duration than many other consonants, more breath is normally required for its production than for the production of any other fricative. On this account, hearing-impaired children who produce the sh inconsistently in their everyday speech are often found to have a more general problem with breath flow. Because the tongue is further back in the mouth for sh than for /s/, the frequency range of the sound is considerably (about an octave) lower. The normal frequency range of the fricative components of sh extends from just under 2000 Hz to well over 12,000 Hz, depending on vowel context. The zh and the sh differ significantly only in that the zh is voiced; it therefore contains low-frequency harmonics in addition to the high-frequency fricative turbulence, and this turbulence is somewhat quieter for zh than for sh, because the involvement of the larynx in voicing absorbs some of the energy present in the breath stream.

Because the sh and zh are louder, and create turbulence that is lower in frequency than that of the /s/ and /z/, children with useful high-frequency hearing find them easier to detect. Most children with hearing levels of up to 110 dB at 2000 Hz can be expected to detect these sounds, as well as discriminate and identify them, when fitted with appropriate hearing aids and earmolds.

Children who have no audition beyond 1000 Hz are unable to detect the sh through audition, but should be able to detect the voicing component of the zh. These sounds can both be detected by most children fitted with a single-channel cochlear implant or single-channel tactile device, but they are more likely to be discriminable, and even identifiable, by those who have been successfully fitted with multi-channel instruments. The reception and production of the voiced-voiceless distinction between these two sounds are dealt with in the following chapter. Here, the sh is treated as the more important member of the pair because it is more frequently used, and because it is important, as a first step, to establish production of the fricative quality that the two sounds share.

Informal learning of the sh can be expected of children who have either hearing aids or other sensory devices that permit them to detect its fricative energy. The sound is rarely produced involuntarily by children, but it is often spontaneously imitated by them in response to a caregivers shhhh signal to be quiet. The sound can frequently be introduced in water play, in which words like *swish* and *splash* abound, and the sh itself can be used to describe the sound of something moving through water, or of air escaping from a balloon or other toy. The sound occurs in *One, Two, Buckle My Shoe*, and in *Hush-A-Bye Baby*, but does not appear frequently in other nursery rhymes or songs. However, such a source of stimulation can be created by caregivers and professionals who like to invent rhymes and create songs. In everyday life, the word *brush* can be introduced as regularly as teeth are cleaned, and as often as rooms are tidied. Other opportunities to present the sound in common activities are offered by such words as *fish*, *wish*, *wash*, *push*, *rush*, *shove*, *show*, *crash*, and *shout*.

Formal teaching of the sh can be attempted through imitation if it can be established that the child is able to detect the fricative energy of the sound, either through the use of aided hearing that extends beyond 2000 Hz, or through the use of a cochlear implant or tactile device. While this speech pattern has features that can often be visually identified, vision alone does not help in its initial production. The tongue placement and the turbulent breath stream are not visible. Hearing and touch are therefore the modalities of choice for providing the child with sensation of these features in formal teaching.

The use of set is also one of the most effective strategies in the formal teaching of the sh. For this sound, the previously acquired unvoiced th and the /s/ most usefully provide it. *First*, have the child produce a long, unvoiced th. *Next*, ask the child to draw the tongue back over the top teeth until the /s/ is produced. *Finally*, repeat the previous step but continue to take the tongue back sufficiently far for the sh to result. If the child has been taught to produce the /s/ through the use of set as described above, there should be no difficulty in obtaining the sh in this manner. Once it has been obtained, immediately draw the child's attention to the sensation created by the production of the sound. Continue to do this as you have the child first use the sound to arrest front vowels, as in the words *hash* and *fish*. Then generalize production and sensation as you have the child use the sound to arrest central vowels, as in the words *hush* and *wash*. When the sound can be produced with ease with front and mid vowels, rehearse the sound in back vowel contexts and, finally, use the sh to release and interrupt vowels as in the words *shoe* and *tissue*. As soon as the sound can be produced with ease in various vowel contexts, its use in everyday speech communication should be encouraged.

If this or any other strategy involving the use of set fails, analyze the possible reasons for failure. If the concept of "pull the tongue back over your top teeth" is not established, for example, teach it as outlined for the development of /s/, and try again. If the sound does not then emerge, have the child repeat the procedure with the tongue being drawn back over the bottom teeth. The strategy can be tried once or twice on several successive days; however, always be stringent in limiting the number of trials that fail. Be prepared to attempt alternative strategies (see below) later on - perhaps another day - so that time can dim the memory of any unsuccessful trials.

The tongue position for the sh is similar to that for the vowel in the words *head* and *get*. However, as mentioned above, the jaw is opened wider for the vowel than for the sh. These facts suggest another strategy: have the child whisper the syllable *esh*, closing the jaw quickly following production of the vowel without moving the tongue. One or two tries usually result in success. The problem with this strategy lies in finding simple ways to explain the required sequence of actions to a child. Explanation is more demanding on both teacher and child than demonstration.

A tactile-visual strategy for eliciting the sh through imitation is to have the child imitate you as you blow on his or her hand, terminating each blowing episode with the sh and a smile. As the smile spreads the lips, it also tends to spread the tongue into the desired position. In practice, this sounds as if one is breathily whispering the word *wish* as the model. The external sensation this produces would be primarily tactile, but the internal (oro-sensory) sensations would be strongly kinesthetic. The strategy can, of course, be used to good effect without directing the breath stream on the hand, providing the child is able to detect the breath stream and turbulence through a sensory aid.

Another tactile-visual strategy that can be used to elicit the sh involves placing the tip of the finger over the lower teeth onto the tip of the tongue, and expelling the breath stream as one smiles. Again, the smile is required to spread and elevate the tongue, while the insertion of the finger tip indicates how far the tongue is to be retracted. This strategy can be combined with the prior production of a front vowel, so that the complete trial would involve the child whispering *hish*.

Yet another tactile-visual strategy is to have the child place a small pencil or tongue depressor across the tongue and between the teeth, and then to expel breath while smiling. When this strategy is successfully used, the sound should quickly be elicited again without such help so that the tactile and kinesthetic information created by the production of the sound will permit the child to repeat it.

As soon as the sh has been elicited in isolation or through arresting a front vowel, its production without aids or prompts should be rehearsed so that the child may become either consciously or unconsciously aware of the resulting sensations. The production of the sound should then be generalized to other vowel contexts, as well as to initial, medial, and final positions in syllables and words. Alternation of syllables containing sh with those containing nasal consonants is particularly helpful in establishing well controlled production of this sound.

Level 1 function words containing the sh include *she* and *short*.

Level 2 function words containing the sh include *should*, *shall*, *sure*, *shortest*, *sharp*, and *sharper*.

Level 3 function words containing the sh include *shallow* and *assured*.

the semi-vowel y

The semi-vowel y, as in the word *you*, can be produced as soon as vowels can be alternated on one breath. Such skill is the only *prerequisite*. It is not one of the most frequently occurring sounds. The letter (grapheme) is more frequent than the sound (phoneme) because y is used in writing at the end of words like *beauty*. The sound we are concerned with here, the semi-vowel y, is found in spoken language at the beginning of words like *yes* and *yet*, in the middle of words like *bayou*, and *kayak*, and sometimes between words like *he ought* or *we owe*. This semi-vowel is really a way of releasing and bridging vowels: it is a sound that begins like an over-tense ee̱, and then moves rapidly and smoothly into the following vowel.

The acoustic character of the y̱ sound is best depicted by means of a spectrogram, such as that shown in Figure 13-1. The first formant rises as the second formant falls. Children with hearing beyond 2000 Hz and children successfully fitted with multi-channel cochlear implants or tactile devices should be able to detect and learn to track these changes in second formant frequency. Those with no hearing beyond 1000 Hz should be able to detect the gradual onset and the glide of the first formant. However, as suggested by Figure 13-1, the two semi-vowels y̱ and /w/ can be confused by such children without the aid of speechreading, because their first formants are similar. The /d/ is commonly substituted for the y̱ by hearing-impaired children who do not have appropriate sensory aids, or have not learned to use them. The substitution is essentially due to visual confusion of the two sounds.

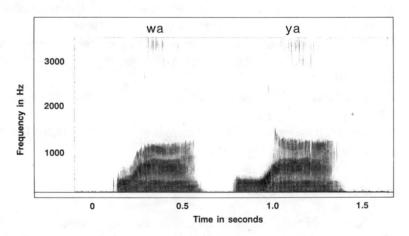

figure 13-1. Spectrograms of the /w/ and j̱ in the context of /a/, indicating the similarity of the F₁ components of these semi-vowels. Children with no aided hearing beyond 1000 Hz may readily confuse them through audition alone. The temporal differences (j̱ as ya being the longer) are not consistent in everyday speech.

Informal learning of the y̱ can best be encouraged in interaction between parent and child (e.g., That's *your* doll. *You* do it! That one's *yellow*). Numerous opportunities for focusing on the sound are also present in table games involving two or more people. Such games permit both caregivers and children to use words like *your* (as in "It's *your* turn!"), *you* (as in "Do you have that card?"), and *yes* (as in "Yes, you do!").

Formal teaching of the y̲ is relatively easy. All one has to do is to have the child alternate the e̲e̲ and any other vowel, progressively shortening the e̲e̲ and lengthening the other sound. To facilitate the production of this speech pattern, begin the alternation process through alternating the e̲e̲ with a central or a back vowel. This procedure most readily conveys the concept of a rapid glide from a high front vowel position. It also maximizes the distance over which the tongue travels, and thus enhances the kinesthetic sensations associated with the sound. The e̲e̲ and the other vowel can be associated with each of the child's hands, or a pair of objects that can be lifted or touched in turn, in order to convey the notion of alternation. As with teaching the /w/, the teacher or clinician can also walk, step by step, in time with the child's alternation of vowels; then, as soon as the alternation has been mastered, have the child shorten one of the vowels so that the rhythm induces the adult to limp. Once the sound has been evoked as a *ya* or *you*, generalize its production to front vowels in words like *yes*, *yeah*, or *year*.

There are relatively few function words that contain the y̲ sound. *Level 1 function words* with the y̲ semi-vowel include *yes, you, your, yet, yellow,* and *yummy.*

Level 2 function words containing this sound include *yours, yourself,* and *young.*

Level 3 function words that include the sound (but not the letter) are *useless* and *useful.*

the plosives /g/ and /k/

To produce the plosives /g/ and /k/, the back of the tongue must be raised to touch the velum about where it joins the hard palate, and thus briefly close off the vocal tract. The sounds are similar in every respect except place of production to the /b/ and /p/, and to the /d/ and /t/. Ability to make these other plosives is an advantage in the formal teaching of the /g/ and /k/. The essential difference between the /g/ and the /k/, is that the /g/ is voiced, and therefore contains harmonics that are not present in the /k/. Developing the /k/ as distinct from the /g/ will be discussed in the next chapter.

The /g/ and the /k/, like most other consonants, are used to release, interrupt and arrest vowel sounds. In word-initial positions, their plosive bursts are released into the vowel, but in word-final positions they are often unreleased. The tongue, in such cases, temporarily stops the breath stream. For example, the /g/ is usually unreleased in the middle of the utterance *big boy*, and the /k/, too, is mostly unreleased between the two words *sick child*. If the sounds are released under such conditions, the rhythm of the speech tends to be abnormal. If released, the /g/ and the /k/ produce noise bursts that vary in frequency according to vowel context. This variation in frequency occurs because the point at which these sounds are made changes from one vowel to another. When made with the front vowels, the point of contact can be as much as seven millimeters further forward on the palate than when it is made with the back vowels.

Children effectively fitted with any type of sensory aid - hearing aids, cochlear implants or tactile devices - should be able to recognize both the /k/ and the /g/ as plosives. This is because their bursts, sudden onset in releasing vowels, and the brief silence they create in the speech stream when interrupting and arresting them, are spread across the frequency range (see Chapters 2 and 3). Thus, their plosive qualities are usually well transmitted by most sensory aids. The identification of the sounds as /g/ and /k/ requires the perception of their high-frequency components. These components are most likely to be detectable by children who have appropriately aided hearing that extends beyond 3000 Hz.

Informal learning of the /g/ and /k/ is usually a slow process. Although most babies babble /aga aga/ around three months of age while lying in the crib, the sound tends to disappear a few months later, to return into production once the child is beginning to talk, and to be used reliably only after the child is talking quite well. Most children, normally hearing or hearing-impaired, confuse the /d/ and the /g/ in the early stages of speech development, and thus say *goggy* for *doggy*. This is a well recognized phonologic process in spoken language acquisition and, unless it persists over an unduly long period, is not to be considered as a target for correction. If children are given enough experience of these sounds during play and everyday living - and they occur frequently in simple words, such as *good, go, gone, get, got, game, come, cup, cake, cow, coat, car*, and *candy* - those with sufficient ability to perceive spectral information will spontaneously acquire them. Learning to gargle may speed up acquisition. Rhymes, such as *Goosey Goosey Gander* help provide stimulation with the sound. Those who habitually substitute

/d/ for /g/ can quickly be taught the sound once an extensive basis of spoken language has been acquired (see below).

Formal Teaching of /g/ is best approached through the use of set. Once /b/ and /d/ have been well established, the /g/ can usually be obtained with a minute or so of work as follows: *First*, have the child repeat a chain of syllables initiated with /b/, preferably /babababa/. *Next*, repeat the procedure using syllables initiated with /d/, namely /dadada/. *Third*, ask the child to try to make more sounds like that with his or her finger holding down the tip and blade of the tongue. This usually leads a child to the immediate production of the /g/. *Fourth*, have the child repeat the production of the /g/ without holding the tongue down with the finger. *Finally*, generalize the production of the /g/ to other vowels and to different verbal contexts. The child should, of course, be reinforced following success at each stage.

Production of the sound is facilitated by working first in the context of the ah vowel. This is because the ballistic movement of the tongue required to make the /g/, and the sensations arising from such movement, are enhanced by the greater distance the back of the tongue has to be elevated from this, rather than from any other vowel. The strategy of using set in this vowel context usually leads to the production of the /g/, because production of both the /b/ and /d/ help define that the target is a voiced plosive; moving from the bilabial /b/ to the lingua-alveolar /d/ indicates that tongue contact with roof of the mouth is desired, and the range and type of tongue movement that results in the production of the /g/ confirms for the child that the sound is distinct from earlier acquired plosives.

An extension of this strategy is to elicit the sounds through reference to a set provided by the nasals - those that have the same place of production. In this strategy the child is encouraged to produce the /m/ and then is taught to terminate the sound with a syllable released with the plosive /b/, as in /mmmmmm-ba/. The next step is to follow a similar path, this time by producing the /n/ and terminating it with a syllable released with the /d/, as in /nnnnnn- da/. The purpose here is to help the child infer that pairs of nasals and plosives have exactly the same place of production. Once one can be sure that sufficient rehearsal has allowed this inference to be drawn, then the final step in the process is to have the child produce a long ng sound and terminate it with /g/, as in ng-ga. Of course, this strategy requires that the child has a previously acquired ng. While strategies to promote the acquisition of ng are provided later in this chapter, there is no reason why it should not precede the development of the /g/. Indeed, some children find it easier to obtain the n͟g first, because they can experiment to find the appropriate tongue position for it as they vocalize for several seconds.

It is possible to teach the /g/ using hand analogy. In this procedure, one hand is employed to represent the roof of the mouth, and the other to represent the tongue. The hand representing the tongue can be used, as shown in Figure 13-2, to indicate that the back of the tongue is to contact the palate in the production of this sound, just as the front of the tongue is used to produce the /d/. This strategy is usually less effective than the one previously described, because it is less direct.

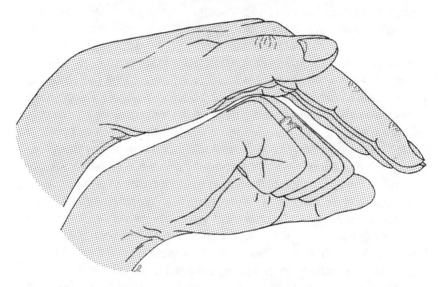

figure 13-2. **The position in which hands can be placed to provide an analogy for teaching the /k/ or /g/. The upper hand represents the palate, and the lower hand, the tongue.**

It is also possible to teach the /g/ through manipulation; that is, by having the child press a finger under his or her chin in order to raise the tongue to the palate. The /g/ is produced as the pressure is suddenly released. This strategy should not be applied to the child by a teacher or clinician: it would be too invasive. Children taught the /g/ in this manner can be prompted in its use from a distance by the professional pointing a finger under the chin, thus to remind the child of the mechanics of its first production.

Models and drawings of the vocal tract's configuration for the production of /g/ have been employed over several centuries as an aid in teaching children who have no useful residual hearing. Along with explanations on how to produce the sound, such strategies rank as only somewhat better than none. Static models and drawings have, of course, been used in attempts to teach many different sounds; but perhaps most frequently the /g/. They have not been discussed in this or earlier chapters, because their frequent mention could have been misconstrued as more than weak encouragement to use them. They are mentioned here mainly in recognition of the need for comprehensive coverage.

The unreleased /g/ can be developed by rehearsing a string of repeated syllables initiated by /g/ - such as /gagaga/ - while having the child initiate each syllable only when he or she is signalled to do so, thus making the production of these repeated syllables arrhythmic. The type of desired timing control is indicated by the number of dots between items in the following series of syllables: /ge.. ge. ge... ge ge/. Once the professional's control of the rhythm has been established, the child will begin automatically and speedily to move the tongue to the /g/ position, and not release it until signalled to do so. This strategy thus inevitably leads to the production of syllables released and arrested by the /g/, as in *geg*, the final sound being the target - the unreleased /g/. It remains to generalize the production of the sound to other contexts and practice it to automaticity, so that words like *egg, big, hug, bug, rug, tug, rag, nag,* and *dog* are pronounced in utterances without breaking their rhythm, or introducing intrusive voicing. Key words of this type including those ending in /k/, such as *back, book,* and *look,* abound in the language. A simple test for natural rhythm using unreleased plosives can be constructed from any set of known vocabulary. For example, one could use some of the above words to construct the sentence "He gave the egg to the big dog." It should normally stress both *egg* and *dog* and contain no more than eight syllables.

Level 1 function words containing the /g/ and /k/ include *can, can't, again, ago, together, cold, cool, big,* and *good.*

Level 2 function words containing these sounds include *ago, could, couldn't, across, close, got, careful, careless, of course, kind,* and *ugly.*

Level 3 function words with /g/ and /k/ include *correct, calm,* and *against.* The construction of a future tense with *going to* also offers many everyday opportunities for practice.

the affricates ch and j

The c̲h̲, as in *chair*, occurs far more frequently in English that the j̲, as in jump. These sounds are often considered to be difficult for hearing-impaired children to pronounce. This is probably because the *prerequisites* for their successful pronunciation have not been sufficiently well recognized. These prerequisites are the mastery of unreleased plosives (stops) and the mastery of the fricative s̲h̲. The difference between the c̲h̲ and the j̲ is simply one of voicing. This feature will be discussed in the next chapter.

Both sounds occur as initial, medial, and final phonemes in words. For example, one has c̲h̲ in the words *cheese*, *itchy* and *hatch*; and the j̲ occurs at the beginning of *jam*, in the middle of *major* and at the end of *wedge*. The c̲h̲ is initiated from the stop /t/, with the impeded breath stream being immediately released through the fricative s̲h̲. Thus, in pronouncing the words *light shoes*, *white sheep*, and *wheat shop* at normal speed, the c̲h̲ automatically occurs. Once pronounced in this way, pronunciation can be slowed to yield *lie choose*, *why cheap*, and *wee chop*, respectively. The c̲h̲ sound is perceptually more salient than the j̲ because the power of its fricative turbulence is stronger. For this reason, and because it occurs more frequently than the j̲, the c̲h̲ may appear first as a result of informal learning by hearing-impaired children. For the same reasons, it is recommended that the c̲h̲ be developed first in formal teaching.

The characteristics of the stop and fricative components of c̲h̲ have been described in earlier sections of this chapter. They will not be repeated here. For the high-frequency components of both the stop and fricative to be perceived, hearing-impaired children must have well-aided high-frequency hearing, effectively fitted single- or multi-channel cochlear implants, or appropriate tactile devices. There is not enough information in the frequency range below 1500 Hz to permit the spontaneous acquisition of these sounds through low-frequency residual hearing. The most common substitution for these sounds among hearing-impaired children is the s̲h̲ which is visually similar to them. The c̲h̲ has been considered by many as one of the most difficult for hearing-impaired children to acquire. More likely, it is one of the hardest sounds for insufficiently skilled professionals to teach. With the use of the strategies outlined below, neither its learning nor its teaching should present undue difficulty.

Informal learning of the c͟h and j͟ can be expected of children who can detect speech energy in the high-frequency range. All of us tend to produce this sound involuntarily when we sneeze, and sneezes amuse young children. It is, therefore, often possible to develop the c͟h through drawing children's attention to it when they sneeze, and having them imitate sneezes. In play, the sound can readily be associated with that made by a train. Rhymes such as *Jack and Jill,* and *Jack be Nimble* will help, but there are an enormous number of everyday words that can be used as key vocabulary. These include *chase, chair, itch, stitch, chalk, chat, catch,* and *watch.* There are also several key words for the j͟ in early vocabulary, including *jump, jam, job, jog, ledge, hedge, jar, ajar, badge* and *jello.* Approximations to these and similar words can be expected of children who focus strongly on speechreading. Their substitutions usually include s͟h for c͟h; for example, they tend to say *wash* for *watch,* and *ships* for *chips.* In treating this problem, unisensory listening experience (not giving visual cues) can profitably be used to help such children whose aided hearing extends beyond 2000 Hz, and those with other types of sensory aids that transmit high-frequency cues. This type of training often permits sufficient focus on the silence preceding the release of the typical high-frequency fricative component for such children to differentiate s͟h and c͟h. Some may consider this strategy formal, but it is certainly not as formal as those described immediately below.

Formal teaching of the c͟h is most simply carried out by using abutting syllables, or adjoining words in which the s͟h follows the stopped /t/. Examples include *at-she, it-shoo, what-share,* and *that-sheaf.* Providing the /t/ is truly stopped, the two component syllables, when produced quickly, should blend to make a c͟h that can be isolated, repeated, and alternated in various vowel contexts, put in words, and used in language.

A similar strategy, one that also relies simply on speeding up pronunciation of the adjacent /t/ and s͟h, is to have a child the child say a word beginning with s͟h and ending with the stopped /t/, such as *shoot,* several times in quick succession. *Shoot-shoot-shoot* rapidly becomes *shoe-choo-choot.* Again, the c͟h thus elicited can only be carried over into communicative speech if its production is systematically generalized. For any of these strategies to be successful, the s͟h and the stopped /t/ must have been practiced to automaticity. Given such automaticity the sound can usually be elicited in three trials or less. Failure to elicit the c͟h by these strategies strongly suggests that the s̲h̲ and stopped /t/ have not been developed sufficiently.

The following strategy is designed to obtain production of the c̲h̲ in a word-initial position from a child like Mary, an eight-year-old girl with aided hearing up to 2000 Hz: *First* obtain a stopped /p/ from Mary in the word *up* each time you raise your finger. *Second*, have her produce a stopped /t/ in the word *at* each time you raise your finger. *Third*, have her say the word *sheep* as you move your hand horizontally. *Fourth*, tell her to produce a well-stopped *at* as you raise your finger and, on the same breath, produce the word *sheep* as you move it horizontally. As these components of the trial are speeded up the words *a cheap* will be produced. *Fifth*, repeat the first part of the previous step silently and then, starting from the unreleased /t/ position, go on to have Mary produce a range of words initiated with c̲h̲, like *cheese, chop, chip, chap,* and *choose*, so that production of the sound is generalized to all vowels. Finally, ensure its carry-over into everyday spoken language.

When the stopped /t/ and the s̲h̲ are not produced with ease by a child, revision of these sounds should be undertaken prior to working on the preceding strategy. For example, in such work with Hope, a similar hearing-impaired child, see that she can produce, on one breath, a syllable final /p/ in spaced but repeated words, such as *up* or *hip*. If there is any release of breath, any confusion with a released plosive, go no further until she has mastered it. *Second*, have her repeat words ending in the unreleased /t/, such as *what* or *it*, several times on one breath at spaced intervals. Ensure that no breath is released between the stop and the beginning of the next word. Indicate the spacing of the intervals required by dropping a finger when you wish the child to produce another syllable. *Third*, have Hope produce the s̲h̲ sound as you move your hand horizontally. *Fourth*, tell her to produce both the well stopped *what* (or *it*) as you drop your finger and the s̲h̲ as you then move it horizontally. At first, the two parts of this trial should be practiced slowly on one breath. Then, when she is really comfortable with the task, speed up the trials, and Hope will produce the word *watch* (or *itch*). Reinforce such productions through repetition in several vowel contexts, have her practice them in other words ending in c̲h̲, and then see that production is generalized. Alternate syllables and words beginning with s̲h̲ and /s/ so that the self-generated sensations associated with each become part of her articulatory code.

Function words containing ch and j are scarce.

Level 1 function words are *how much?*, *not much*, and *each*.

Level 2 function words are *which, cheeky, chilly*, and *cheap*.

Level 3 function words such, just, cheerful, gentle, and *adjacent* are available.

the nasal ng

In order to produce this sound, the *prerequisites* are that a talker is able to elevate the back of the tongue to the palate, open the velopharyngeal port so that the breath stream is expelled through the nose, and simultaneously produce voice. This sound is to the nasals what /g/ is to the plosives. The ng is commonly found in medial and final positions in words, such as *bingo* and *thing*, but is never used at the beginning of a word. It is most commonly met in present participles and gerunds, such as *walking, wishing*, and *being*, and in expressing future intent through the use of *going to*. The ng is rarely stressed in these contexts, so it is, on average, one of the quieter sounds in the language. It is sometimes stressed in the context of verb stems such as *bang* and *hang*, and in nouns, such as *wing, string*, and *fang*.

Like other nasals, the ng is characterized by a low-frequency murmur at about 300 Hz, and some fairly weak higher formants. It is often impossible for normal listeners to tell the ng from other nasals when the sound is presented in isolation; so, for the most part, its identification rests on the listener's ability to perceive formant transition cues that lie mainly above 1500 Hz (see Chapter 2). Their frequency varies according to vowel context.

Hearing-impaired children fitted appropriately with any available sensory aid should be able to detect the low-frequency murmur of the ng. Children with low-frequency hearing who are not provided with sufficient amplification at 250 Hz may be unable to detect this speech sound. Only children who can perceive the high-frequency components of ng and the vowel transitions related to it can be expected to be able to identify the sound as such. These would include children with well-aided hearing up to at least 3000 Hz, and possibly some children fitted with multi-channel cochlear implants or multi-channel electro-tactile devices.

Informal learning of the ng can be promoted in play through pretending to cry like a baby, or growl like a dog with the mouth not fully open. Nursery rhymes, like *Ding Dong Bell* and *Sing a Song of Sixpence*, can also help focus on the sound. Most important for informal learning, however, is for caregivers to provide ample opportunity for the child to hear the sound in the course of meaningful verbal interaction involving verb + ing contexts (for example, walking, running, hopping), and words like *bang, sing, ring, wing, thing,* and *think.* The ng is usually one of the latest sounds to be acquired. Providing the child is approximating more and more mature patterns, and is marking the present tense with at least the right number of syllables (e.g., *walk-i* for walking, *go-i* for going, and *eat-i* for eating), there is no need to consider formal teaching until after age five.

Formal teaching is best undertaken using the set provided by the previously acquired nasals, /m/ and /n/. Indeed this sound was used to provide an example of set at the beginning of this chapter. Let us work this time with Dawn, a profoundly hearing-impaired six-year-old child who has good hearing for the low-frequency nasal murmur at about 300 Hz. *First,* have Dawn produce a long /m/. *Second,* ask her to produce a long /n/. *Third,* ask her to make a sound like the /n/ while holding down the front of the tongue with a finger. With Dawn, as in the vast majority of cases, this strategy is immediately effective. *Fourth,* following appropriate reinforcement for desired responses, have Dawn rehearse the ng in single words or syllables with the sound arresting different vowels (e.g., *bing, bang, bong*). *Fifth,* as soon as she is comfortable in this, have her practice alternating loud and quiet syllables, making the syllable ending with ng the quieter one of each pair.

Alternation of a stressed syllable followed by an unstressed *ing* is an essential step towards mastery of the present and past continuous verb endings and the pronunciation of gerunds, like *going, coming,* and *having.* This step helps a child to acquire the necessary motor speech skills, and also to recognize the tactile and kinesthetic sensations that are produced as this pattern is used. The association of the first of the two syllables with one step, and the ng with another step taken by the clinician or teacher, and then limping towards the child as he or she repeats words like *walking, jumping,* and *swimming* will usually help to develop the concept of stressed and unstressed syllables. *Finally,* when the ng has been rehearsed, promote the child's use of the sound in everyday discourse.

Another reliable strategy is to have children feel the pressure of the tongue against the palate as they are vocalizing and expelling the breath through the nose. The pressure and placement required can be learned directly by having the child place his or her finger on the adult's tongue. Alternatively, and less directly, as this may not be regarded as sufficiently hygienic and acceptable practice unless hands are really clean, or surgical gloves are worn, one may teach the sound by using hand analogy similar to that illustrated for the /g/. In this case, the adult would shape a hand to represent the palate and the child would be helped to shape a hand to represent the tongue, and to press it upwards against the adult's in the required position and with appropriate pressure. One may sometimes avoid all of the above formal strategies simply by asking the child to vocalize with the mouth open and to feel the breath emerging from the nostrils. However, unless the child can also visualize the tongue position, this strategy may yield /n/ instead of ng.

Most strategies for eliciting the ng are similar to those described for the /g/ and /k/. One can use description, illustration and manipulation to encourage the child to put the tongue in the right place. None of these yields results as accurately and as quickly as the utilization of set.

Regardless of which strategy is used to elicit the ng there is always a danger that, because its duration is not important when it is produced in isolation, sufficient attention will not be paid to developing the child's production of the sound with the accuracy, speed, economy of effort, and flexibility that are necessary for its incorporation into everyday phonology. This is, of course, a requirement for all speech sounds taught formally (see Chapter 8), but a particularly important one for the ng.

There are relatively few *function words* at any level involving the ng. One is the word *angry*. Others include those that center around the word *thing*; namely, *nothing, something, anything,* and *everything*.

the consonantal /r/

The /r/ can be made by retroflexing (turning back) the tip of the tongue, or by raising the back of the tongue. The *prerequisites* for production are the ability to make one or other of these adjustments to the tongue so that the breath flow is diverted to either side of it. The retroflexed /r/ is probably easier to elicit should formal teaching be required. In the production of this sound, the under side of the tongue usually touches the palate just behind the alveolar ridge, but an acceptable /r/ can be produced with the tongue tip simply pointing up and back, and not actually touching. The /r/ sound is often made in association with lip-rounding. Like the /l/, the consonantal /r/ is a lateral sound; one that is made by expelling the breath stream around the sides of the tongue rather than over the top of it. Confusions between the /l/ and /r/ are common among many talkers of Asiatic origin because their native languages have a sound that is neither one, but lies in between the two. Such confusions rarely occur among hearing-impaired talkers. Lip-rounding and tongue retroflexion each serve to lower formant frequencies, and there are, therefore, both motor (lip-rounding) and perceptual (formant-lowering) reasons for the /w/ to be commonly substituted for the /r/ in young children. This substitution often persists and becomes permanent in a substantial proportion of hearing-impaired speakers who have learned to focus attention more on the lips than on the tongue.

The /r/ takes many forms. In releasing a vowel it is voiced. In blends, when it follows unvoiced consonants, as in the words *pray* and *trap*, it becomes unvoiced, whereas in between and following vowels it usually takes on some vowel-like qualities. Most North American talkers raise part of the tongue and direct some of the breath stream around (rather than just over) the tongue when pronouncing final vowels in words like *fur* and *mother*. This results in such words receiving substantial /r/ coloring.

To hear the /r/ a child must have aided hearing up to at least 1000 Hz. To differentiate the /r/ and the /l/ one has to be able to be able to perceive the changes in the frequency of its formants - particularly F_3. To understand what these changes sound like, contrast two syllables produced with a forced whisper: *lee* and *ree*. Readers with normal hearing who do this will find that the /r/ leads to a much greater glide in pitch than the /l/. To be able to perceive the /r/ and its effects on the vowels that follow it through audition, hearing-impaired children must be able to detect the glides it produces in the frequency range 1500 - 3000 Hz. This is feasible only for those with sufficient aided high-frequency hearing. Such glides, which vary in frequency according to vowel context, cannot be heard by children having only low-frequency residual audition, or by most of those using single-channel sensory aids. Multi-channel cochlear implants and multi-channel electro-tactile devices may permit something of the glide to be detected. All appropriately prescribed sensory aids should permit at least detection of the voicing components of the different /r/ sounds.

Informal learning of the /r/ can be encouraged in many play situations. The trilled /r/, heard when children play with toy racing cars or motor cycles, is a useful basis for production of the /r/ in spoken language, although it does not normally occur in the speech of North American talkers. Using the /r/ in guessing games provides opportunities for children and caregivers to take turns in declaring each other *right* or *wrong*. The sound also occurs in rhymes, such as *Ring-a-Ring o' Roses* and *Rain, Rain, Go Away*, as well as in songs, such as *Row, Row, Row Your Boat* and *Run Rabbit, Run*. In everyday life, words with /r/ are common, and many such words form part of children's basic vocabulary. Those with consonantal /r/ include *rag, real, reach, read, rice, ride, ring,* and *run*. Many more early words also begin with the /br/, /tr/, /pr/, and /str/ blends that will be discussed in the next chapter. An excellent, informal way to encourage the production of /r/ and prevent its confusion with the /w/ is to whisper words such as these in occasional "secrets" when close to children who are known to have sufficient sensory reception of high frequencies. Because reduction of distance increases the intensity of speech at the listener's ear, a forced whisper from three inches is louder than a shout from eight feet; and, because forced whispering enhances perception of the glide, this "secret" recipe for providing emphasis to the /r/ family of sounds can be suprisingly effective, not only for certain hearing-impaired children, but also for their normally hearing peers who are having trouble in developing them.

Formal teaching can be undertaken through the provision of set involving the /l/. While the /l/ requires the tip of the tongue to be raised to the alveolar ridge, the retroflexed /r/ requires that it be turned back so that it points to, or touches, a location just behind it. The most direct strategy by which a child can be helped to accomplish such tongue placement is a tactile one. *First*, have the child imitate the vowel ah. *Second*, have him or her repeat /lalala/. *Third*, ask for /lalala/ to be repeated slowly, saying /l/ as you raise your finger and ah as you lower it. *Fourth*, have the child push back the tip of the tongue with the finger from the /l/ position before releasing each of three more similar syllables, bringing the finger out from the mouth to release each vowel. (You may add to the power of this strategy by demonstrating how you want this done before asking them to do it.) *Fifth*, have the child rehearse the production of this sound without using the finger. The ah vowel offers the most appropriate facilitating context for teaching this vowel in this manner, for in this context, the tongue is not so widely spread that lateral breath flow for the /r/ is inhibited, the lips are not so rounded that confusion between the /w/ and the /r/ is encouraged, and there is adequate room for insertion of the little finger into the mouth. As soon as the sound can be produced in this context, it should be used with other vowels and in words.

Another formal teaching strategy, one that is appropriate only for children like Dalin, who can perceive the high-frequency (F_3) /r/ glides, is to work from an unvoiced th. *First*, have him imitate a long unvoiced th. *Second*, have him imitate the word *three*, taking the tongue back rapidly from the th position. By emphasizing the rapid retraction of the tongue, the /r/ position is usually reached within a few trials. *Third*, once the /r/ has been obtained, have Dalin rehearse *three-three-three-ree* until the /r/ alone releases the syllable. *Fourth*, generalize the sound to other vowels. The ee vowel is facilitative in this strategy because it maximizes the acoustic glide and, at the same time, prevents lip-rounding that could lead to visual confusion with /w/. As with all other formally taught sound patterns, its phonologic use should be immediately encouraged. As stated in Chapter 7, carry-over may be enhanced by immediately following up with informal strategies.

Level 1 function words containing the /r/ include *round*, *rainy*, *ready*, and *red*.

Level 2 function words containing this sound include *right*, *wrong*, *around*, *really*, *rude*, *rough*, and *real*.

Level 3 function words containing the /r/ include *rapid*, *ripe*, *rotten*, *rusty*, *rich*, *rare*, and *rid*.

Linguistically based practice of the consonantal /r/ can be provided through the use of the prefix *re*, as in *renew* and *redistribute*. Practice with the vocalic /r/ can be given in suffixes that are formed with the er to create nouns from verbs, as in *run - runner* and *talk - talker*.

suggestions for further reading

The most extensive treatment of the material presented in this chapter is to be found in Ling (1976). Some suggestions for speech practice materials suitable for work with adolescent children and young adults is provided by Subtelny and Lieberth (1985). See References, pp. 433 ff.

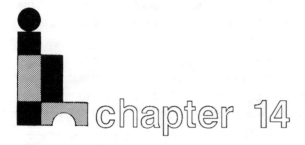

chapter 14

development of the voiced-voiceless distinctions and consonant blends

the voiced-voiceless distinction

Nasals (such as /m/), semi-vowels (such as /w/), and glides (such as /l/ and /r/) are all known as voiced sounds because the vocal cords usually vibrate as these sounds are produced in everyday conversational speech. In contrast, some consonants, such as the plosives /p/, /t/, and /k/, the fricatives /f/, /s/, and sh, and the affricate ch are voiceless; that is, made without vocal cord vibration. Most plosives, fricatives, and affricates can, however, be made with or without voicing. They are members of cognate pairs, such as /b/ and /p/, /v/ and /f/, and j and ch. The first part of this chapter is concerned with various ways in which the voiced-voiceless distinctions among cognate pairs can be achieved, and the strategies that can be used to help children develop the skills required to make such distinctions. The second part deals with the production of voiced and unvoiced consonants in blends.

In *word-initial consonants* voicing is perceived when vocal cord vibration begins at about the same time as all other components of the sound. In contrast, voicelessness is perceived when the onset of vocal cord vibration follows the release of other components by about thirty- to forty-thousandths of a second (msec). Readers with normal hearing can easily hear the difference in the timing of voice-onset by listening to the delay in vocal cord vibration as they say /pa/ and then /ba/. The voiced-voiceless distinction they perceive will be due to differences in what is known as *voice onset time* (VOT).

In *word-final consonants* the voiced-voiceless distinction is sig- nalled as much by the duration of preceding vowels and continuants as by the presence or absence of vocal cord vibration. This is most clearly demonstrated by whispering two words that usually differ in this regard, such as "his" and "hiss." To signal the /z/ sound in "his" the vowel is lengthened and the consonant shortened, whereas the process is reversed to signal the /s/ in "hiss." Of course, vocal cord vibration is featured in voiced consonants that appear in word-final position, but it is not an essential feature.

In *medially placed consonants*, such as the /b/ in "rubbing" or the /p/ in "report", the duration of the preceding vowel, the duration of lip closure, and the relative intensity of voice and bursts all signal whether sounds are voiced or unvoiced. Compared with the medial /b/, the medial /p/ is typically preceded by shorter vowels, has a greater duration of closure, and is followed by vowels and plosive bursts having greater intensity. Most of these effects appear to be mechanically rather than linguisitically based, essentially because some of the energy present in the breath stream is absorbed by voicing. Similar timing features lead to the differentiation of all other manners of production in medially placed con- sonants.

perceptual aspects

As the above discussion suggests, the ability to perceive voice- voiceless distinctions depends to a very large extent on a child's capacity to detect and discriminate temporal (time) differences between speech sounds. The ear is normally much better than the eye in dealing with the duration of vowels and consonants, and any gaps between them. The skin is not as good as the ear - but better than the eye - in the transmission of temporal information. Much of the timing that underlies the production of voiced-voiceless distinctions affects the frequency range below 1000 Hz. All things considered, then, hearing aids, cochlear implants, touch, and tactile devices are all likely to provide more information on voiced-voiceless distinctions than speechreading, although some types of hearing impairment can adversely affect the auditory perception of sounds that differ in time.

productive aspects

Of the three aspects of speech production - manner, place, and voicing - voicing may be the hardest for hearing-impaired children to master at an early stage in speech acquisition, because such fine control of duration is involved. In part, this is why it is left until the later stages in the Ling system (see Chapter 8). By leaving the acquisition of the voiced-voiceless distinction in cognate pairs of consonants until manner and place of consonant production have been developed, the system ensures that children receive a great deal of incidental experience which leads, without conscious effort, to gradually refined control of vocal duration (see Chapter 8). To be explicit, the most basic aspect of control of vocal duration is introduced in the first stage of development, when speech-breathing and vocalization are established. During the second stage, gross differences in vocal duration (long, short, and varied production) are produced, and voiced sounds are contrasted with whispered ones. These differences are practised during the third stage (vowel production), but are refined in the fourth and fifth stages when consonants differing in manner and place of production are developed. In these stages, unvoiced fricatives are contrasted and alternated with voiced consonants of all other types, and used to release, interrupt, and arrest vowels. Meaningful speech with appropriate rhythmic properties is to be expected as soon as a few vowels and consonants have been acquired. Laryngeal control should, therefore, be well-practiced and largely established by this, the sixth, stage in which the voiced-voiceless distinction is to be mastered. Progress through the previous stages of the system provide all of the prerequisites for the acquisition of sufficient mastery to ensure the use of voiced-voiceless distinctions in communicative speech.

informal learning strategies

Informal strategies include abundant exposure to speech communication, and the provision of positive reinforcement when untaught distinctions are spontaneously acquired (for example, when /p/, /t/, and /k/ are used in words like *pop*, *tiptoe*, and *kitten* when only /b/, /d/, and /g/ have been specifically taught, or when these distinctions have not been encouraged in previous stages).

Voiced-voiceless distinctions can be encouraged by playing a game like musical chairs, in which children continue to walk around some chairs while the syllable /ta/ is being repeated, and to sit down as soon as a string of /da/ syllables is produced. For variety, the consonants in such a game can be varied from one cognate pair to another, and placed either at the beginning or at the end of syllables. For example, strings of syllables changing from /pa/ to /ba/, /iss/ to /iz/, or *chee* to *jee* can also be used. Once children know the game, and can play it reliably through the discrimination of several different cognate pairs, they can become the leader whose job it is to produce the syllables and control the game. Interestingly, the breathing patterns, heart rate, or some other aspect of behavior in very young babies changes as one syllable is substituted for another in a series of syllables presented in this way. The same sort of game can be played with a single child, who can be asked to start drawing a line, or taking things from a box as soon as the change from voiced to voiceless consonants (or the reverse) is made. If appropriate hearing aids (or other sensory aids) are used, most children should be able to discern the essential differences between the two speech sounds in any cognate pair, and to participate effectively in games such as these.

formal teaching strategies

Voiced-voiceless distinctions occur in three manners of consonant production: plosives, fricatives, and affricates. If the procedures so far suggested in this book have been followed, children will have developed all of the voiced plosives, and all of the unvoiced fricatives and affricates. Most, by this stage will, through communicative experience, also have developed further voiced- voiceless distinctions spontaneously. The task at this stage will then, at most, be to develop /p/, /t/, and /k/ through reference to their cognates /b/, /d/, and /g/, to develop voiced fricatives and affricates, and to ensure that voiced-voiceless distinctions are used appropriately in communicative speech.

Formal auditory strategies for teaching production of voiced and voiceless pairs of consonants should begin with discrimination training. The same type of training can be provided for children wearing cochlear implants. For example, in the *first* step, associate /ba/ with a picture of a sheep, and /pa/ with a picture of a man. To do this, ask the individual to listen carefully and point to the one of the pair that you say. Use as many prompts or cues as required to establish the required association. On each trial, be sure to provide knowledge of correctness. In the *second* step repeat this task until the child can do it correctly five times out of six with eyes shut. *Finally*, once the child can discriminate between the pair, the child and the professional reverse roles so that the child say the words, and the teacher or clinician makes the appropriate response and seeks approval. If a clear distinction is not made, repeat the discrimination training and try again. If the auditory procedure is not effective, go straight to an auditory-visual-tactile discrimination procedure, because the visual differences between voiced and voiceless pairs are minimal.

The same steps as those outlined above can be used in the prior training of discrimination skill when a child is to be taught to produce a voiced-voiceless distinction through the use of a cochlear implant or a tactile device. Similar procedures can also be followed when neither of these instruments is available, and direct touch has to be employed.

Set is important in the formal teaching of voicing distinctions just as it is in teaching other speech patterns. For example, *Item A* of a set might be the prior production of the voiced or voiceless cognate of the target sound having the same manner and place of production. *Item B* of the set would be production of a whispered vowel to prepare a child for the production of a voiceless plosive, or the production of a voiced vowel to prepare a child for the production of a voiced fricative. The sound's manner and place (A), as well as its voicing (B) characteristics, can thus be specified, and the set should lead most easily to *Item C*, the target pattern. Set is implicit in the formal teaching strategies outlined below.

Voiceless plosives in word-initial position require that vocal cord vibration follows burst release by about 20 to 30 msec. Such a delay in voice onset time (VOT) must be both perceived and produced by a child if unvoiced plosives are to be developed. When there are some unvoiced plosives in a child's repertoire, it can be assumed that at least some voiced-voiceless distinctions can be perceived. In such a case, the best formal strategy is to generalize the existing distinctions to other cognate pairs.

The perception of the voiced-voiceless distinction can be trained through a formal strategy - one that requires the child to discriminate between initially long (over 100 msec) VOTs (as in /p^{h-} ⁻a/), and then increasingly shorter ones until the normal 20 to 30 msec range for /pa/ is reached. The child's ability to produce the distinction is then trained in the same way. This strategy is effective, but can be very time-consuming because perception and production are trained sequentially rather than jointly. The strategy described below, as used with a profoundly hearing-impaired girl, is suggested as a speedier alternative.

First, have the child produce the syllable /ba/ in a strong whisper and, as he or she does this, draw a finger down the upper part of the child's arm, above the elbow. (This should pose no problems if whispering has been used, as suggested, from the second stage of the system.) *Second*, repeat the first step until the strongly whispered syllable and the tactile component are clearly associated. *Third*, have the child say a normally voiced a̲h̲ vowel, and, as she does this, draw a finger down the lower part of her a̅r̅m̅, from the elbow to the wrist. *Fourth*, repeat the third step until the voiced vowel and the tactile component are clearly associated. *Fifth*, explain that you now want both the whispered /ba/ and the voiced vowel produced without a pause between them and, by producing the whispered /ba/ and voiced a̲h̲, and drawing a finger down your own arm as you do it, you provide the child with a model of the required behavior. *Sixth*, have her imitate your model, repeating the procedure until it is done with ease. *Finally*, speed up production of the sequence until, without the tactile prompt, the utterance takes on the quality of a /pa/ rather than a /ba/.

The above strategy can be used, if necessary, to teach both the /t/ from the /d/, and the /k/ from the /g/. It can also be used to generalize production of each of these unvoiced plosives to other vowel contexts.

Word-final stops involving the voiced-voiceless distinction are, as stated above, signalled more by durational cues than by the presence or absence of vocal cord vibration. The most important prerequisite for the development of the distinction in word-final position is the ability to produce /b/, /d/, and /g/ as unreleased stops. Once this is achieved, one can ensure acquisition of the distinction by varying the duration of the vowels, and the rate of closure in various syllables containing them - very short vowels and rapid closure in the case of unvoiced stops, and longer vowels and less rapid closure in the case of voiced stops. To promote such production, the following steps may be followed. *First*, have the child make a long vowel, such as e̲e̲e̲e̲, and arrest it gently with a bilabial. It will sound like a /b/. *Second*, have the child make a short e̲e̲ vowel and arrest it sharply with a bilabial. It will sound like a /p/. *Third*, have the child produce a long eeee vowel and arrest it sharply with a bilabial. The /p/ quality will persist. *Fourth*, have the child make a short ee vowel and arrest it gently. It will be a /b/. *Fifth*, have the child listen (with hearing aids or cochlear implant) or feel (with a tactile device or through direct touch) in order to discriminate between words containing two-voiced plosives, two unvoiced plosives, and words differing in word-final cognates, such as *lap* and *lab*, *fat* and *fad*, and *Dick* and *dig*. If this type of training is needed at all, then it will also be important to ensure that as soon as the distinction can be made in one vowel context, its production is generalized to all others.

The bilabials /b/ and /p/ provide the most facilitating context for the development of the voiced-voiceless distinction in the word-final position. This is because the timing of labial closure can be most readily heard, seen, and felt. (The lower frequency of F_1 of all vowels with bilabials make them easier for hearing-impaired people to detect through audition, the lips are the most visible of the speech organs, and they are also the most sensitive part of the vocal tract.)

Generalization from syllables to words and discourse are important steps in the development of the voiced-voiceless distinction. As soon as a child can produce the distinction in syllable-initial plosives, practice in the discrimination and production of the distinction should be afforded in pairs of words, such as *pea-be, pail-bail, to-do, tore-door*, and *cane-gain*. Similarly, when the distinction can be made in the discrimination and production of syllable-final stops, the distinction should also be practised in pairs of words, such as *cup-cub, rip-rib, rope-robe, lap-lab, cap-cab, hit-hid, hurt-heard, hat-had, back-bag, luck-lug, pick-pig*, and so on. Also, as a further step towards the integration of the distinction into everyday communicative speech, it is advisable to ensure that it is first mastered in commonly used phrases that occur in everyday life, such as *That's too big, It's time to go home*, and *I don't want to do that*. Specially constructed sentences to highlight the distinction in running speech, such as *Daddy asked Peter to pick up the big red bag*, that have no meaning or relevance to a child are quite unnecessary and their use should be avoided.

Repetition of syllables containing the various plosives is the only formal teaching strategy that is recommended for developing voiced-voiceless distinctions in word-medial positions, providing that sufficient practice has been given to developing them in the other positions as described immediately above. It cannot be overstressed that extensive use of the formal strategies described above is rarely necessary if spoken language has been developed systematically through all previous stages (see Chapters 9-12), and if consistent use has been made of well-adjusted modern communication aids of the type discussed in Chapters 4 and 5.

Voiced fricatives and affricates can be formally taught through the use of one simple strategy. *First*, ask the child to produce a string of syllables, such as /fafafafa/ or /afafafaf/, releasing or arresting each syllable with the unvoiced cognate. (This task should not be a serious problem, because the unvoiced fricatives and the affricate ch will have been mastered at previous stages as described in Chapters 9 through 12.) *Second*, ask the child to produce the vowel used in step one, making it about three to five seconds long, and having the child feel the continuity of its vibration as he produces it. *Third*, ask him to repeat the string of syllables rehearsed in the first step, while voicing and, at the same time, feeling the continuity of the utterance as rehearsed in the second step. (In short, step three is the addition of steps one and two.) Successful completion of this task leads to voicing of all the syllables. (For example, /ususus/ becomes /uzuzuz/ and /sasasa/ becomes /zazaza/.) *Fourth*, once the third step can be achieved with ease, isolate single syllables from the string of syllables used (for example, /uz/ on its own should be produced following /uzuzuz/). *Finally*, syllables containing the voiced fricatives; or voiced affricate j, as in judge, should be rehearsed in everyday words, and then used in meaningful sentences and discourse.

The most important aspect of formal training in the production of voiced fricatives is ensuring that sufficient turbulence is present in each. Voicing detracts from the overall energy of the high-frequency turbulent components typically present in unvoiced fricatives and affricates. Children who are profoundly or near totally deaf may need extensive use of a tactile strategy - such as feeling the breath flow on the fingers - to ensure from the outset that such turbulence is strongly associated with each of the voiced fricatives, and with the voiced affricate. This strategy is most effective when such sounds are rehearsed in word-final position. Strategies to enhance continuous breath flow may also be required to avoid confusion of alveolar and palatal fricatives with nasals or plosives. They should therefore be used until the characteristics of the sounds are firmly established.

Function words, such as *the, this, that, these, those, there, with, of, have, as, is, was, has,* and *does,* being among the most frequently used in English, are the words that provide the most practical entry for voiced fricatives into spoken language. Function words tend to contain a larger proportion of voiced than of unvoiced fricatives, whereas the reverse is true of content vocabulary. Probably because of this, most hearing-impaired children tend to acquire a range of voiced fricatives spontaneously. When this is the case, formal teaching can, providing the fricative turbulence associated with such sounds is adequate, be largely restricted to the use of generalization strategies that ensure their production in all vowel contexts. The final step in the teaching of voiced fricatives is, of course, to ensure their use in speech communication.

the development of blends

Blends, sometimes known as clusters, are formed when two or more consonants occur in abutting positions in or between words. The perception and production of blends is largely determined by how well each of their elements can be perceived and produced. The most common elements in word-initial blends are /l/ and /r/ as in the words *blue, brown, play, pray,* and *street.* The most common elements in word-final blends are the /s/ and /z/ that provide the plural and possessive markers for nouns. Any phoneme can abut and blend with another between adjacent words, but some such blends occur more commonly than others, because words most frequently end in sounds such as /n/, /t/, /d/, and /k/, and begin with /b/, /k/, /p/, and /s/. Blends are so common in spoken language that if one is unable to recognize and produce them with reasonable accuracy, the intelligibility of speech can suffer enormously.

Unless hearing-impaired children use appropriately selected sensory aids - hearing aids, cochlear implants or tactile devices - they are likely to experience considerable difficulty in the perception of blends. Research on speechreading has shown that a given blend can be visually confused with other blends, or with single consonants, in up to 90 percent of trials. All types of single- and multi-channel sensory aids transmit sufficient time and intensity cues to resolve many such confusions in speechreading. Most children with residual hearing that extends beyond 2000 Hz, and who wear appropriate hearing aids, can also receive spectral information that will permit them to identify most blends through audition alone, or through the combined use of audition and vision. Most children successfully fitted with multi-channel cochlear implants or multi-channel tactile devices should also be able to identify most blends when speechreading is supplemented by the spectral information these instruments provide.

The perception and production of blends is complicated by the changes that can result when two or more consonants occur together, particularly in word-initial position. For example, the /l/ and the /r/ are produced with voice when, as single sounds, they release vowels in words like *low* and *rake*. However, both of these sounds tend to become voiceless when they follow unvoiced consonants in blends, as in the words *slow*, *play*, *pray*, and *try*. Moreover, they tend to influence the sounds they follow, sometimes so strongly that the two are compounded into something quite unlike either alone. For example, the /t/ and /r/ in a word like *try* form a sound that is similar to the ch in *child*. At the same time, some sounds that are normally unvoiced, like the /p/ and /t/ are pronounced with such short VOTs when they follow the /s/ in words like *spot* and *star* that they are much more like their cognates /b/ and /d/. Indeed, when one compares the pronunciation of *spot* with *sbot*, and *star* with *sdar*, differences cannot normally be detected. The importance of this in the process of developing blend production is clear: blends have to be specifically developed as such, but they cannot usually be acquired or taught until each of their elements has been mastered. Thus, in general, children are unlikely to be able to produce the /kr/ blend as in *creep* before they have mastered the production of the /k/ and the /r/ in simpler words like *key* and *read*. It follows that hearing-impaired children will often delete one of the phonemes in a blend or cluster, just as young normally hearing children do, not necessarily because they cannot perceive them sufficiently clearly, but because they have not achieved adequate prior mastery over the production of both elements.

In general, word-initial and word-final blends can be taught, and are usually learned, at about the same time. Certain word-initial blends, however, are harder for a child to produce than others. Five levels of difficulty can be identified among such blends, as indicated below.

The least difficult of word-initial blends are those made with the tongue and the lips that occur in words like *smile*, *spot* and *swim*. Once the /s/ is mastered, these are the easiest of blends for a child to acquire, because the elements of the blend are produced sequentially, and because the /s/ must be completed before the next element can be formed.

Slightly more difficult are blends of two sequentially produced elements that both involve the tongue - blends found in words like *stop, skip, slap* and *snug.*

Third in order of difficulty are blends in which the elements are formed simultaneously with the tongue and lips - those found in words like *blink, brought, fly, fruit, quick, play, prod,* and *twice.* (To check that the elements in such blends are formed simultaneously, poise yourself to say these words and you will find that the second element is prepared before the first is released. Note, for example, that the tongue is touching the alveolar ridge ready for the /l/ before the /b/ is released in the word *blink.*

Even more difficult are the word-initial blends that mainly involve creating complex configurations of the tongue in order to prepare simultaneously for the production of the two consonants. Examples of such blends occur in words like *dry, glad, great, cry, shrink,* and *trip,* in which the tongue has to form the first of the consonants while assuming an appropriate position for the immediate production of the second. The degree of difficulty involved can again be demonstrated by poising oneself to say the words *die* and *dry,* or *gad* and *glad.* The contrasts in tongue position required to initiate them clearly illustrates the extent to which the two elements are simultaneously prepared.

Among the most difficult of word-initial blends are those containing three adjacent consonants. They are present in words such as *scrape, squeeze, spring,* and *string.*

Word-final blends do not vary so much in difficulty as in type. Five types of blends can be identified. These are briefly described below:

- Blends consisting of two continuants (sounds that can be prolonged and yet retain their character), such as those in the words *tiffs, pills,* and *film.* (Most are formed as plurals.)

- Blends consisting of a stop and a continuant as in the words *cabs, hats, pigs, bottle,* and *button.* (Again, most are formed with plurals.)

- Blends consisting of a continuant and a stop as in the words *lift, cold, camp, hand,* and *wasp.*

- Blends formed with two stops as in the words *act, apt,* and *bagged.* (These include the past tense of many verbs ending in *ed.* The final element in these blends is produced as an isolated sound)

- Combinations of the above, as in the words *ample*, *asked* and *kittens*.

Regardless of how easy or difficult blends may be to produce, they occur quite frequently in English - much more frequently than in romance languages - and must be mastered if intelligible speech is to be achieved. One should not be daunted by the task. Providing children have acquired the prerequisite skills by completing previous stages in the system, the application of simple strategies will ensure the rapid development of consonant blending ability.

informal learning strategies

The spontaneous development of blends can be expected only if a hearing-impaired child is known to be capable of perceiving them through aided audition, or through speechreading supplemented by the use of sense modalities other than vision. Informal learning can be encouraged by using blends while playing with a child under optimal conditions for speech reception. For example, playing with colored toys or paints provide opportunities to use words like *blocks*, *green*, *grey*, *blue*, *black*, and *brown*. Activities call for instructions, such as *smile*, *smell*, *break*, *bring*, *brush*, *blow*, *stop*, and *start*. Setting table requires words like *bread*, *glass*, *plate*, *place*, *gravy*, *tray*, and *spoon*. These are examples of blends that occur in word-initial position. Using plurals and possessives in the course of everyday life provides opportunities for the child to perceive and to use certain blends that appear in word-final position. Using regular verbs in the past tense calls for yet another type of word-final blend (see above).

formal teaching strategies

In order for blends to be produced with ease, awareness of the feedback associated with each, but particularly that provided by the kinesthetic and tactile sensations produced in speaking, must be developed by the child. To develop sufficient conscious or unconscious awareness of sensation, adequate time must be allocated and a generous quantity of experience provided.

The first two sorts of initial blends described above - those that permit the sequential production of each element and appear in words such as *small*, *space*, *sweet*, *ski*, *slide*, *snap*, and *stone* - can be developed by separating the /s/ from the rest of the word (or syllable) and then alternating the two parts slowly at first, and then faster and faster until they do, indeed, blend into the original word. Thus *ski* would be separated into /s/ and /ki/ and the child asked to say s-ki-s-ki-s-ki-s-ki-s-ki. It sometimes helps to associate one part of the word with the child's left hand, and the other part with his or her right hand, and then signal the speed of alternation by lifting and lowering each of the child's hands in turn.

The formal strategy described immediately above would have disastrous results if one tried it with blends that require simultaneous preparation of the speech organs for their production - those that appear in words like *black, brown, play, quick, dream,* and *glad.* Because plosives are not sounds in their own right, but only ways of releasing, interrupting or arresting vowels, blends such as these cannot be separated into two parts to form words like *b-lack, p-late,* and *g-lad.* The idea looks fine in writing, but in speech the words would come out as *b^u-lack, p^h-late,* and *g^u-lad.* An intrusive vowel would have been introduced between the plosive and the rest of the word. Intrusive voicing - sometimes introduced in this way - is a common fault among certain groups of hearing-impaired children, one that finally leads to a breakdown in the natural rhythm of speech and to reduced intelligibility. To illustrate how best to teach these sorts of blends, study the several different steps described below that will be used in teaching such blends to Sarah.

First, ensure that Sarah can produce word-final, unreleased stops in words such as *up, tub, hit, hid, lick,* and *dog.* Have her repeat each word several times, ensuring that none of the final phonemes is aspirated (released). *Second,* target a particular CCV (consonant blend + vowel) for development - for example, a CCV, such as *bla* from *black. Third,* placing the first element of the blend at the end of the syllable to form a CVC sequence (so that *bla* becomes *lab*) have her slowly repeat the syllable, ensuring that the final stop is unreleased. *Fourth,* have Sarah increase her speed of repetition, allowing no pause between syllables. (This will result in a sequence such as *lablablab* that contains the desired blend.) *Fifth,* having established the sensory-motor patterns required for the accurate production of the blend in this way, have her initiate similar sequences with the target blend. *Finally,* have her use the blend in other vowel contexts, words, words in sentences, and in discourse. The same basic strategy can be used for teaching all other blends of this type for inclusion in words like *brown, flew, fright, quick, please, prowl, twice, drop, glad, grip, cry, shrink,* and *tramp.*

The most effective strategy for teaching all sorts of blends is, without question, the one described above for teaching certain initial blends to Sarah. Simply expressed, it can be considered as a two-step procedure:

First, place the first element in the blend at the end of the syllable (so, for example, /sma/ becomes /mas/, /sta/ becomes /tas/, /pla/ becomes /lap/ and /stra/ become /tras/); and *Second*, have the child rehearse the resulting sequence slowly at first and then faster and faster until the targeted blend appears (/masmasmas/, said quickly, requires the same sensory-motor components as /smasmasma/). This strategy will usually work with all word-initial and word-final blends from the simplest to the most complex. However, it is always worth while having alternative procedures available for the more complex sound patterns so further strategies are provided below.

An alternative for teaching CCV blends is to ask the child to form the second element of the blend (for example, the /l/ in the word *black*) and, while holding the tongue in the /l/ position, form the /b/. The blend is then produced as the child releases the two together. This strategy can be quite effective, but because it requires the child to understand explanation (even if it is accompanied by demonstration), a satisfactory outcome may not be easily achieved.

To teach complex blends, such as *spr* in *spray*, the best strategy - one to be employed with Sam - is as follows. *First* ensure that the /pr/ blend is mastered. If it is not, then teach it by means of the strategy used with Sarah, above. *Second*, ensure that the /s/ has been mastered. If it has not, teach it by means of one of the strategies described in Chapter 12. *Third*, ask Sam to produce a long /s/ sound, and then, after a brief pause, the syllable *pray*. Repeat this step until he has no difficulty in producing a series of the two items on one breath. (This will result in repetitions of *s-pray*.) *Fourth*, have him say the complete word several times on one breath, joining the elements of the blend and pausing between each word. *Fifth*, generalize the production of the blend to other words, such as *sprint*, *sprat*, and *spring*, and then ensure its use in words in sentences and in meaningful discourse. Follow the same basic strategy in teaching other blends of a similar nature, such as those found in words like *scrape*, *squeeze*, and *string*.

Word-final blends can, if necessary, be developed through much the same sorts of strategies as discussed above. It cannot be overemphasized that the amount of formal teaching required to develop blends of either type will decrease in direct proportion to the amount of information a child can receive through his or her hearing aids (or other types of sensory aids), and the amount of effective communicative experience in which the child is engaged. Most final blends contain predominantly high-frequency energy. Even so, single-channel cochlear implants and tactile devices can be very helpful in signalling the presence of certain elements, for example, the released plosive at the end of regular verbs in the past tense in words such as *shopped*. The strategies presented below are for use with those children who need special help in acquiring word-final blends in spite of (or in addition to) a history of using appropriate sensory aids and having abundant experience of communicative interaction.

Word-final blends ending in two continuants can be taught simply by teaching the final element (such as the /s/ sound in *muffs* or the /z/ sound in *comes*) and asking the child to add it to the first part of the word. If necessary, the main part of the word can be associated with a sticker or star on one hand, and the final sound in the blend with another star or sticker on the other. The child is then being asked to produce the appropriate elements when the hands are raised and lowered. This strategy is effective with teaching not only how to signal all plurals and possessives, but how to produce words like *film*, and *listen*.

Words ending in continuant and a stop, such as *lamp, help, laughed, cold, thank* and *ask*, all require the production of the unvoiced sounds /p/, /t/ and /k/ rather than their voiced cognates. This is true even when the word in question is spelled with a final /d/ (as in regular past tense verbs). In citation form (saying the word on its own rather than in the stream of speech), the final consonant is released and such pronunciation can be developed simply by teaching the final element in isolation (one of the rare cases in which isolated plosives occur in English), and adding it to the first part of the word. For example, in the word *lamp* the blend would be developed by *first* teaching the released /p/, *second* having the child say *lam*, *third* asking for the production of *lam - p*, and *fourth* asking for the whole word *lamp*. This strategy has to be used with caution because words containing these blends rarely appear in citation form in running speech, and to teach them as if they do can lead to habitual errors that cause breakdown in normal speech rhythms leading to a reduction of intelligibility. In running speech, these plosives are either released into the vowels that follow them, blended with some subsequent consonants and stopped (produced without release) ahead of other plosives or fricatives.

In words ending with a stop and a continuant, such as *cabs, lips, lids, hits, bags, feeble, supple, tickle*, and *button*, all stops are released through the final continuant. It is extremely important to ensure that intrusive voicing and intrusive aspiration are not introduced in these blends - faults that would, for example, lead to the production of *bags* as *bag*ᵃ*s*, and *lips* as *lip*ʰ*s*. To avoid the risk of such error, the stops ending the first part of the word should be unreleased, and the last part of the word added to the unreleased stop. Thus the stages in helping a boy named Gordon, for example, to develop these word-final blends would be: *first* to ensure that he can produce the final continuants (the /s/, /z/, /l/, and /n/) in word-initial and word-final position in syllables; *second*, to have him arrest the first part of the word with an unreleased stop; *third*, have him produce the word with a brief pause between the unreleased stop and the continuant (for example *bag-s*, *feeb-l*, and *but-n*); and *fourth* ask him to repeat each word several times on one breath, pausing only between complete words. Once the blends are produced normally, words containing them should be used accurately in practice sentences of the type used in everyday life and in meaningful discourse.

Words ending in two stops, such as *apt*, *act*, *bagged*, and *stabbed*, are quite common. They include the past tense of all regular verbs ending in /b/, /p/, /g/, and /k/. The first of the two stops has to be unreleased, and the final stop (usually the /t/, even following voiced sounds) is produced in citation form as an isolated sound (as in *ac-t*). Like continuant-stop blends, the final /t/ can be released through a vowel, or blended with a continuant in running speech (as in *act or get off the stage*, and *she can act really well*). Strategies for teaching stop-stop word-final blends should include a step ensuring that unreleased stops can be properly produced. Complex word-final blends found in words such as *rifts*, *acts*, *asked*, *apples*, and *kittens* are best broken down into components syllables as a first step in formal teaching. Thus one can treat *rifts* as *rift* + *s*, *asked* as *ask* + *t*, and *kittens* as *kit* + *n* + *z*. Providing all other word-initial and word-final blends mastered, complex word-final blends do not pose a serious problem in formal teaching.

suggestions for further reading

Ling (1976), and Calvert and Silverman (1983) deal with teaching the voiced-voicelss distinction at some length. Very few books or articles have covered the teaching of blends to hearing-impaired children. Further information about both the structure and teaching of blends is contained in Ling (1976). See References, pp. 433 ff.

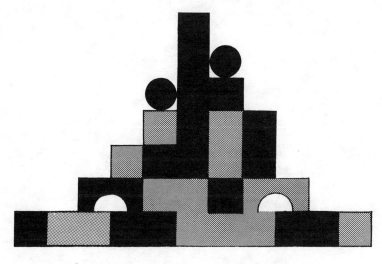

appendices

a. some speech communication guidelines

b. some basic requirements of
   hearing-impaired children and their parents

c. sample questions for students

d. glossary

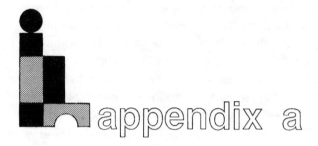

some speech communication guidelines

The material provided in this book suggests a number of important guidelines that may be used by students, professionals, or parents to remind them of the key issues in developing speech communication, and to serve as discussion points in lectures and workshops. Two dozen of them are listed below.

1. Ensure that your hearing-impaired child is wearing appropriate hearing aids (one for each ear), and/or other instruments as prescribed, in order to optimize contact with the acoustic environment; in particular, speech reception and sensory feedback relating to speech production during all waking hours.

2. Talk to a hearing-impaired child clearly, at a normal conversational level, and at close range to ensure optimal speech reception.

3. Be aware of a young child's direction of regard, and talk to him/her about the features in the objects and events that are of interest while he or she is observing them.

4. Follow a child's interests and be alert to his or her focus of attention. Do not constantly try to lead, or exert control over topics of discussion.

5. Talk to children within and about the routine situations in their lives. Such situations offer important and frequently repeated opportunities for communication development, particularly in the early years. The emotional climate of such routines can afford security and pleasure - conditions that are optimal for learning verbal skills.

6. Talk about events and objects that relate to shared experiences. It is only through communication within shared contexts that infants can begin to perceive the significance of language. The context of an interaction can endow an utterance with meaning.

7. Use different voice patterns, particularly intonation, to indicate significant aspects of the speech you address to hearing-impaired children. Tone of voice (prosody) conveys information about the speaker's emotional state and can sometimes convey meaning more effectively than the words in an utterance.

8. Use intonation to mark important elements in utterances. It is a typical feature of the speech of mothers to children (motherese). How clearly a speech pattern can be heard and/or seen (perceptual salience) is a major factor in learning. Function words, prefixes, such as *in*, at the beginning of the word *inadequate*, and suffixes at the end of words, such as the *ed* in *wanted*, and the *ing* in the word *waiting*, can be rendered all the more salient by using prosody appropriately.

9. Allow a child sufficient time to respond in conversational situations. Turn-taking and other conversational skills have to be learned, and a child may not have acquired the skills that permit speedy responses in the early stages of communication growth.

10. Accept the responsibility for understanding the child in the early stages of spoken language acquisition, but gradually shift the responsibility for being understood onto the child. Be aware of the narrow line that separates demanding too little and demanding too much.

11. Talk mainly in complete sentences. An intellectually normal child who is exposed mainly to two-word utterances or simple language is being denied optimal opportunity to deduce the rules governing more complex constructions.

12. Ensure that hearing-impaired children acquire as much as possible of their spoken language in the context of activities provided by normal home life.

13. Provide hearing-impaired children with optimal opportunities for the development of spoken language communication through the close collaboration, and joint commitment of professionals and parents.

14. Be prepared, if you are a parent, to undertake the initial development of your hearing-impaired child's spoken language skills. Others can never give the same amount or quality of time and attention to your child as you can.

15. Be prepared, if you are a professional, to offer support and be a source of information and encouragement to parents. Do not advocate formal teaching of a speech skill to a young child until he or she has failed to acquire that skill following adequate provision of informal learning opportunities.

16. Work as much as possible in one-on-one situations until children have acquired reasonable communication skills.

17. A child who has received mainly one-on-one attention has to learn a different range of speech communication skills if he or she is to interact effectively in a group.

18. Put aside time to play with (rather than work with) your hearing-impaired child. Just enjoying a child will offer an abundance of opportunities to communicate. It will also help everyone to keep things in perspective.

19. Do not begin formal teaching of vowels and consonants until informal learning of spoken language has been given fair trial. It is unproductive to spend time trying to elicit specific speech sounds from children before they are energetically attempting to communicate vocally and verbally with those around them.

20. Remember the complexities of speech production and speech reception, and give hearing-impaired child sufficient time to grasp them before you conclude that he or she is not able to handle them.

21. Use meaningful communication as your base for developing spoken language. It is your only guarantee that you are not attending to one aspect of speech at the expense of other equally important aspects.

22. Optimize children's contact with their hearing peers in order to enhance natural developmental of their spoken language skills.

23. Motivate your child to talk by ensuring that he or she experiences success in the acquisition of spoken language skills, and makes meaningful use of them in speech communication.

24. Adopt an alternative communication system only when experience with good quality perceptual-oral programming has shown it to be necessary. They may impede rather than enhance a given child's development of spoken language.

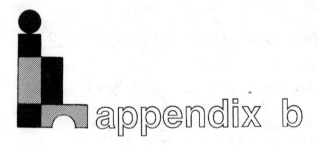

appendix b

some basic requirements of hearing-impaired children and their parents

introduction

Many individual differences are to be found among normally hearing children. On account of hearing problems and their effects, even more individual differences exist among hearing-impaired children. These differences can be adequately catered for only through the provision of different communication modes and various educational methods. No one method or collection of methods can meet the communication and educational needs of all those who are born with or acquire significant degrees of hearing impairment. However, we live in an oral society and, recognizing this, exponents of all methods advocate that hearing-impaired children should learn spoken language. The teaching and learning of perceptual-oral skills is, therefore, at least a part of most programs for such children; whether or not it is a successful part depends on the nature of the diagnostic and treatment programs that are provided. It is commonly held throughout our society that children should be given a fair chance to attain the objectives we set for them. The following points, and the brief discussions on them are centered on the conditions that should exist *if learning to communicate effectively through spoken language is an accepted objective for hearing-impaired children.*

requirements relating to hearing-impaired children

1. *Hearing-impaired children should have access to early and accurate diagnosis of their auditory problems, so that they can have the benefit of early intervention programs.* Significant hearing impairment affects about one child in a thousand at birth and during early infancy. Efficient procedures can lead to detection and diagnosis of such impairment in the first few months of life, and to the early initiation of habilitative treatment. Such early treatment can enhance most hearing-impaired children's potential to become adults who are fully independent members of society at large. It remains to ensure that programs employing such procedures become generally available in all areas where the population is sufficiently large to support them.

2. *Hearing-impaired children require the services and devices that are necessary to promote optimal development of their potential for speech reception and speech production.* Otological and audiological services, and technological devices can do much to enhance the reception of spoken language by most hearing-impaired children. Optimal use of devices for speech reception can, however, be promoted only in perceptual-oral programs. Sign and Cued Speech do not generate acoustic signals that can be transmitted by such devices and children's attention to visual modes of communication can detract from the reception of spoken language.

3. *Hearing-impaired children who have the potential to learn how to communicate fluently through speech require the type of habilitation and educational services that will permit them to achieve that potential.* The greatest opportunities for communicative interchange, personal-social growth and independence, educational achievements, and advancement in employment are open to those who have the best command of spoken language.

4. *Each hearing-impaired child requires the type of treatment that permits him or her to achieve educational and communication skills at an optimal rate.* This requirement implies that no child should be placed in an educational setting that has the potential to hinder the development of spoken language.

5. *Hearing-impaired children require the type of education that permits them to be integrated to the fullest possible extent with their normally hearing peers.* To the extent that they have been segregated from the mainstream of educational endeavor and have had limited contact with their normally hearing peers as children, hearing-impaired individuals are less able than their normally hearing peers to achieve normal socio-economic standing as adults.

6. *Hearing-impaired children attending regular schools as integrated pupils should be provided with such support services as are necessary to maintain their optimal performance in such educational settings.* Support services for hearing-impaired children attending regular schools as integrated pupils is essential if they are to succeed in their school work, avoid undue frustration, and make optimal progress towards competence in spoken language. Such services should include continued audiological management, tutoring in academic subjects that prove to be difficult for them, and specialist assistance to overcome any problems relating to spoken language development.

7. *Hearing-impaired children should be placed in programs that feature ongoing review and revision of their habilitative and educational progress, so that the suitability of the chosen communication mode and the adequacy of their academic achievements is ensured.* In order to ensure that children who are hearing-impaired are learning to communicate as effectively as possible through the use of spoken language, and are progressing academically at optimal rates, habilitative or educational programs must have a diagnostic component, so that factors that hinder or enhance a child's communication skills and educational achievements can be identified, and any necessary remedial support or reinforcement can be provided. Such reviews should include consideration of conditions that could inhibit or enhance carry-over (see Chapter 8).

8. *Hearing-impaired children should be taught by professional personnel who are adequately prepared for the task.* Demographic studies show that the standards of education and speech communication generally achieved by profoundly hearing-impaired children remain abysmally low. Such findings appear to be related to widespread deficits in professional preparation. Specialist teachers of the hearing-impaired should receive more instruction on most aspects of spoken language development and audiological management, particularly as they pertain to early intervention; most speech pathology programs should provide more information and experience relating to the specific problems of hearing-impaired children; and most audiology programs should be somewhat more concerned with auditory management in relation to spoken language development. Professional preparation programs that are specifically geared to the production of specialists with a wider range of skills are required.

9. *Hearing-impaired children who are sufficiently mature should be able to choose the communication mode that best suits their own philosophies and needs as they perceive them.* Unless programs ensure that children develop effective speech communication skills by the time they are mature enough to choose a mode of communication for themselves, they will be deprived of the chance to do so, because, unlike sign language that can be learned at any stage in life, effective spoken language can only be learned in childhood. Those who become most fluent in both sign and speech usually have normal hearing, are hard of hearing, or are adventitiously deafened individuals. Those who most frequently fail to acquire both sign language and spoken language are profoundly hearing-impaired children. The option to choose to communicate through spoken language is, therefore, one that is most often closed to them when their early treatment has been through total communication programs in which sign has predominated over speech.

10. *Hearing-impaired children require access to age-appropriate programs and materials including access to college and university-level programs and specialist training for employment.* Hearing-impaired children are assured of an education in the least restrictive environment by PL 94-142 in the United States and by similar laws in many other countries.

11. *Children with handicaps in addition to hearing impairment require educational placement that is appropriate both for the hearing impairment and the additional handicap.* The proportion of hearing-impaired children who are known to have handicaps in addition to hearing impairment appears to have risen steadily over the past few decades. This apparent increase is due both to the use of better diagnostic procedures that permit recognition of the additional problems and to actual increases related to the causes of hearing impairment and other disabilities. Not all hearing-impaired children with additional disabilities require special education settings. Similarly, not all children with additional disabilities require sign language instruction. Generally, if children are low performers in one communication mode, they are likely to be so in any other mode.

12. *Hearing-impaired children require appropriate special educational help regardless of the difficulties that may be encountered by local education authorities in adjusting provisions to respond to fluctuations in the incidence of hearing impairment.* Individualized educational instruction for certain hearing-impaired children, and appropriate help for their parents are constantly jeopardized by the variation in the numbers of children who require them. This is particularly true in areas where there are small populations. No child should be deprived of optimal educational opportunities because it is administratively inconvenient for an educational authority to provide them.

13. *All hearing-impaired children should have access to appropriate educational help and not be denied it simply for financial reasons.* Children from lower socio-economic groups tend to have much poorer communication skills and educational achievements than children from wealthier families. Their impoverished attainments are in great part due to the limited opportunities afforded them. The cost of providing alternative options, particularly those that feature spoken language acquisition, has led many education authorities to restrict the choices open to parents. The cost of providing optimal opportunities for spoken language acquisition by hearing-impaired children is too often assessed on the basis of the immediate cost of education without regard to the long-term benefits of ensuring that children acquire skills that will lead to them becoming productive adults, able to contribute maximally to society rather than becoming a long-term charge to it.

requirements relating to parents of hearing-impaired children

14. *Parents require fully documented reports on the hearing impairment of their child and should have such reports explained in terms that they can understand, so that they can make informed decisions that affect their child.* Professionals should ensure that parents understand the facts relating to their child's hearing status and amplification needs, and provide them with copies of documented test results. Failure to do this violates the parents' autonomy and prevents them from giving truly informed consent to any form of treatment for their child.

15. *Parents should receive a complete and impartial explanation of the communication modes that can be used with their child, and what procedures are involved in their development, so that they can choose wisely on behalf of themselves and their child.* It must be made clear to parents that: **a)** successful oral education requires appropriate hearing aids or alternative sensory devices, and that attention be given to factors outlined in Chapter 7; **b)** successful Cued Speech programs require most of the family to learn how to cue (a six-to-eight-hour task to learn the cues, plus several weeks to practice them to fluency), and that attention be given to the details provided in Chapter 5; **c)** successful total communication programs require most of the family to learn how to sign (a six-to-twelve-month task to master basic signing, plus several years to become as fluent in sign as most people are in speech).

16. *Parents should have a complete and impartial review of, and should be given the opportunity to study, the types of habilitation or educational settings that might be considered for their child, so that they have the knowledge that permits them to choose the type of program that will have the least restrictive effects on their child's development.* This requirement implies that parents be provided with a clear understanding of, and opportunity to investigate for themselves, the likely implications of choosing a particular mode of communication for their child. They should be encouraged to determine the effects that each mode of communication has had on the development of other hearing-impaired children with similar histories and similar hearing impairments (see Chapter 1).

17. *Parents of young hearing-impaired children require access to parent-infant programs in which they can learn to serve as the primary agents in the habilitation process.* Intervention involving parents and children on a one-to-one basis through the first few years of life can, regardless of the mode of communication chosen, lead to higher levels of overall development than intervention initiated at a later stage.

18. *Parents should be able to select habilitation and educational programs that offer treatment using the mode of communication they prefer for their hearing-impaired children.* Parents should be assured of their children's access to educational settings that employ the mode of communication of their choice. The necessary variety of programs is not yet available in all areas, even where the population is sufficiently large to support them with ease. Oral options are not offered in some localities on the grounds that speech skills can be developed optimally if their children are placed within a total communication setting. Such grounds for limiting the range of options open to parents are not acceptable. Children learn spoken language best in environments where they and their peers use speech as their main means of communication. Available evidence indicates that the simultaneous use of sign and speech tends to impoverish both.

19. *Parents who are unable, for whatever reason, to participate in early habilitation programs as the primary agents of intervention should be helped to place their hearing-impaired children in suitable child-oriented programs.* Hearing-impaired children's early years must be constructively used to promote their spoken language and general development. Parents who are not in position to be at home with their young children should be able to place them in child-centered programs. Child-centered total communication and Cued Speech programs are often less advantageous for children whose parents cannot be the primary agents of habilitation because these modes of communication are usually confined to the habilitation setting. Even over a period of several years, most working parents acquire insufficient signing skills to communicate with their children at any but the most elementary levels.

20. *Parents should be helped to ensure that their children are not assigned to a particular educational setting simply on the basis of their hearing levels.* Many hearing-impaired children in North America who have the potential to remain, or to become, speaking individuals able to function in a hearing society, are assigned to schools where they are taught to regard themselves as "deaf" and unnecessarily, unwillingly, or involuntarily become part of a deaf subculture. Even totally deaf individuals can learn to use spoken language.

recommended further reading

Some of the studies relating to the use of sign language as an alternative, or as a potential supplement, to spoken language communication appear in journal articles rather than books. Bornstein, Saulnier, and Hamilton (1980) record the difficulties that family members have in learning sign and communicating with their hearing-impaired children. Cokely and Baker (1980), Marmor and Pettito (1979), and Huntingdon and Watton (1986), among others, show that high rates of inaccuracy in both speech and sign tend to occur during their simultaneous presentation. Jensema and Trybus (1978) show that sign language is negatively correlated with academic attainments and spoken language skills, and Subtelny and Snell (1988), as well as Schildroth and Karchmer (1986), have found negative correlations between aural-oral skills and sign language. These studies are but a few of the many that indicate that the acquisition of oral skills, and to a lesser extent educational achievements, are by and large incompatible with the use of sign language. However, hearing-impaired children of hearing-impaired parents appear to be an exception, probably because their parents are fluent in the use of the language that is addressed to them from the earliest days of their infancy (see Geers, Moog, and Schick, 1984; Geers and Schick, 1988). More discussion and a wider perspective on the relative merits and problems of early intervention through both spoken language and total communication are provided by the various contributors to two books edited by the writer (Ling, 1984a; 1984b). See References, pp. 433 ff.

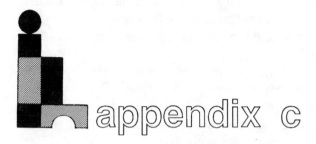

sample questions
for students

The sample questions in this appendix have been used as the basis of discussions in lectures and workshops. They are a useful guide to the range of introductory-level knowledge that is required in order to promote the development of spoken language in hearing-impaired children of different age levels. The following questions, and variations on them, can be answered simply from reading this particular text. However, a more extensive study of the various topics discussed is strongly recommended. Such study might involve further reading (of the materials suggested at the end of each chapter, and of new texts as they become available), discussions, and guided practical experience. More advanced questions, are, of course, also recommended for the more advanced student.

chapter 1.

1. List ten of the activities that are involved in producing and perceiving spoken language.

2. What are the differences between speech and language?

3. Discuss the various conditions that best promote perceptual-oral language skills.

4. In what ways are pre-verbal behaviors important to the later development of spoken language?

5. What guidelines would you adopt to ensure that parents make a wise choice of communication mode for their child?

6. What are some of the most important components of early auditory-verbal programs?

7. In what ways may spoken language development be affected by the new environmental conditions a child may meet as he or she becomes older?

8. What range of professional activities are appropriate for a school-based speech communication specialist?

9. Discuss the principles and practices that underlie the effective promotion of carry-over of spoken language skills from lessons to life.

10. What factors may inhibit the development of spoken language, and how may the obstacles they pose be overcome?

chapter 2.

1. Describe the three dimensions of sound.

2. List the frequencies of the ten lowest harmonics of a voice having a fundamental frequency of 125 Hz.

3. Briefly describe the vocal tract, and state which organs contribute most to the differentiation of speech sounds.

4. How are formants produced, and how important are they to intelligibility?

5. How could knowing the formant frequencies of the vowels assist professional personnel in the selection of sensory aids for hearing-impaired children?

6. What are formant transitions, and how do they help in consonant recognition?

7. What are the main acoustic cues differentiating consonants by their manner of production, and over what frequency range do they occur?

8. How does place of consonant production affect the frequency characteristics of speech?

9. Coarticulation is the production of strings of adjacent sounds in the stream of speech. Say why skills in the articulation of isolated sounds are less important for speech intelligibility than coarticulation skills.

10. What forms of feedback on speech production are available to all hearing-impaired children?

chapter 3.

1. Briefly describe the components of the auditory system.

2. Give a simple account of how the components of the auditory system act to transmit speech signals in ways that permit their perception.

3. State how malfunction of the various parts of the auditory system can result in different forms of hearing impairment.

4. Specify four levels of processing in the perception of speech and describe how each level can be affected by different levels of hearing impairment.

5. Compare and contrast the major effects of prelingual and postlingual hearing impairment.

6. What is an air-bone gap, and what does its presence signify?

7. In which frequency band does the nasal murmur occur? What steps would you take to ensure that a child is able to detect the nasal consonants in conversational speech?

8. Discuss variations in the intensity levels of speech sounds. State why they occur, and use differences between particular speech sounds to illustrate your answer.

9. Give five examples showing how The Five-Sound Test can be used to advantage in the context of a habilitation program.

10. Construct four typical audiograms having widely different configurations, and specify the range of sounds that children with such audiograms would be unable to detect without amplification.

chapter 4.

1. What do you consider to be the goals of hearing aid selection?
2. Describe the various sorts of personal hearing aids that are currently available.
3. What effects may the various types of earmolds have on the transmission of speech, and how should they be taken into account in hearing aid selection?
4. Provide an account of the hearing aid selection procedures used by audiologists in your locality.
5. For what reasons may the amplification needs of prelingually hearing-impaired children differ from those of adventitiously hearing-impaired adults with similarly severe hearing levels?
6. Discuss the concepts *dynamic range of hearing* and *dynamic range of speech* in relation to the process of hearing aid selection.
7. What outcome measures or observations might lead you to accept or reject the assertion that a hearing aid selection procedure had resulted in the provision of optimal amplification for a hearing-impaired child?
8. Explain how aided audiograms could help you determine whether selected hearing aids permit a child to detect particular components of speech.
9. Discuss the advantages of charting audiograms in dB SPL rather than dB HL.
10. In what ways have the growth and the products of technology over the past few decades led to new ways of thinking about the acquisition of auditory skills by hearing-impaired children?

chapter 5.

1. One has to perceive speech as it is spoken by others, and also as one produces it oneself (through feedback) in order to learn to talk. Indicate how the various senses might be used to promote the perceptual aspects of perceptual-oral skills.
2. Discuss the concept of speechreading as (a) a primary, and (b) a supplementary speech communication channel.

3. Describe the advantages that Cued Speech might offer a totally deaf child who could not benefit from a cochlear implant.

4. Select six speech patterns that can be visually confused through speechreading, and suggest how the direct, natural use of touch could be employed to resolve each of the ambiguities.

5. What factors would encourage you to select a tactile device as a communication aid for a child?

6. What factors would encourage you to select a cochlear implant as a communication aid for a child?

7. How might different modes of communication affect a child's acquisition of skill in using either a tactile device or a cochlear implant?

8. How could one judge whether the use of a tactile device or a cochlear implant is actually benefitting the child for whom it was selected?

9. What do you consider to be the most important ethical issues relating to the selection of the various technological aids to speech reception?

10. What sense modalities can be used to ensure that a child develops control over the suprasegmental aspects of speech?

chapter 6.

1. Suggest ten good reasons for generally using complete sentences in talking to hearing-impaired children. What exceptions would you make to such usage?

2. Define phonemes and morphemes and say how they relate to spoken language.

3. Why are function words important components of a language? Suggest a half-dozen reasons for the difficulty some hearing-impaired children might have in acquiring them.

4. Discuss the acquisition of syntax by hearing-impaired children, and describe some of the steps you would take to ensure the development of syntactic abilities in: a) a preschool, b) an elementary school and, c) a high school child.

5. How can you determine whether a hearing-impaired child's language is developing in semantically appropriate ways?

6. Suggest ways in which educational programs can encourage the pragmatic integrity of young, hearing-impaired children's language.

7. Discuss the ways in which parents can encourage the development of a hearing-impaired child's skill in understanding and producing narratives.

8. Write a short play that records the sequences and types of interaction that might take place between a clinician or teacher and a hearing-impaired eight-year-old girl over a ten-minute period. The objective of the play is to illustrate the adult's use of effective strategies for developing the child's conversational skills.

9. (a) Suggest a half-dozen different, meaningful contexts that would permit a parent to focus on developing a young child's ability to formulate a particular type of question. **(b)** Repeat the exercise to indicate how at least five other question forms could also be developed within contexts that are meaningful to the child.

10. List a dozen of the most important things that parents should do in order to encourage a two-year-old child's acquisition of spoken language.

chapter 7.

1. Explain why strategies for both formal teaching and informal learning are likely to be required to develop high standards of spoken language among profoundly hearing-impaired children.

2. Outline the factors that influence the acquisition of perceptual-oral skills by hearing-impaired children. Explain why each factor is important.

3. How would you evaluate (or obtain evaluations of) each of the factors influencing a hearing-impaired child's progress in the acquisition of perceptual-oral skills?

4. Using the algorithm depicted in Figure 7-2, and the rationale presented for promoting informal learning, describe the steps you would take to help different children develop and employ in their communicative speech: a) an intonation pattern, b) a vowel, c) an alveolar consonant, and d) a consonant blend.

5. How may the promotion of informal learning be affected by the extent of a child's hearing impairment and the nature of particular speech patterns? Give examples using different children and different speech patterns to illustrate your points.

6. Examine a dozen aspects of language that can become meaningful to a child only when the concepts underlying them are developed through social experience and social interaction. *Or* discuss the possibilities and limitations of computer-aided instruction in developing knowledge and meaningful use of various aspects of spoken language in hearing-impaired children.

7. Discuss the acquisition of reading skills and the acquisition of language. In what ways might the one enhance, fail to enhance, or even inhibit the other?

8. Discuss the concrete-abstract dimension of language, and describe a half-dozen of the ways in which you would seek to help hearing-impaired children develop the ability to comprehend, generate, and express abstract notions.

9. Discuss the formal spoken language teaching that you have observed, and examine the steps that were taken by clinicians, teachers, or caregivers to ensure that skills taught were carried over from lessons into everyday life. How would you rate the adequacy of the steps taken, and what would you do to ensure that such carry-over is achieved?

10. Using the algorithm depicted in Figure 7-3, and the rationale presented for the use of formal speech teaching, describe the formal strategies that you would use to help different children develop and employ in their communicative speech: a) an intonation pattern, b) a vowel, c) an alveolar consonant, and d) a consonant blend.

chapter 8.

1. Specify the seven stages in Ling's model of speech acquisition, and evaluate the model as a guideline for sequencing the development of both phonologic and phonetic-level skills.

2. Phonologic-level evaluation is a criterion referenced procedure that provides more useful information for the purposes of developing spoken language than tests of speech intelligibility. Discuss this statement, and examine the view that the information yielded by a phonological evaluation is sufficiently important to justify the time spent in doing it.

3. On what basis would you select the sense modality that you would employ to develop a particular speech pattern? To what extent and in what ways could tactile and kinesthetic cues contribute to the learning and maintenance of any such pattern?

4. To what extent do you consider the selection and use of a particular sense modality for enabling a given aspect of spoken language to be perceived to be an intrinsic part of a speech development program? Why may it not be realistic to rely on auditory-oral instruction or explanation in sign language to develop the necessary perceptual-oral skills?

5. On what basis would you select the sense modality that you would employ to develop a particular speech pattern, and to what extent could tactile and kinesthetic sensation contribute to the development and maintenance of any such pattern?

6. It has been said that teaching and learning involve proceeding from the known to the unknown, the easy to the difficult, and the simple to the complex. Discuss this statement in relation to the provision of anticipatory set.

7. Should syntactic, semantic, and pragmatic aspects of language, as well as the phonologic aspects of speech, be developed to high levels of automaticity? Justify your views in relation to the four components of automaticity: accuracy, speed, economy of effort and flexibility.

8. Speech skills that are acquired in lessons or clinical sessions must be carried over into meaningful spoken language if they are to be used effectively in everyday perceptual-oral communication. What conditions would you seek to establish in order to ensure that skills acquired by a profoundly hearing-impaired child at the phonetic level become an integral part of his or her spoken language?

9. A profoundly hearing-impaired girl has somewhat nasal speech and, on this account, you predict that she will have difficulty in producing consonants, particularly fricatives in running speech. You decide that immediate action should be taken to overcome the problem. Outline the steps you would take to ensure that the prerequisites for later speech acquisition are acquired by the child.

10. How many target behaviors would you include in a spoken language lesson, and how would you determine what they should be?

chapter 9.

1. Describe the speech errors of an eight-year-old, hearing-impaired girl that you might meet in a special class for the deaf, and say what remedial measures you would consider using to help her overcome them.

2. How might (a) a six-year-old girl and (b) a sixteen-year-old girl, both profoundly hearing-impaired, be motivated to improve their spoken language?

3. What steps could you take to ensure that a two-year-old, profoundly hearing-impaired boy who is just beginning to talk, would maintain normal breathing for speech as he continued to develop spoken language?

4. A six-year-old boy joins the class you teach. He smacks his lips as he attempts to produce plosives. You (rightly) consider poor oral breath flow to be the major problem. He has no organic deficits. How would you treat him?

5. Make notes on the many ways in which you, as the parent of a profoundly hearing-impaired baby boy, would encourge him to vocalize and to acquire a wide range of voice and speech patterns.

6. When, and for what reasons, might you consider introducing formal teaching strategies to develop a hearing-impaired child's breath and voice control? You are currently promoting spoken language development with this child through the use of informal learning strategies in a parent-infant program.

7. Why would you want to spend time on the development of control over intensity, duration, and fundamental frequency when a child's vowels, diphthongs, consonants, and consonant blends are not clearly produced?

8. What influences might currently available aids, devices, or instruments have on the development of prosody among hearing-impaired children?

9. How might a child be helped to learn how to whisper and to produce utterances in a quiet, moderate, and loud voice?

10. Outline the remedial steps that you would take to help a ten-year-old profoundly hearing-impaired child with a monotonous voice acquire acceptable intonation patterns, and to use them in communicative speech?

chapter 10.

1. Complete an aided audiogram for each of the children whose unaided hearing levels are shown in Figure 10-1. Assume that each has optimal binaural amplification. State what vowels might be detected, confused, or identified by each of the three children through aided audition alone.

2. What vowel errors have hearing-impaired children typically acquired in traditional educational programs. State how modern perceptual-oral provision might prevent their occurrence.

3. (a) In what ways are back, central and front vowels acoustically different? (b) For what reasons might speechreading be regarded as providing inadequate information for the acquisition of vowels by profoundly hearing-impaired children?

4. Why are oo, ah, and ee such important vowels for children to develop?

5. What teaching strategies that have been used, or are currently being used, with hearing-impaired children might lead to inappropriate tongue movements in vowel production?

6. Suggest several ways in which the acquisition of front vowels by hearing-impaired children can be encouraged. Consider both formal and informal strategies.

7. The F_2 transitions associated with the various vowels are important to a listener's perception of consonants. Say why this is so, and how you would attempt to ensure that such transitions would be optimally perceived and produced by severely hearing-impaired children.

8. Why may back vowels provide the best physical and acoustical context for the teaching of certain consonants to profoundly hearing-impaired children?

9. Discuss the means by which diphthongs can be developed and later employed in discourse by children with different levels of hearing impairment.

10. Discuss (a) generalization and (b) carry-over in relation to the acquisition and the use of vowels in spoken language.

chapter 11.

1. Can most manner distinctions usually be acquired through informal learning by profoundly hearing-impaired children? Give the reasons for your positive or negative response to this question.

2. What manners of consonant production are: (a) most likely and (b) least likely to be confused through speechreading alone?

3. Discuss the difficulties profoundly hearing-impaired children have in the acquisition of the nasal /m/, and suggest reasons for the frequency with which remedial work on nasality is needed. Say how you would approach the task of: (a) preventing and (b) overcoming problems with the nasal/non-nasal distinction among such children.

4. Why is it regarded as important that certain children acquire the unvoiced th in the early stages of consonant acquisition?

5. Describe a simple developmental and remedial strategy that can be used to prevent or overcome intrusive plosion in nasals and fricatives.

6. Discuss the merits and the problems associated with the use of direct (natural) touch in teaching manner distictions among consonants to profoundly hearing-impaired children.

7. Suggest activities that could help promote carry- over of the production of manner distinctions among consonants from speech lessons into everyday life.

8. What phonetic and phonologic skills are prerequisites for the formal teaching of manner distinctions among consonants?

9. How would you determine whether further phonetic level or phonologic level teaching might be required in order to automatize a child's production of consonants differing in manner of production?

10. (a) What sort of spoken language would you expect of a child who is in the process of learning to produce manner distinctions in consonants? (b) What phonologic targets might be considered for a child at this stage of speech acquisition?

chapter 12.

1. Specify the acoustic cues that permit the perception of place distinctions among consonants. To what extent, and in what ways, might profoundly hearing-impaired children be made aware of such cues?

2. Describe a half-dozen ways in which set could be used to teach some aspect of grammar, or develop some aspect of discourse.

3. State how you would seek to integrate previously learned aspects of spoken language with the informal learning of various alveolar sounds by young, hearing-impaired children.

4. Fricatives and nasals in word-initial position are habitually followed by intrusive plosion in the speech of a severely hearing-impaired eight-year-old girl. What steps would you take to deal with the problem?

5. Describe some of the generalization procedures you would use to ensure that fricatives differing in manner and place of production, once elicited, could be produced with all vowels at a phonetic level?

6. What sort of strategies might be used to exploit available sense modalities in order to elicit alveolar sounds from a totally deaf child, and to develop their use in spoken language communication?

7. In what ways would you seek to enhance carry-over of the alveolar consonants? Are there both similarities and differences between the carry-over strategies you would employ for these and for other consonants?

8. Assume that a severely hearing-impaired child has begun to use the /s/ in some of the function words listed in Chapter 12, but does not use the /s/ morpheme in everyday speech. How would you set about ensuring the carry-over of the /s/ to all aspects of spoken language?

9. Discuss the possibilities and limitations of using the sense of touch in the teaching of place distinctions in consonant production by severely and profoundly hearing-impaired children.

10. Rank order the consonants discussed in Chapter 12 in relation to the difficulty profoundly hearing-impaired children might have in acquiring and using them in discourse. Justify the decisions you make in carrying out this task.

chapter 13.

1. In what ways can the auditory, visual, tactile, and kinesthetic sensations experienced by a profoundly hearing-impaired child assist in the acquisition and use of plosive consonants differing in place of production?

2. Some consonants can be more easily elicited from hearing-impaired children in certain contexts than in others. Discuss the idea that facilitating contexts may exist for every consonant. Give examples that illustrate your points.

3. What differences are there between the informal learning strategies and the formal teaching strategies that you would use in promoting the acquisition of palatal and velar consonants by profoundly hearing-impaired children?

4. What are some of the major problems that a teacher or clinician might meet in developing the use of fricatives by hearing-impaired children? What are the common causes of such problems, and what remedial procedures would you adopt to treat them?

5. What are the prerequisites for the production of the sounds discussed in Chapter 13? How would you verify that they are present before you set out to elicit such speech patterns?

6. You have elicited the ng from a profoundly hearing- impaired, six-year-old child by means of a tactile strategy. What steps would you take to generalize production of the ng, and to ensure its carry-over into everyday communication?

7. Under what conditions might it be helpful to suppress speechreading cues in order to promote a severely hearing-impaired child's perception of sh through other sense modalities?

8. What sort of spoken language skills would you expect a child to have acquired by the time that he or she has mastered the production of consonants differing in place of production?

9. Discuss the concept of speech correction, and state how you would deal with a situation in which a child produces all speech sounds clearly at a phonetic level, but uses barely intelligible speech in everyday life.

10. You attempt to elicit a target pattern through imitation, but although the profoundly hearing-impaired girl you are teaching tries to respond appropriately, her attempt to reproduce the speech pattern is unacceptably off target. Describe your immediate response to the child, say how you would analyze the problem, and specify the principles on which you would base further attempts to elicit that target pattern.

chapter 14.

1. Describe the ways in which the voiced-voiceless distinction among consonants may be influenced by adjacent sounds.

2. How would you integrate the child's acquisition of the voiced-voiceless distinction and blends with the skills that a child had acquired at all previous stages of spoken language devlopment?

3. For what reasons may formal teaching of the voiced-voiceless distinction be left until manner and place of consonant production have been developed?

4. Rank order as many strategies as you can for evoking the voiced-voiceless distinction on a scale of relative difficulty. Include strategies that are known to you but not included in this book. Provide a rationale for arranging the strategies in the selected order.

5. You have just evoked a voiced th from a profoundly hearing-impaired child. Describe the steps you plan to take in order to generalize its phonetic level production.

6. You have worked with a profoundly hearing-impaired, six-year-old girl, and she has successfully generalized productions of voiced-voiceless distinctions at the phonetic level. Describe the strategies that you would have in place to ensure the carry over of such distinctions into everyday discourse.

7. Describe formal strategies that can be used to evoke and develop production of all types of blends. Which of these do you prefer using, and why?

8. Outline the possible reasons for severely hearing- impaired children aged three, six, and nine years of age omitting some of the final consonants in word-final blends, and say what steps you would take to deal with this problem.

9. What levels of spoken language skills would you expect to find among children who had acquired a few word-initial and word-final blends?

10. How would you determine whether a hearing-impaired child had achieved adequate mastery of all blends, and on what grounds would you decide that no further teaching of consonant blending skills is necessary?

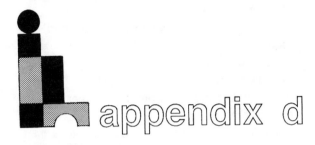

appendix d

glossary

This glossary contains explanations of the uncommon or technical words that are used in this text. So far as possible, they are also explained as they appear. All of them are necessary for adequate understanding of the material presented here, as well as for the appreciation of other books and articles relating to perceptual-oral development in hearing-impaired children. Effective perceptual-oral habilitation and education involve making optimal use of hearing-impaired children's senses and cognitive skills in developing their perception and production of spoken language. Those concerned with such children must be familiar with the vocabulary used by other individuals who write about, talk about, or work with them. The vocabulary presented below is likely, therefore, to prove useful not only to students and parents as an aid in reading this book, but as a help in communicating with various professionals about childhood deafness.

allophones: different forms of the same sounds.

alveolar ridge: the ridge just behind the top teeth.

anoxia: lack of oxygen.

approximation: an intelligible, but inaccurately pronounced utterance.

articulation: movement of tongue lips and jaw to create sounds.

articulatory: to do with the movements involved in talking.

audiogram: a graph showing an individual's hearing levels.

audiometer: the instrument used to measure hearing.

audiometric: measures of hearing.

bimodal: the use of two senses - e.g., hearing and vision.

binaural: of or for both ears.

blend: two or more adjacent consonants produced together.

caregiver: any person caring for a child.

clavicle: the collar-bone.

clavicular: (breathing): using the upper chest rather than the diaphragm.

coarticulation: preparing and producing more than one sound at a time.

cochlea: the inner ear (see Figure 3-1).

cochlear: belonging to the cochlea.

conjoining: adding two sentences to make them one (often with *and*).

cutaneous: pertaining to the skin.

CV syllable: syllable made up of a consonant and a vowel.

CVC syllable: syllable made up of a consonant, vowel, and consonant.

decibel (dB): one tenth of a Bel; the unit of sound measurement.

diaphragm: the muscle separating the chest and abdomen.

diphthongs: two vowels making a single sound, like /au/ in *cow*.

discourse: purposeful use of several sentences in an utterance.

dyad: two individuals treated as a pair; usually mother and child.

earmold: the plastic form coupling the hearing aid and the ear.

electro-cochlear: electrical stimulation of the inner ear.

electro-tactile: stimulation of the skin by an electric signal.

ellipsis: deliberate omission of a word or words in a sentence.

ERA	electrical response audiometry.
formants:	peaks of vocal resonance.
frication:	turbulence created by forcing air through a narrow space.
fricative:	sounds that have turbulent breath flow such as /f/ and s<u>h</u>
function words:	relational words that clarify the meaning of sentences.
glottal:	originating at the vocal cords.
glottis:	the space between the vocal cords.
grapheme:	a written letter of the alphabet.
interlexical:	between words.
intervocalic:	between vowels; as /r/ in *hurrah*.
kinesthesis:	sensation arising from movement.
kinesthetic:	pertaining to kinesthesis.
labial:	pertaining to the lips.
labio-dental:	a sound made with involvement of the lips and teeth.
LDL:	Loudness discomfort level: when sound just becomes too loud.
lipreading:	understanding speech by watching the lips.
meatal:	pertaining to the ear canal.
meatus:	(me-ey-tus) the ear canal.
microPascals:	(abb. μPa); the units used for specifying sound pressure.
modality:	a sensory channel such as hearing, vision, or touch.
monaural:	of or for only one ear.
morpheme:	the smallest unit of meaning (word or part of a word).
morphophonemic:	relating to the the form and meaning of words.
Motherese:	the style of speech many mothers use with their children.
neural:	relating to the nerves.(neural damage = nerve damage).
non-verbal:	not related to words.
operant:	something acting to encourage particular behavior.

ossicles:	small bones (e.g., those in the middle ear).
otitis media:	inflammation of the middle ear.
otolaryngologist:	a physician specializing in ear, nose, and throat.
otoscope:	the instruments used to look into the ear canal.
pharyngeal:	pertaining to the pharynx.
pharynx:	the area at the back of the mouth.
phoneme:	the smallest sound in a language that carries meaning.
phonemic:	pertaining to phonemes.
phonologic:	pertaining to phonology, the sounds of meaningful speech.
pinna:	the outer ear.
plosive:	a sound with explosive quality such as /p/, /d/ and /k/.
post-vocalic;	after a vowel; e.g., the er in *mother*.
pragmatics:	the purpose-related aspects of language.
probe-tube:	small tube with microphone for measuring in-the-ear SPL (sound pressure level).
proprioception:	awareness of self-generated sensations.
prosody:	the tune and rhythm of utterances.
retroflexion:	turning the tongue tip up and back, as for /r/.
segmental:	consonants and vowels are segmental elements of speech.
semantics:	the meaning-related aspects of language.
sensori-neural:	involving the cochlear and/or the auditory nerve.
spectrogram:	a chart showing speech intensity, frequency and duration.
spectrographic:	pertaining to making, displaying or analyzing spectrograms.
speechreading:	understanding speech by watching the talker.
SPL:	sound pressure level (measured in microPascals).
suprasegmental:	prosodic - relating to the tune and rhythm of speech.
supra-threshold:	the range of hearing above threshold.
syntax:	the system of rules governing the creation of sentences.
tactile:	pertaining to touch. (Tactile devices work through touch).

transducer:	a device that changes one form of energy to another.
transformation:	operation changing a sentence form, but retaining its meaning.
tympanometry:	measuring ear drum movement.
tympanus:	the ear drum.
unimodal:	involving only one of the senses.
unisensory:	involving only one sense - usually hearing.
velar:	the sounds made with the tongue at or near the velum.
velo-pharyngeal port:	the opening between the velum and the pharynx.
velum:	the soft palate - the movable part at the back.
vibro-tactile:	stimulation of the skin by means of vibration.
vocalic:	in the context of vowels.
VRA:	visual response audiometry.
word-final:	the position of the last sound or sounds in a word.
word-initial:	the position of the first sound or sounds in a word.

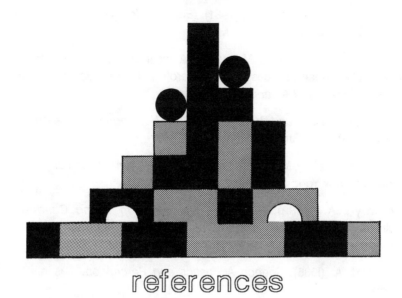

references

Baer, T. Sasaki, C. and Harris, K. (1987). (Eds.) *Laryngeal Function in Phonation and Respiration*. Boston: Little, Brown and Company.

Beasley, D.S. (1984). (Ed.) *Audition in Childhood*. San Diego: College-Hill Press.

Berg, F.S. (1987). *Facilitating Classroom Listening: A Handbook for Teachers of Normal and Hard-of-Hearing Students*. San Diego: College-Hill Press.

Berger, K.W. (1972). *Speechreading: Principles and Methods*. Baltimore: National Educational Press.

Berliner, K.I. and House, W.F. (1981). Cochlear implants: An overview and bibliography. *American Journal of Otology, 2, 277-282.*

Berliner, K.I. and House, W.F. (1982). The cochlear implant program: An overview. *Annals of Otology, Rhinology and Laryngology Suppl. 91, 11-14.*

Bess, F.H. (1988). *Hearing Impairment in Children*. Parkton: York Press, Inc.

Bess, F.H., Freeman, B.A., and Sinclair, J.S. (1981). *Amplification in Education.* Washington, D.C.: A.G. Bell Association for the Deaf.

Bess, F.H. and McConnell, F.E. (1981). (Eds.) *Audiology, Education, and the Hearing-Impaired*. St. Louis: Mosby.

Blamey. P.J. and Clark, G.M. (1985). A wearable multiple-electrode electrotactile speech processor for the profoundly deaf. *Journal of the Acoustical Society of America, 77, 1619-1621.*

Blank, M., Rose, S.A. and Berlin, L.J. (1978). *The Language of Learning*. New York: Grune & Stratton.

Bloom, L. and Lahey, M. (1978). *Language Development and Language Disorders.* New York: John Wiley and Sons.

Boothroyd, A. (1982). *Hearing Impairments in Young Children.* Englewood Cliffs: Prentice-Hall, Inc. Washington, D.C.: A.G. Bell Association for the Deaf.

Boothroyd, A. (l986). *Speech Acoustics and Perception*. Austin, TX: Pro-Ed.

Bornstein, H., Saulnier K.L., and Hamilton, L.B. (1980). Signed English: A first evaluation. *American Annals of the Deaf, 125, 467-481.*

Breeuwer, M. and Plomp, R. (1985). Speechreading supplemented with formant-frequency information from voiced speech. *Journal of the Acoustical Society of America 77, 314-317.*

Bricker, W. and Bricker, D. (1970). A program of language training for the severely handicapped child. *Exceptional Children 37, 101-111.*

Bromwich, R. (1981). *Working with Parents and Infants*. Baltimore: University Park Press.

Bronfenbrenner, U. (1975). Is early intervention effective? in M. Guttentag and F. Steunig (Eds.) *Handbook of Education Research, Vol. 2* Beverly Hills: Sage Publications.

Bullowa, M. (1979). *Before Speech*. Cambridge: Cambridge University Press.

Bunch, G.O. (1987). *The Curriculum and the Hearing-Impaired Student.* San Diego: College-Hill Press.

Calvert D.R. and Silverman S.R. (1983). *Speech and Deafness* (Revised Edition). Washington, D.C.: A.G. Bell Association for the Deaf.

Carney, A.E., and Beachler, C.R. (1986). Vibrotactile perception of suprasegmental features of speech: A comparison of single-channel and multi-channel instruments. *Journal of the Acoustical Society of America, 79, 131-140.*

Chomsky, N. (1957). *Syntactic Structures.* The Hague: Mouton.

Chomsky, N. (1981). *Lectures on Government and Binding.* Dordrecht, Holland: Foris.

Clark, G.M. et al. (1987a). *The University of Melbourne-Nucleus Multi-electrode Cochlear Implant.* Basel: Karger.

Clark, G.M., et al. (1987b). Preliminary results for the cochlear corporation multielectrode intracochlear implant in six prelingually deaf patients.*The American Journal of Otology, 8, 234-239.*

Clark, H.H. and Clark, E.V. (1977). *Psychology and Language.* New York: Harcourt Brace Jovanovich, Inc.

Cokely, D. and Baker, C. (1980). Problems with rate and deletions in simultaneous communication. *Directions, 1, 22.*

Cole, E. and Gregory, H. (1986). (Eds.) *Auditory Learning.* Washington, D.C.: A.G. Bell Association for the Deaf.

Cornett, R.O. Cued Speech. (1967). *American Annals of the Deaf, 112, 3-13.*

Crystal, D. (1981). *Clinical Linguistics.* New York: Springer-Verlag.

Crystal, D., Fletcher, P., and Garman, M. (1976). *The Grammatical Analysis of Language Disability: A Procedure for Assessment and Remediation.* London: Arnold.

DeFilippo, C.L. (1984). Laboratory projects in tactile aids to lipreading. *Ear and Hearing, 5, 211-227.*

DeFilippo, C.L. and Sims, D.G. (Eds.) (1988). *New Reflections on Speechreading. Monograph of the Volta Review* Washington, D.C.: A.G. Bell Association for the Deaf.

Dodd, B. and Campbell, R. (Eds.) (1987). *Hearing by Eye: The Psychology of Lip Reading.* Hillsdale, NJ: Erlbaum.

Erber, N.P. (1985). *Telephone Communication and Hearing Impairment.* San Diego: College-Hill Press.

Ewing, A.W.G. and Ewing, E.C. (1964). *Teaching Deaf Children to Talk.* Manchester: Manchester University Press.

Fey, M. (1986). *Language Intervention with Young Children.* San Diego: College-Hill Press.

Fletcher, P. and Garman, M. (1986). *Language Acquisition (2nd Ed).* Cambridge: Cambridge University Press.

Forner, L.L. and Hixon, T.J. (1977). Respiratory kinematics in profoundly hearing-impaired speakers. *Journal of Speech and Hearing Research, 20, 373-408.*

Gallagher, T.M. and Prutting, C.A. (1983). (Eds.) *Pragmatic Assessment and Intervention Issues in Language.* San Diego: College-Hill Press.

Geers, A.E., Moog, J.S., and Schick, B. (1984). Acquisition of spoken and signed English by profoundly deaf children. *Journal of Speech and Hearing Disorders 49, 378-388.*

Geers, A.E. and Schick, B. (1988). Acquisition of spoken and signed English by hearing-impaired children of hearing-impaired or hearing parents. *Journal of Speech and Hearing Disorders, 53, 136-143.*

Gerber, A. (1973). *Goal: Carryover.* Philadelphia: Temple University Press.

Grant, J. (1987). *The Hearing-Impaired: Birth to Six.* San Diego: College-Hill Press.

Halliday, M.A.K. and Hasan, R. (1976). *Cohesion in English.*London: Longman.

Haycock, G.S. (1933). *The Teaching of Speech.* Washington, D.C.: A.G. Bell Association for the Deaf.

Hixon, T.J. and collaborators (1987). *Respiratory Function in Speech and Song.* San Diego: College-Hill Press.

Hochberg, I, Levitt, H., and Osberger, M.J. (1983). (Eds.) *Speech of the Hearing-Impaired.* Baltimore, MD: University Park Press.

Huntingdon, A., and Watton, F. (1986). The spoken language of teachers and pupils in the education of hearing-impaired children. *The Volta Review, 88, 5-19.*

Hyams, N.M. (1986). *Language Acquisition and the Theory of Parameters.* Dordrecht: D. Reidel Publishing Company.

Jeffers, J. and Barley, M. (1971). *Speechreading.* Springfield, IL.: Charles C Thomas.

Jensema, C.J. and Trybus, R.H. (1978). *Communication Patterns and Educational Achievement of Hearing-Impaired Students.* Washington DC.: Office of Demographic Studies.

Jerger, J. (1984). (Ed.) *Pediatric Audiology.* San Diego: College-Hill Press.

Jung, J.H. et al. (1989). *Genetic Syndromes in Communication Disorders.* Boston: Little Brown and Company.

Killion, M.C. (1981). Earmold options for wideband hearing aids. *Journal of Speech and Hearing Disorders, 46, 10-20.*

Kintsch, W. (1974). *The Representation of Meaning in Memory.* Hillsdale, NJ: Lawrence Erlbaum.

Kretschmer, R. (1985). (Ed.) *Learning to Write and Writing to Learn.* Monograph of *The Volta Review.* Washington, D.C.: A.G. Bell Association for the Deaf.

Kretschmer, R.R. and Kretschmer, L.W. (1978). *Language development and intervention with the hearing-impaired.* Baltimore: University Park Press.

Lack, A. (1955). *The Teaching of Language to Deaf Children.* London: Oxford University Press.

Lauter, J.L. (1985). (Ed.) Proceedings of the Conference on the Planning and Production of Speech in Normal and Hearing-Impaired Individuals: A Seminar in Honor of S. Richard Silverman. *ASHA Reports, 15.*

Lieberman, P. (1972). *Speech Acoustics and Perception.* Indianapolis: Bobbs Merrill.

Ling, D. (1976). *Speech and the Hearing-Impaired Child: Theory and Practice.* Washington, D.C.: A.G. Bell Association for the Deaf.

Ling, D. (1984a). (Ed.) *Early intervention for Hearing-Impaired Children: Oral Options.* San Diego: College-Hill Press.

Ling D. (l984b). (Ed.) *Early Intervention for Hearing-Impaired Children: Total Communication Options.* San Diego: College-Hill Press.

Ling, D. and Ling, A.H. (1971). *Basic Vocabulary and Language Thesaurus for Hearing-Impaired Children.* Washington, D.C.: A.G. Bell Association for the Deaf.

Ling, D. and Ling, A.H. (1978). *Aural Habilitation: The Foundations of Verbal Learning.* Washington, D.C.: A.G. Bell Association for the Deaf.

Luterman, D. (1987). *Deafness in the family.* Boston: Little, Brown and Company.

Lybarger, S.L. (1985). Earmolds. In J.Katz (Ed.) *Handbook in Clinical Audiometry* (3rd Ed.) Baltimore, MD: Williams and Wilkins, pp 885-910.

MacNeilage, P.F. (1983). (Ed.) *The Production of Speech.* New York: Springer-Verlag.

Markides, A. (1983). *The Speech of Hearing-Impaired Children.* Manchester: Manchester University Press.

Marmor, G.S. and Pettito, L. (1979). Simultaneous communication in the classroom.: How well is English grammar represented? *Sign Language Studies,* 23, 99-136.

Martin, F.N. (1981). (Ed.) *Medical Audiology.* Englewood Cliffs, NJ: Prentice-Hall, Inc.

Martin, F.N. (1986). (Ed.) *Introduction to Audiology* (3rd Ed.). Englewood Cliffs, NJ: Prentice-Hall, Inc..

McLean, J.E. and Snyder MacLean, L.K. (1978). *A Transactional Approach to Early Language Training.* Columbus: Charles Merrill Publishing Co.

Mencher, G.T. and Gerber, S.E. (1981). (Eds.) *Early Management of Hearing Loss.* New York: Grune and Stratton.

Minifie, F.D., Hixon, T.J., and Williams, F. (1973). (Eds.) *Normal Aspects of Speech, Hearing, and Language.* Englewood Cliffs, NJ: Prentice-Hall.

Moog, J.S. and Geers, A.E. (1975). *Scales of Early Communication Skills for Hearing-Impaired Children*. St. Louis, MO.: Central Institute for the Deaf.

Moog, J.S. and Geers, A.E. (1979). *Grammatical Analysis of Elicited Language-Simple Sentence Level*. St. Louis, MO.: Central Institute for the Deaf.

Moog, J.S. and Geers, A.E. (1980). *Grammatical Analysis of Elicited Language - Complex Sentence Level*. St Louis. MO.: Central Insitute for the Deaf.

Moog, J.S. and Geers, A.E. (1983). *Grammatical Analysis of Elicited Language - Pre-sentence Level*. St Louis, MO.: Central Institute for the Deaf.

Nicholls, G.H. (1979). *Cued Speech and the Reception of Spoken Language*. Washington DC.: Cued Speech Office, Gallaudet College.

Northern, J.L., and Downs, M.P. (1984). *Hearing in Children* (3rd Edition). Baltimore, MD: Williams and Wilkins.

Owens, E., and Kessler, D.K. (1988). *Cochlear Implants in Young Children*. San Diego: College-Hill Press.

Owens, R.E. (1988). *Language Development*. Columbus: Merrill Publishing Company.

Pappas, D. (1985). *Diagnosis and Treatment of Hearing Impairment in Children*. San Diego: College-Hill Press.

Perigoe C.B. and Ling, D. (1986). Generalization of speech skills in hearing-impaired children. *The Volta Review, 88, 351-366.*

Pickett, J.M. and McFarland, W. (1985). Auditory implants and tactile aids for the profoundly deaf. *Journal of Speech and Hearing Research, 28, 134-150.*

Pinker, S. (1984). *Language Learnability and Language Development*. Cambridge: Harvard University Press.

Pollack, M. (1988). (Ed.) *Amplification for the Hearing-Impaired.* Orlando: Grune and Stratton, Inc.

Proctor, A. (1984). Tactile aids for the deaf: a comprehensive bibliography. *American Annals of the Deaf, 129, 409-416.*

Quigley, S.P. (1978). Effects of hearing impairment on normal language development. In F.N. Martin (Ed.) *Pediatric Audiology.* Englewood Cliffs, NJ.: Prentice-Hall, Inc., pp 35-63.

Quigley, S.P. and Paul, P.V. (1984). *Language and Deafness.* San Diego: College-Hill Press.

Reed, M. (1984). *Educating Hearing-Impaired Children.* Milton Keynes: Open University Press.

Rees, R.J. (1984). *Parents as Language Therapists.* San Diego: College-Hill Press.

Ross, M. and Giolas, T.G. (1978). (Eds.) *Auditory Management of Hearing-Impaired Children: Principles and Prerequisiters for Intervention.* Baltimore, MD.: University Park Press.

Sanders, D. (1977). *Auditory Perception of Speech.* Englewood Cliffs: Prentice-Hall, Inc.

Schildroth, A.N. and Karchmer, M.A. (1986). (Eds.) *Deaf Children in America.* San Diego: College-Hill Press.

Sherrick, C.E. (1984). Basic and applied research on tactile aids for deaf people: progress and prospects. *Journal of the Acoustical Society of America,* 78, 78-83.

Snow, C.E. and Ferguson, C.A. (1977). (Eds.) *Talking to Children.* Cambridge: Cambridge University Press.

Stickler, K. R. (1987). *Guide to analysis of Language Transcripts.* Eau Claire, WI: Thinking Publications.

Stovall, D. (1982). *Teaching Speech to Hearing-impaired Children.* Springfield, IL: Charles C Thomas.

Stremel, K. and Waryas, C. (1974). A behavioral psycholinguistic approach to language training. In L. McReynolds (Ed.) *Developing Systematic Procedures for Training Childrens' Language.* ASHA Monograph No. 18. Washington, D.C.: ASHA

Stubbs, M. (1983). *Discourse Analysis: The Sociolinguistic Analysis of Natural Language.* Chicago: The University of Chicago Press.

Subtelny, J. and Lieberth, A.K. (1985) *Speech and Auditory Training: A Program for Adolescents with Hearing and Language Disorders.* Tucson, AZ: Communication Skill Builders.

Subtelny, J. and Snell, K.B. (1988). Efficacy of a distinctive feature model of therapy for hearing-impaired adolescents. *Journal of Speech and Hearing Disorders, 53, 194-201.*

Tate, G.M. (1972). *Oral English.* Sydney, Australia: South Pacific Commission.

Van Uden, A. (1980). *A world of language for deaf children* (P.I). Amsterdam: Swets and Zeitlinger, 1977.

Vaughan, P. (l976). (Ed.) *Learning to Listen.* Don Mills, Ontario: General Publishing Co. Ltd.

Wilbur, R.B. (1987). *American Sign Language.* San Diego: College-Hill Press.

Wood, D., Wood H., Griffiths, A. and Howarth, I. (1986). *Teaching and Talking with Deaf Children.* New York: John Wiley and Sons.

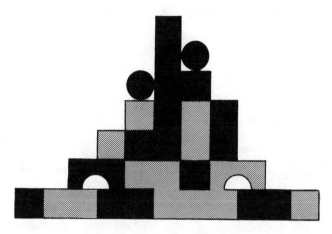

index of subjects